Communications in Nursing

Susan Smith

Communicating

Assertively and

Responsibly

In

Nursing: A

Guidebook

SECOND EDITION

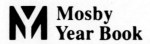

Mosby
Year Book

St. Louis   Baltimore   Boston   Chicago   London   Philadelphia   Sydney   Toronto

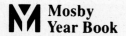
Mosby
Year Book

Dedicated to Publishing Excellence

Editor: Linda Duncan
Developmental Editor: Kathy Sartori
Project Manager: Mark Spann
Production Editor: Tim Furnish
Designer: Julie Taugner

Printed in the United States of America.

Mosby–Year Book, Inc.
11830 Westline Industrial Drive
St. Louis, MO 63146

Library of Congress Cataloging-in-Publication Data

Smith, Susan, 1946-
    Communications in nursing : communicating assertively and
  responsibly in nursing : a guidebook / Susan Smith.— 2nd ed.
        p.   cm.
    Includes bibliographical references and index.
    ISBN 0-8016-6357-1
    1. Communication in nursing.   2. Nurse and patient.   I. Title.
    [DNLM: 1. Communications—nurses' instruction.
2. Interprofessional Relations—nurses' instruction.   3. Nurse
-Patient Relations.   WY 87 S6661c]
RT23.S65   1992
610.73′069′9—dc20
DNLM/DLC
for Library of Congress   91-32701
                                                                      CIP

  92 93 94 95 96   C/DC/DC   9 8 7 6 5 4 3 2 1

To my loving parents-in-law:
Jim and Aileen Smith
and
To my terrific nephews:
Todd and Sean Beresford.

Preface

This book is written for you, a nursing student who is learning about communicating effectively in the context of a helping relationship. This textbook adheres to the Standards of Nursing Practice developed by the American Nurses' Association, which advises a systematic approach to nursing practice: the assessment of the client's status, the plan of nursing actions, the implementation of the plan, and evaluation. You will learn how to apply these steps of the nursing process in your interpersonal communication with clients and colleagues. The approach fostered in this textbook derives from Standards V and VII, which press for client participation in decision-making about progress related to health promotion, maintenance, and restoration (ANA, 1973).

You will be introduced to a humanistic approach for interacting with clients and colleagues. In addition to acquiring a conceptual understanding of communicating in a helpful way, you can practice handling difficult client-nurse and nurse-colleague interpersonal situations in a caring way. Too often nurses are able to discuss theoretical notions about communication, but not able to apply this knowledge in their clinical practice. This book is designed to help you integrate the essential communication behaviors into your nursing skill repertoire.

Each of the essential interpersonal communication behaviors is described, and how each augments client well-being and collegial relationships is articulated. Exercises incorporating real-life nursing situations are included to help you gain confidence and competence in your communication. You are encouraged to expand your awareness of alternative styles of communicating by comparing approaches with your colleagues. Supervised feedback is a useful shaper of effective communication. You will learn how to seek, receive, and give feedback about communicating in assertive and responsible ways.

How This Textbook Will Help You Become an Effective Helper in the Client-Nurse Relationship

An important ability you require as a nurse is that of communicating effectively with your clients and colleagues. Whether you are teaching a client, carrying out a nursing treatment, completing a health assessment, managing a life-threatening crisis, or handling a client's irritation, you must be able to relate in a humane and helpful way. To contribute to a positive and safe work environment you need to be able to communicate clearly with your colleagues. Whether you are reporting to a colleague about a client, making a referral or suggesting an alternative nursing approach to your health care team, you must have the communication skills to convey your message accurately and with conviction.

The following overview outlines how each chapter in this book will contribute to your potency as an assertive and responsible nurse communicator.

PART ONE: COMMUNICATION COMPETENCE

CHAPTER	WILL HELP YOU
1. Communicating assertively and responsibly in nursing	• Appreciate the significance of assertiveness and responsibleness as fundamental approaches for communicating in a caring way.
2. The client-nurse relationship: a helping relationship	• Develop a communication approach which has the interests of your client at heart.
3. Mutual problem-solving in nursing	• Collaborate and validate with your clients at each phase of the nursing process.
4. Warmth	• Demonstrate to your clients in concrete ways that you are concerned and interested in them.

PART TWO: POSITIVE COMMUNICATION AFFECT

18. Positive self-talk

• Keep your internal dialogue supportive so that you are encouraged to communicate with confidence.

PART THREE: COMMUNICATION SKILL

CHAPTER

WILL HELP YOU

19. Overcoming

• Use a rational approach to feel more confident in nursing situations that make you feel anxious.

20. Communicating assertively and responsibly with distressed clients and colleagues

• Reverse your negative reactions to distressed behavior so that you can relate compassionately with distressed clients and colleagues.

21. Communicating assertively and responsibly with aggressive clients and colleagues

• Overcome your blocks to aggression so that you can cope with aggressive clients and colleagues in helpful ways, and feel confident doing so.

22. Communicating assertively and responsibly with unpopular clients

• Become aware of your biases to clients and surmount them so that you can carry out helpful nursing care with unpopular clients.

23. Managing team conflict in assertive and responsible ways

• Use a systematic problem-solving approach to deal effectively with intercollegial conflict.

REFERENCE

American Nurses' Association. (1973). *Standards of nursing practice.* Kansas City, Mo.: The Association.

ACKNOWLEDGMENTS

It has been a pleasure to work with the editorial staff of the Nursing Division of Mosby-Year Book. Linda Duncan, Senior Editor, and Kathy Sartori, Developmental Editor, have been exceptionally helpful in their generous support and encouragement. I am thankful to my husband Bob, who has skillfully contributed his computer knowledge and feedback. I have been inspired by the interest and competence in interpersonal communication demonstrated by students I have taught and learned from in the past 10 years at the University of Victoria School of Nursing.

Contents

READER PLEASE NOTE

Throughout this book the pronoun "she" is used to denote the hypothetical nurse, and the hypothetical client is referred to as "he" in most instances. This plan does not reflect how things are in reality, but it facilitates smoother writing and avoids some of the more cumbersome non-sexist writing techniques.

Communications
in Nursing

COMMUNICATION COMPETENCE

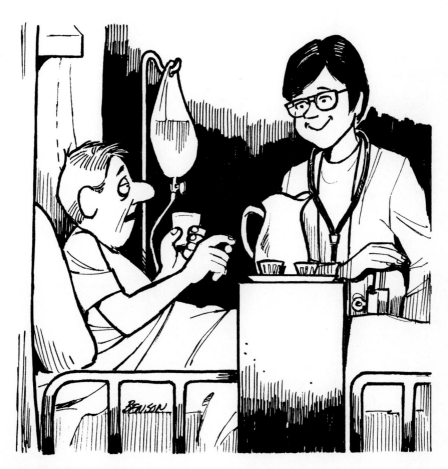

"The great communicator."

INTRODUCTION TO PART 1: COMMUNICATION COMPETENCE

The first step to becoming a better nurse communicator is to build a sound knowledge base about the essential communication behaviors. Your valuing and emotional preference for each of the communication behaviors grows hand in hand with this intellectual understanding. A clear conceptualization of each communication behavior, including the ability to articulate its benefits and knowledge about when to employ each one, shapes your communication repertoire.

You are already familiar with some of the essential interpersonal communication behaviors you will learn about in Part One. You can add to your knowledge base, enhancing your communication competence, by actively studying each chapter in this section. You are encouraged to assess your level of understanding of each communication behavior, noting your strengths and weaknesses, and to work at maintaining areas that are satisfactory and improving those that do not yet meet the objectives outlined at the beginning of each chapter.

Developing your communication competence in this way will mean that you can demonstrate knowledge and defend the employment of the appropriate communication behaviors required in interactions with clients and colleagues. This cognitive understanding of the various communication behaviors builds the foundation for your ability to communicate effectively with clients and colleagues.

CHAPTER 1

Communicating Assertively and Responsibly in Nursing

*"Caring is one of life's essential ingredients;
it may be the most essential ingredient."*

E.O. Bevis

This book is designed to help you, a student in nursing, to improve your ability to communicate assertively and responsibly with your clients and colleagues.

Before going any further you need to understand the meaning of three important concepts used in the opening sentence: communicate, assertively and responsibly. These concepts are significant because they form the framework for the direction of the textbook.

THE MEANING OF INTERPERSONAL COMMUNICATION

Communication involves the reciprocal process of sending and receiving of messages between two or more people (Smith & Williamson, 1981; Haney, 1979; Hein, 1980; Weaver, 1981; Bradley & Edinberg, 1986). In this book the focus will be on the communication exchange between you, as the nurse, and your clients and colleagues. Communication can either facilitate the development of a therapeutic relationship or create barriers between you and your clients and colleagues (Stuart & Sundeen, 1991).

Any message has two parts: the verbal expression of the sender's thoughts and feelings, and the nonverbal expression of the sender's thoughts and feelings. Verbally, cognitive and affective messages are sent through words, voice inflection, and rate of speech; nonverbally, they are conveyed by eye movements, facial expressions, and bodily posturing.

4

The sender determines what message he wants to transmit to the receiver, and he encodes his thoughts and feelings into words and gestures. The sender's message is transmitted through sound, sight, touch, and occasionally through smell and taste, to the receiver.

The receiver of the sender's message has to decode the verbal and nonverbal transmission to make sense of the thoughts and feelings communicated by the sender. After decoding the sender's words, speech patterns, facial and body movements, the receiver encodes a return message. He encodes his thoughts and feelings verbally into words and nonverbally into gestures and transmits them to the original sender.

In an interaction between two people (i.e., a nurse and her client, or a nurse and her colleague) each person is both a sender and a receiver and alternates between these two roles. When a sender is speaking he is also receiving messages from the person who is listening to him. The listener is not only receiving the speaker's message, but also simultaneously sending a message to him. Figure 1-1 illustrates this reciprocal nature of the sending and receiving roles in communication.

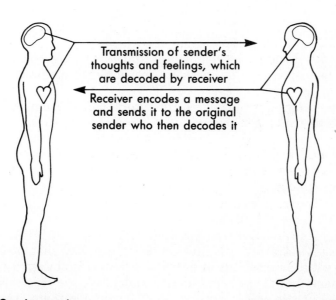

Sender-receiver

The sender encodes his thoughts and feelings into words and gestures and transmits them to the receiver via sound, touch, sight, and smell. At the same time the sender is receiving messagees from the person with whom he is communicating.

Receiver-sender

The receiver deciphers the sender's transmission. He determines what request the sender is making of him, after he decodes the sender's cognitive and affective messages. Simultaneously the receiver is sending messages to the other person.

Figure 1-1 Reciprocal nature of interpersonal communication

At any point in an interpersonal communication we send and receive verbal and nonverbal messages about thoughts and feelings.

With little prompting you know that the complex process of interpersonal communication is influenced by many variables that affect how messages are sent and received (Stuart & Sundeen, 1991; Knapp, 1980; Levine & Adelman, 1982; Northouse & Northouse, 1985). Take a few minutes to think of the variety of factors that you know from experience affect the exchange of messages between people. Add your ideas to the following list of some of the factors influencing interpersonal communication:

- Environmental factors: formality, warmth, privacy, familiarity, freedom or constraint, physical distance between people, climate, mood, architecture, arrangement of furniture
- Territory and personal space: crowding, seating arrangements, power and dominance characteristics of participants, including roles, status, and position; physical characteristics of interaction participants, including size, height
- Physical appearance and dress: body shape, body color, body smell, hair, sex, body movements, body adornments, posture, age, touching
- Nonverbal cues: facial expressions, eye movements, vocal cues; emotions or mood conveyed by eye gazing, facial movements, and paraverbal sounds; cultural interpretation of such cues
- Intrapersonal factors: developmental stage, language mastery, differences in perception, differences in decision-making processes, differences in values, self-concept

When these factors are considered the interpersonal communication process looks something like Figure 1-2.

Note that any of the above factors has the potential to facilitate communication or act as a barrier to effective communication, depending on the context of the situation.

A function of communication is to transmit messages from one person to another. The real purpose of communication is to create meaning (Lewis, 1973; Berger & Bradac, 1982): the sender of a message wishes to convey a meaning to the receiver, and vice versa. With this intent the sender chooses certain words and gestures in a way that he believes is congruent with his intended message. The sender's objective is to transmit a message that is clear and understandable to the receiver.

But the purpose of communication does not stop there. The real purpose of creating understanding in another person is to influence the other person to effect some change (Lewis, 1973, p. 10). One such change is to influence another to respond to a request. Gerrard, Boniface & Love (1980, p. 115) stated that the sender attempts to persuade the receiver to respond to his requests. Requests from clients and colleagues may be for:

- Understanding
- Action
- Information and/or
- Comfort

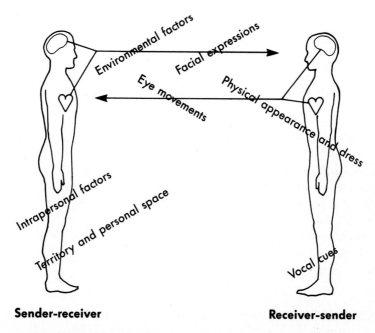

Sender-receiver   **Receiver-sender**

Figure 1-2 Factors influencing interpersonal communication

Requests may be stated in obvious or indirect ways. The following examples illustrate what is meant by direct and indirect requests.

A client has postoperative pain. His physiological need is for pain relief. He asks you: "When is the last time I had my pain killer?" (He winces and holds his wrist.) His obvious request is for information about the time of his last analgesic. His indirect request is for information about the next time he can have more. He is anticipating action (you giving him the medication) so that he will be comforted.

A nursing assistant says at the beginning of the shift: "I have a terrible headache. I was up for 3 hours last night with my sick daughter. Do you have an aspirin I could have?" Her physiological need is for rest and pain relief. Her obvious requests are for understanding (that you will empathize with her pain), and action (that you will give her an aspirin). She is possibly hoping that you will comfort her by making allowances for the fact that she is not her usual perky self.

A nurse, newly hired to a unit, needs to feel that she belongs and fits in. When she asks you to show her around the unit she is indirectly asking you to understand that she feels alone and unsure. She is directly asking you to take action to orient her, and provide her with information about procedures and policy. She is likely hoping that you will make her feel welcome (comforted).

In your interpersonal relationships as nurses, you will act as sender and receiver. The purpose of this book is to help you develop your clarity as senders and your comprehension as receivers of messages. You will learn how to deliver assertive and responsible messages, and to accurately decode messages from your clients and colleagues. You will become confident interpreting both direct and indirect requests from your clients and colleagues, and make responsible decisions about how to respond assertively.

This summary encapsulates the important functions of interpersonal communication in nursing: "First, communication is the vehicle for establishing a therapeutic relationship, since it involves conveying information and exchanging thoughts and feelings. Second, communication is the means by which people influence the behavior of another. Thus it is critical to the successful outcome of nursing intervention. Finally, communication is the relationship itself, since without it, a therapeutic nurse-patient relationship is impossible" (Stuart & Sundeen, 1991, p. 108).

THE MEANING OF ASSERTIVENESS

Assertiveness is the ability to confidently and comfortably express your thoughts and feelings while still respecting the legitimate rights of others (Adler, 1977; Jakubowski & Lange, 1978; and Herman, 1978). Assertiveness is distinguished from passive behavior, in which individuals disregard their own needs and rights, and aggressive behavior, in which people disregard the needs and rights of others (Sundeen, Stuart, Rankin, & Cohen, 1989).

"Assertion is not continual confrontation, but making a conscious choice about what to say, when, how, and to whom. The assertive professional nurse consciously makes decisions regarding social and work encounters and determines responses pertinent to each situation. . . . While not allowing others to take advantage of her, the assertive nurse does not withdraw, but remains involved in interactions with people. This behavior demonstrates respect for herself and for others involved" (Herman, 1978).

Communicating assertively means:
- Being skilled in a variety of communication strategies for expressing your thoughts and feelings in a way that simultaneously protects your rights and those of others
- Having a positive attitude about communicating in a forthright and fair way
- Feeling comfortable and in control of negative feelings such as anxiety, tenseness, shyness, or fear
- Feeling confident that you can conduct yourself in a self-respecting and other-respecting way; and
- Keeping your rights and those of others equally paramount

Assertiveness refers to a style of communicating that has positive benefits for you and others (Herman, 1978; Jakubowski & Lange, 1978). Communicating assertively solidifies an attitude of mutual respect. It builds your self-confidence to know that you can treat others fairly while taking care of your own needs. This experience builds a healthy attitude of mutual respect. Speaking out about your thoughts and feelings provides others with clear, direct messages that are easier to receive than wishy-washy or assaultive ones. Assertiveness helps build trust between people.

Some authors suggest that there are certain assertive skills (such as expressing opinions or saying "no") or special circumstances that call for assertive behavior (such as meeting someone, being evaluated, or confronting others). The notion emphasized in this book is that we can be assertive every time we communicate. With each person we encounter in any situation, we have the choice of communicating in an assertive or a nonassertive style. The words we choose and the way we express them can be assertive, unassertive, or aggressive.

Unassertiveness is a failure to stand up for our legitimate rights and possibly those of others. It means communicating in an uncertain or uncomfortable way. When we are unassertive we lose out because we fail to show respect for ourselves, which lowers our self-esteem. "We see ourselves as a doormat the world walks on and we don't reach our goals or get our preferences respected. Instead nonassertive behavior invites others to infringe upon us and take advantage of us" (Jakubowski & Lange, 1978, p. 11).

Aggressiveness is that bulldozing, loud, forceful way of trying to get what we want, even at the expense of others. When we act aggressively, our rights are responded to out of all proportion to those of others. Although we may temporarily gloat at our achievement, the experience is short-lived when we realize how we may have embarrassed ourselves or, worse, hurt another in our determination to get what we wanted. In an aggressive approach mutual respect is lacking; others are treated as objects standing in the way of getting what we want.

Table 1-1 differentiates between assertive communication and unassertive or aggressive styles of relating to others.

This book is intended to foster an assertive style in your communication with your clients and colleagues.

THE MEANING OF RESPONSIBLE COMMUNICATION

As defined in Webster's dictionary, 1986 edition, *responsible* means, "likely to be called upon to answer; able to respond or answer for one's conduct and obligations . . ." As nurses, this accountability may be described as being personally responsible for the outcome of our own professional actions (Open University, 1984). To act this responsibly means that our nursing care is based on knowledge, not tradition or myth (Open University, 1984, p. 22).

Table 1-1 ASSERTIVE AND NONASSERTIVE STYLES OF COMMUNICATION

Characteristics	Assertive	Nonassertive style:	
		Unassertive	Aggressive
Attitude toward self and others	I'm OK You're OK	I'm not OK You're OK	I'm OK You're not OK
Decision making	Makes own decision	Lets others choose for her	Chooses for others
Behavior in problem situations	Direct, fair confrontation	Flees, gives in	Outright, assaultive
Verbal behaviors	Clear, direct statement of wants; objective words; honest statement of feelings	Apologetic words; hedging; rambling: failing to say what is meant	Loaded words; accusations; superior, haughty words; labelling of other person
Non-verbal generally	Confident, congruent, messages	Actions instead of words (not saying what you feel); looking as though you don't mean what you say	Air of superiority; flippant, sarcastic style
Voice	Firm, warm, confident	Weak, distant, soft, wavering	Tense, shrill, loud, cold, demanding, authoritarian, deadly quiet
Eyes	Warm, in contact, frank	Averted, downcast, teary, pleading	Expressionless, cold, narrowed, staring
Stance	Relaxed	Stooped; excessive leaning for support	Hands on hips; feet apart
Hands	Gestures at appropriate times	Fidgety, clammy	Fists pounding or clenched
Pattern of relating	Puts herself up without putting others down	Puts herself down	Puts herself up by putting others down
Response of others	Mutual respect	Disrespect, guilt, anger, frustration	Hurt, defensiveness, humiliation
Consequences of style	I win, you win; strives for "win-win" or "no lose" solutions	I lose, you lose; only succeeds by luck or charity of others	I win, you lose; beats out others at any cost

Adaptation of "Characterological Lifechart of Three Fellows We All Know" by Gerald Piaget from THE ASSERTIVE WOMAN by Stanlee Phelps and Nancy Austin © 1975. Reproduced for Susan Smith with permission of Impact Publishers, Inc., P.O. Box 1094, San Luis Obispo, CA 93406. Further reproduction prohibited; and Gerrard B., Boniface W. & Love B., (1980). *Interpersonal skills for health professionals.* Reston, Virginia: Reston Publishing Company, Inc., p. 185.

To communicate responsibly means to communicate in a logical, systematic way based on the facts presented in the situation and your nursing knowledge. Responsible communication demonstrates accurate problem-solving behavior for the particular situation. Griffith-Kenney & Christensen (1986, p. 4) stated that the nursing process is a systematic means for nurses to demonstrate accountability and responsibility to clients. The American Nurses' Association Standards of Nursing Practice, (1973) based on the nursing process, are designed to help nurses fulfill their obligation of responsibility and accountability for the nursing care their clients receive. In the interpersonal communication process, here is how the steps of the nursing process are followed to ensure responsible communication:

1. **Collection of data.** You must collect the essential verbal and nonverbal data about your client's (or colleague's) thoughts and feelings.
2. **Assessment of the data.** After ensuring that you have secured the necessary data you must analyze the information. This step includes determining what request your client (or colleague) is making of you.
3. **Establishing expected outcomes (objectives).** At this point you decide whether it is reasonable to meet your client's (or colleague's) request. You must indicate what you hope to achieve by your communication.
4. **Planning your communication strategy.** This is where you decide what you will say, how you will phrase it, and what nonverbal gestures you will use to transmit your message. Your plan should be congruent with your expected outcomes.
5. **Implementing your plan.** At this point you respond to your client or colleague. This textbook encourages you to respond assertively and responsibly.
6. **Evaluation.** Here is where you check whether your response was assertive and responsible, and whether your objectives (expected outcomes) were achieved.

This whole problem-solving process takes place during every client-nurse (or nurse-colleague) interaction. While you are receiving a message from your client or colleague you are trying to determine its meaning. You decide whether you will meet his request, then transmit an assertive and responsible message congruent with your decision. As you send your message you observe the effects of your words and gestures on your client or colleague. You are sending and receiving messages continuously.

This textbook will help you apply the nursing process in your interactions with clients and colleagues.

ABOUT CARING

In her opening remarks on caring published in the proceedings of the 1989 Wingspread Conference on Caring, Leininger predicted that caring will become the central and major focus in substantiating and legitimizing the discipline and profession of nursing by 2010. "Consumers will seek caring behaviors, decisions, and actions that reflect respect for human beings, active listening, and many other care attributes that are only limitedly known in nursing today. Consumers will have a growing antipathy for being treated like machines with body parts, or merely persons to perform sundry tasks on" (Leininger, 1990, p. 28).

Caring is not an abstract concept; there are explicit ways we can communicate as nurses to show we care. Encompassed in caring is a commitment to the preservation of common humanness and an unrelenting respect for the uniqueness and human dignity for each of the clients and colleagues we encounter (Delaney, 1990, p. 603). "Caring is one of life's essential ingredients; it may be the most essential ingredient" (Bevis, 1981). In the realm of nursing, Corless and Riordan (1990, p. 61) stated emphatically that for client care activities to be nursing, caring must characterize that interaction between the nurse and client.

Caring is the moral ideal that guides nurses through the caregiving process, and knowledgeable caring is the highest form of commitment (Watson, 1988, p. 2). Watson noted that we are beginning to recognize that nurses can have an extensive command of scientific facts and theories and be technically an expert without being caring professionals. Nurses can be technically and scientifically correct but still make moral errors. Corless and Riordan (1990) forewarn nurses that while there is satisfaction in being technically proficient, such satisfaction alone is short-lived. Nursing care is a modality that is scientifically based and humanistically oriented, and nursing actions that are perceived as caring include both expressive and instrumental behaviors (Tripp-Reimer & Cohen, 1990). Caring communication holistically takes into account the whole person, demonstrating respect for clients as people, not just bodies requiring nursing interventions.

The question you are likely asking yourself is: "How can I ensure that my communication is *caring?*" Some nurse researchers would say that this is one of the key nursing research questions to be answered. If we as nurses consciously desire to generate the feeling of being cared for in our clients, and intend our behavior to convey this desire to our clients, we must remember that not all intended caring on our part is perceived as caring by our clients (Larson, 1987). In an extensive review of care research derived from qualitative research methodology, Tripp-Reimer and Cohen (1990) discovered discrepancies between nurses' and clients' perceptions of the importance of expressive and instrumental behaviors in caring. Nurses identified more expressive behaviors (such as listening, touching, and presence) as indicators of caring. In contrast, clients identified more instrumental behaviors (such as accessibility and monitoring) as indicative of caring. There may be discrepancies in the care nurses consider optimal and that which clients consider important (Tripp-Reimer & Cohen, 1990, p. 85). Caring is situation-specific. "Caring must encompass knowledge and skills in the ability to identify care needs and nursing actions that will bring about positive change; that is, movement toward the protection, enhancement, and preservation of human dignity" (Delaney, 1990).

The implications are clear. We must find out what is perceived to be important to our clients in their return to health, validate the effect our caring actions are having on them, and adjust our actions in keeping with their needs. Taking these actions is responsible nursing. This book will convince you of the importance of validating at each step of the nursing process, and enhance your ability to communicate in a respectful, mutual way with both clients and colleagues. It is equally important to communicate caringly with colleagues as well as clients. If there is caring between colleagues at work, nurses supported in that environment will likely pass on that caring to their clients. Conversely, if there is little caring between colleagues, then nurses are unlikely to feel complete and satisfied enough to demonstrate caring with their clients. This book will help you enhance your skills for contributing to a supportive workplace, one in which there is clear and direct communication between work colleagues.

Caring involves being assertive and responsible. If you let others walk all over you by being unassertive, or invade others' rights by being aggressive, you cannot act in a caring way with others. If you care enough for yourself by being assertive, you will know how to care for others. Our clients and colleagues trust that we have the skills and knowledge to act with good judgment. Using the problem-solving process increases the probability of communicating responsibly. Whatever we are doing (taking a history, discussing a new nursing technique, changing a dressing, teaching a class, or proposing a new policy), we can accomplish it in an assertive, responsible, and caring way.

HOW CAN YOU LEARN TO COMMUNICATE ASSERTIVELY AND RESPONSIBLY?

This book is based on the belief that effective and caring nurse communicators are not born; they are made (Gerrard, 1978; McCroskey, 1984). You can learn to communicate in competent, caring, and confident ways with clients and colleagues. You can replace ineffective and untherapeutic communication habits with helpful interventions. You can continually add to your communications repertoire so that you develop confidence in your ability to communicate in a caring way in a variety of situations with your clients and colleagues.

The view of educational psychologists that learning involves three domains is one that is endorsed in this textbook (McCroskey, 1984; Meichenbaum, 1977; Woodruff, 1961). This book attends to the cognitive (understanding and meaning), affective (feelings, values and attitudes), and psychomotor (physical capability of doing) aspects of your communication learning process.

McCroskey's framework (1984) for learning to communicate effectively by attending to all three domains is the approach adopted in this book. You will improve your communication competence (cognitive domain), positive communication affect (affective domain), and communication skill (psychomotor domain).

Cognitive Domain: Communication Competence

Communication competence is your ability to demonstrate knowledge of the appropriate communicative behavior in any situation. Communication competence is demonstrated by identifying behaviors that would be appropriate or inappropriate in an observed interpersonal situation.

Affective Domain: Positive Communication Affect

A positive communication affect is that of liking and wanting to produce appropriate communication behavior. You value effective communication and have the attitude that you want to be a skillful communicator.

Psychomotor Domain: Communication Skill

Communication skill is your ability to perform appropriate communication behaviors in any given situation. To be considered a skilled nurse communicator you must be able to successfully implement communication strategies that are assertive and responsible.

Figure 1-3 denotes that to become a caring nurse communicator you need to develop in all three domains. The negative consequences of incomplete development in all three aspects are illustrated.

HOW THIS BOOK WILL HELP YOU BECOME A BETTER NURSE COMMUNICATOR

This book is designed to improve your communication competence, positive affect and skill in the variety of interpersonal situations you will encounter as a nurse.

Part One: Communication Competence

To help you develop your communication competence chapters 2 and 3 set the stage by outlining the nature of the client-nurse helping relationship and the benefits of mutual problem-solving with clients. Chapters 4 through 14 describe the basic interpersonal communication behaviors you require to communicate with clients and colleagues. Guidance is provided to help you implement them in assertive and responsible ways.

In chapters 19 through 23 you will be presented with difficult interpersonal situations and learn which communication behaviors would be most appropriate in those situations. A rationale for correct and incorrect responses is provided to help you crystallize your knowledge of assertive and responsible communication in each situation.

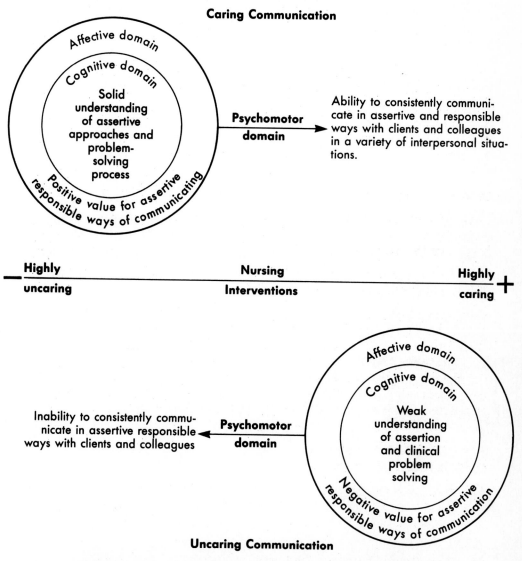

Figure 1-3 Differences between caring and uncaring communication

Part Two: Positive Communication Affect

To develop your confidence and pleasure in communicating effectively, you will benefit from the following chapters:

- In Chapter 15, Feedback, you will learn how to seek, receive and give feedback on your communication performance so that you improve and help colleagues to improve.
- In Chapter 16, Relaxation, you will learn how to release tension, concentrate, and feel in control when you are communicating.

- In Chapter 17, Imagery, you will learn how to envision yourself communicating successfully. This technique acts as a rehearsal and creates a positive attitude.
- In Chapter 18, Positive Self-Talk, you will learn how to keep your internal dialogue positive and realistic.

    At the end of every chapter there is opportunity for supervised feedback sessions in which you can receive comments on your successes in communication, as well as areas where you can make improvements.

Part Three: Communication Skill

Most of the chapters have several practice exercises to assist you in developing proficiency in communicating. By completing these assignments you can try out and perfect the communication behavior you are learning.

    In chapters 19 through 23, you will get supervised practice communicating in situations that are difficult for nurses. The opportunity to compare your suggested responses with correct and incorrect choices is pro-

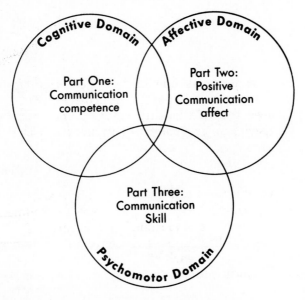

Figure 1-4 Interrelationships of the three parts of this book
The cognitive, affective, and psychomotor learning in this book are interrelated
Each part influences the other two parts
If you understand a communication behavior (C), you feel more confident (A) and eager to implement it (P)
If you feel positive about the value of a communication behavior (A), you are more likely to learn more about it (C) and attempt to use it (P)
If you successfully master implementation of a communication behavior (P), then you likely feel more confident (A) and you immediately learn about the usefulness and importance of the communication behavior (C)

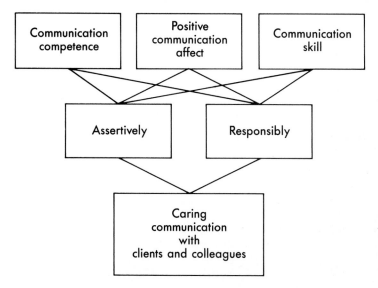

Figure 1-5 Relationship between the concepts forming the framework for this book

vided. Supervised feedback is one of the most important shapers of positive change in communication skill (McCroskey, 1984).

Figure 1-4 shows the relationship between the cognitive, affective, and psychomotor aspects of this communications textbook.

In Summary

This textbook is structured to enhance your interpersonal communication competence, positive communication affect, and communication skill in all client-nurse and collegial relationships. Figure 1-5 illustrates the framework of this book. The focus is on communicating assertively and responsibly when you employ each of the communication behaviors, with every client and colleague, in any situation.

REFERENCES

Adler, R.B. (1977). *Confidence in communication: A guide to assertive and social skills.* New York: Holt, Rinehart and Winston.

American Nurses' Association. (1973). *Standards of nursing practice.* Kansas City, Mo.: The Association.

Berger, C.R., & Bradac, J.J. (1982). *Language and social knowledge: Uncertainty in interpersonal relations.* Bungay, Suffolk: Richard Clay (The Chaucer Press) Limited.

Bevis, E.O. (1981). Caring: A life force. In M.M. Leininger (Ed.), *Caring: An essential human need: Proceedings of Three National Caring Conferences* (pp. 49-59). Thorofare, N.J.: Charles B. Slack, Inc.

Bradley, J.C., & Edinberg, M.A. (1986). *Communication in the nursing context* (2nd ed.). New York: Appleton-Century-Crofts.

Corless, I.B., & Riordan, J.J. (1990). Nursing care: A user-friendly approach—identifying the cutting edge questions. In J.S. Stevenson & T. Tripp-Reimer (Eds.), *Knowledge about care and caring: State of the art and future developments* (pp. 53-64). Kansas City, Mo.: American Academy of Nursing.

Delaney, C. (1990). Computer technology: Endangering the essence of nursing? In J.C. McCloskey & H.K. Grace (Eds.), *Current issues in nursing* (3rd ed.) (pp. 601-606). St. Louis: Mosby–Year Book.

Gerrard, B.A., Boniface, W.J., & Love, B.H. (1980). *Interpersonal skills for health professionals.* Reston, Va.: Reston Publishing Company, Inc. A Prentice-Hall Company.

Gove, P.B. (Ed.) (1986). Webster's Third international dictionary of the English language, unabridged. Springfield, Mass.: Merriam-Webster Inc.

Griffith-Kenney, J.W., & Christensen, P.J. (1986). *Nursing process: Application of theories, frameworks, and models.* St. Louis: Mosby–Year Book.

Haney, W.V. (1979). *Communication and interpersonal relations: Texts and cases* (4th ed.). Homewood, Ill.: Richard D. Irwin, Inc.

Hein, E.C. (1980). *Communication in nursing practice* (2nd ed.). Boston: Little, Brown and Company.

Herman, S.J. (1978). *Becoming assertive: A guide for nurses.* New York: D. Van Nostrand Company.

Jakubowski, P., & Lange, A.J. (1978). *The assertive option: Your rights and responsibilities.* Champaign, Ill.: Research Press Company.

Knapp, M.L. (1980). *Essentials of nonverbal communication.* New York: Holt, Rinehart and Winston.

Larson, P.J. (1987). Comparison of cancer patients' and professional nurses' perceptions of important nurse caring behaviors. *Heart & Lung,* 16(2), 187-193.

Leininger, M. (1990). Historic and epistemologic dimensions of care and caring with future directions. In J.S. Stevenson & T. Tripp-Reimer (Eds.) *Knowledge about care and caring: State of the art and future developments* (pp. 19-31). Kansas City, Mo.: American Academy of Nursing.

Levine, D.R., & Adelman, M.B. (1982). *Beyond language: Intercultural communication for English as a second language.* Englewood Cliffs, N.J.: Prentice Hall Regents.

Lewis, G.K. (1973). *Nurse-patient communication* (2nd ed.). Dubuque, Iowa: Wm. C. Brown Company, Publishers.

McCroskey, J.C. (1984). The communication apprehension perspective. In J.A. Daly & McCroskey, J.C. (Eds.), *Avoiding communication: Shyness, reticence and communication apprehension* (pp. 13-38). Beverly Hills, Calif.: Sage Publications.

Meichenbaum, D. (1977). *Cognitive-behavior modification: An integrative approach.* New York: Plenum Press.

Northouse P.G., & Northouse, L.L. (1985). *Health communication: A handbook for health professionals.* Englewood Cliffs, N.J.: Prentice-Hall, Inc.

Open University Centre for Continuing Education. (1984). *A systematic approach to nursing care: An introduction.* Walton Hall, Milton Keyes, Great Britain: The Open University Press.

Smith, D.R., & Williamson, L.K. (1981). *Interpersonal communication: Roles, rules, strategies and games* (2nd ed.). Dubuque, Iowa: Wm. C. Brown Company, Publishers.

Stuart, G.W., Sundeen, S.J. (1991). *Principles and practice of psychiatric nursing* (4th ed). St. Louis: Mosby–Year Book.

Sundeen, S.J., Stuart, G.W., Rankin, E.A., & Cohen, S.A. (1989). *Nurse-client interaction: Implementing the nursing process.* St. Louis: Mosby–Year Book.

Tripp-Reimer, T., & Cohen, M.Z. (1990). Qualitative approaches to care: A critical review. In J.S. Stevenson & T. Tripp-Reimer (Eds.), *Knowledge about care and caring: State of the art and future developments* (pp. 83-96). Kansas City, Mo.: American Academy of Nursing.

Watson, J. (1988). A case study: Curriculum in transition. In National League for Nursing *Curriculum revolution: Mandate for change* (pp. 1-8). New York National League for Nursing.

Weaver, R.L. (1981). *Understanding interpersonal communication* (2nd ed.). Glenview, Ill.: Scott, Foresman & Company.

Woodruff, A.D. (1961). *Basic concepts of teaching* (concise edition). Scranton, Pa.: Chandler Publishing Company: An Intext Publisher.

SUGGESTIONS FOR FURTHER READING

Chenevert, M. (1991). *Mosby's tour guide to nursing school: A student's road survival kit* (2nd ed.). St. Louis: Mosby-Year Book.

This practical guidebook presents a candid, humorous, and helpful description of the experiences all nursing students are likely to encounter. In addition to describing the difficulties and stresses confronting nursing students, the book provides sound advice for coping with these problems.

Forsyth, D., Delaney, C., Maloney, N., Kubesh, D. & Story, D. (1989). Can caring behavior be taught? *Nursing Outlook,* 37(4), 164-166.

This article concisely summarizes what the authors consider to be the essential behaviors of caring and describe how they can be successfully taught to nurses.

Knapp, M.L. (1980). *Essentials of nonverbal communication.* New York, Holt, Rinehart & Winston.

For nurse readers interested in learning more about all aspects of nonverbal communication, this comprehensive text delineates the various features of nonverbal communication and expounds on each, incorporating extensive literature and research.

Morse, J.M., Solberg, S.M., Neander, W.L., Bottorff, J., & Johnson, J.L. (1990). Concepts of caring and caring as a concept. *Advances in Nursing Science,* 13(1), 1-14.

Although there has been a "significant but rather slow cultural movement" in revitalizing, revaluing, and reestablishing care as central to nursing (Leininger, 1990, p. 31) over the past 3 decades, Morse and colleagues advise that theory development needs to keep pace by focusing on the client and client outcomes of caring; otherwise caring will remain an inadequate and only partially useful concept for nursing.

Northouse, P.G. & Northouse, L.L., (1985). *Health communication: A handbook for health professionals.* Englewood Cliffs, N.J.: Prentice-Hall, Inc.

The authors include an overview of the various models of communication as well as an historical recall of the changing definitions of communication.

Stevenson, J.S., & Tripp-Reimer, T. (Eds.), 1990 *Knowledge about care and caring: State of the art and future developments.* Kansas City, Mo.: American Academy of Nursing.

For nurses interested in reading about care and caring in nursing this up-to-date summary of the proceedings of the 1989 Wingspread Conference on Caring is an excellent resource on the current conceptualization and research of caring in nursing.

CHAPTER 2

The Client-Nurse Relationship: A Helping Relationship

"Let people realize clearly that every time they threaten someone or humiliate or unnecessarily hurt or dominate or reject another human being, they become forces for the creation of psychopathology, even if these be small forces. Let them recognize that every person who is kind, helpful, decent, psychologically democratic, affectionate, and warm, is a psychotherapeutic force, even though a small one."

A. Maslow

OBJECTIVES

Encounters we have with our clients can be harmful or helpful. As a compassionate and caring nurse you will want your interactions with your clients to be helpful and pleasant. This chapter has information that you can integrate and apply to ensure that you relate effectively with your clients.

The nature of the client-nurse relationship is described so that you can explain how it differs from social, collegial, and kinship relationships. The responsibilities of the nurse in the client-nurse relationship have been outlined so that you will be able to articulate your roles and interventions at each stage of the helping relationship. You are invited to discover the extent to which you foster a helping relationship in your interactions with clients.

THE NATURE OF THE HELPING RELATIONSHIP

There is a set of pre-established rules and expectations that directs the course of client-nurse interactions. There may be some overlap in these interactions with those involving friends and family, but one factor in particular differentiates helping from social relationships. *A helping relationship is established for the benefit of the client,* whereas kinship and friendship relationships are designed to meet mutual needs. In particular, the client-nurse relationship is established to help the client achieve and maintain optimal health.

"A successful helping relationship between nurse and client represents a different order of interaction than that which occurs in a friendship. This is not because of any superiority in the nurse, but because of the mutual trust and the responsibilities for assisting others that characterize true professional relationships. . . . There is an underlying purpose in helping relationships that is beyond mutual enjoyment" (Jette, 1983, p. 200). Nursing actions are planned to promote, maintain, and restore the client's/patient's well-being and health (Congress for Nursing Practice, American Nurses' Association [ANA], 1973).

Professional practitioners of nursing bear primary responsibility for the nursing care clients/patients receive (Congress for Nursing Practice, ANA, 1973). The client-nurse relationship is entered for the benefit of the client, and although it is not undertaken primarily for mutual benefit, it is preferable if it is mutually satisfying. The client is satisfied when his health care needs have been met and he senses he has been cared for. The nurse feels a sense of accomplishment when her interventions have had a positive influence on her client's health status, and when her conduct has been competent and caring. The client-nurse relationship may be a mutual learning experience, but in general the goals of the therapeutic relationship are directed toward the growth of the client (Stuart & Sundeen, 1991, p. 93).

Never assume that in the client-nurse relationship the client plays the role of passive receiver awaiting the soothing administrations of an influential nurse. Both the client and nurse bring their respective knowledge, attitudes, feelings, skills, and patterns of behaving to the client-nurse relationship. Calling it a relationship indicates a sense of affiliation that bonds the client and the nurse, and an interdependency and reciprocity between them.

They each come to the relationship with unique cognitive, affective, and psychomotor abilities that they use in their joint endeavor of enhancing the client's well-being. The nurse is responsible for encouraging this interchange of ideas, values, and skills. In an effective helping relationship there is a definite and guaranteed interchange between the client and nurse in all three dimensions.

Standards V and VII of the American Nurses' Association Standards of Nursing Practice (1973) articulate the importance of the client's participation in his health care.

Standard V. Nursing actions provide for client/patient participation in health promotion, maintenance, and restoration. The client/patient and family are continuously involved in nursing care.

Standard VII. The client's/patient's progress or lack of progress toward goal achievement is determined by the client/patient and the nurse. The quality of nursing care depends on comprehensive and intelligent determination of nursing impact upon the health status of the client/patient. The client/patient is an essential part of this determination.

Cognitive, Affective, and Psychomotor Abilities in the Therapeutic Encounter

The following figure outlines some of the cognitive, affective, and psychomotor abilities that the client and the nurse bring to their therapeutic encounter. Figure 2-1 illustrates that both client and nurse come with notions and expectations that will influence the course and outcome of their relationship.

Cognitive

Both client and nurse know something about health and illness in general, and about the client's health concerns in particular. The client has definite notions about what has made him ill, and what might improve his health; in turn, the nurse has her views, based on her knowledge and beliefs about what will help her client. To prevent them from operating in isolation or at cross-purposes, they must exchange the information essential for the client's improvement.

Besides having different ideas, clients and nurses both have preferred ways of observing their worlds and making decisions about what they see. Each of us has a preferred mental process, the one we have developed most highly, the one we use best, that forms the core of our personalities (Lawrence, 1982, p. 8). Clients and nurses have different ways they prefer to use their minds, specifically the way they choose to perceive and make judgments (Myers, 1980, p. 1). Perceiving includes becoming aware of things, people, occurrences, and ideas. Judging includes reaching conclusions about what has been observed.

For example, some clients and nurses are primarily practical. They are attuned to immediate experiences, the literal facts at hand, and the concrete realities. Other clients and nurses prefer to think about what could be, rather than what is. Their intuitive imagination fills their minds with ideas and explanations that do not always depend on the senses for verification.

Consider this situation for understanding of the differences in these two ways of perceiving, and how they would affect the client-nurse relationship.

Mr. Zabrick is an 80-year old resident of a senior citizens' apartment complex where he lives with his retired, widowed sister, age 70. In the past 9 months he has had chemotherapy and radiation treatments for lung cancer. His tumor has vanished and his blood

What the client brings to the client-nurse relationship

COGNITIVE

- Preferred ways of perceiving and judging
- Knowledge and beliefs about illness in general and his illness in particular
- Knowledge and beliefs about health promotion and maintenance in general, and information about his own health care activities
- Ability to problem solve
- Ability to learn

AFFECTIVE

- Cultural values
- Feelings about seeking help from a nurse
- Attitudes towards nurses in general
- Attitudes towards treatment regime
- Values toward preventing illness
- Willingness to take positive action about own health status at this time with this particular nurse

PSYCHOMOTOR

- Ability to relate and communicate with others
- Ability to carry out own health care management
- Ability to learn new methods of self-care

INTERCHANGE

What the nurse brings to the client-nurse relationship

COGNITIVE

- Preferred ways of perceiving and judging
- Knowledge and beliefs about illness in general
- Knowledge about her clinical specialty
- Knowledge and beliefs about health behaviors which prevent illness and promote, regain, and maintain health
- Ability to problem solve
- Knowledge about factors which increase client compliance with treatment regimen

AFFECTIVE

- Cultural values
- Feelings about being a nurse-helper
- Attitudes towards clients in general
- Biases about nursing treatment regime
- Value placed on being healthy
- Value placed on people actively preventing illness or enhancing well-being
- Willingness to help client take positive action to improve his well-being

PSYCHOMOTOR

- Ability to relate and communicate with others
- Proficiency in administering effective nursing interventions
- Ability to teach nursing interventions to client

Figure 2-1 Interchange of knowledge, attitudes, and skills between client and nurse in the helping relationship

work is stabilized, yet to his disappointment he feels lethargic and anorexic.

Eight days ago his sister awoke in the night and found Mr. Zabrick in the bathtub, where he had fallen after mistaking it for the toilet. She noticed that her brother is unsteady on his feet and is losing weight.

Clients (or family members) and nurses who prefer details would perceive Mr. Zabrick's situation by focusing on the concrete, visible evidence that might account for his deterioration. They would notice the lack of saliva under, and the brown furry nature of, the tongue, as well as the unpleasant taste and odor in the mouth. They would see the small, hard stools and the abdominal distention. They would feel the decreased turgor of his skin and the muscle weakness. They would count the amount of fluids and quantity of food consumed by Mr. Zabrick.

Next, the client or nurse who prefers detailed, sensing information would put these pieces together and likely come to the conclusion that Mr. Zabrick is dehydrated. Obviously, this way of perceiving prefers things that are measurable, and the thinking process is systematic, taking one step at a time.

Clients (or family members) and nurses who prefer a more intuitive perceiving process might not gather all these data before jumping to a conclusion about what is happening to Mr. Zabrick. They are likely to look for patterns in the data (as opposed to discrete pieces of information); they would start thinking about the possible explanations and then work back to get the facts. For example, they might notice that Mr. Zabrick has said, "Why bother with trying any more? If I had a chance to do it again, I'm not sure I'd take the treatments", and wonder if his fatigue and grief are consuming him. They might remember that Mr. Zabrick's daughter-in-law died despite rigorous chemotherapy, and that his life-long friend was diagnosed with brain cancer 3 weeks ago, and wonder if Mr. Zabrick's symptoms reflect his doubt about living with such losses. Another theme that intuitive individuals might focus on is the relationship between the assault on Mr. Zabrick's body from treatments, changes in diet, exercise, and sleep deprivation, and the impact of the severe heat and humidity of the past 7 weeks.

These two perceptive processes are very different, and it is important for nurses to understand their preferred way of perceiving, and to try to discover which process the client prefers. You will also note that both ways of seeing the world are valuable—one is not better than the other; they simply pick out different information on which to focus.

Judging, the way of making decisions about the information collected through perception, is the other mental process where clients and nurses may differ. Some persons will have logical, orderly, analytical decision-making processes and treat the world objectively (Myers, 1980). Decision-makers like these prefer to fit all experience into logical mental systems.

The other way of judging uses mental processes to achieve harmony and protect human values above all else. These clients and nurses prefer to tune into the subjective world of feelings and values, and are alert to the human issues in any situation.

Each of us prefers one of these decision-making processes over the other (Myers, 1980). Consider this situation to get more understanding of the two judging processes.

Jossie is a 19-year-old first-year university student who is 8 weeks pregnant and unmarried. She is receiving counseling about her options. She sees three choices and will soon decide whether to have an abortion, continue with the pregnancy and give up her baby for adoption, or carry her baby to term and raise him.

Clients and nurses who prefer a rational, objective way of making decisions would invite Jossie to consider all the facts and then make the only logical decision based on them. They would look at the consequences of any decision Jossie might make and judge it using their heads, not their hearts. They would be able to remain emotionally uninvolved. They have the ability to see the "long view" and would likely invite Jossie to look logically into her future, and act on the most sensible decision (Myers, 1980; Page, 1983).

Clients, family members, and nurses who prefer to consider effects on the people in the situation would likely explore how Jossie feels about each of the choices and how each fits with her values. Such people would likely emphasize the benefits of any plan Jossie considers, rather that criticizing it; they would also likely support Jossie's personal convictions (Page, 1983).

This glimpse at two different methods for using our minds alerts us to the misunderstandings that could arise in the client-nurse helping relationship. We cannot assume that clients' minds are guided by the same principles as our own. Clients, their family members, and your colleagues in the workplace may reason the same as you, or they may prefer using different ways of perceiving and judging. They may not value the things you value, or show interest in the same things you do (Myers, 1980).

We all use different combinations of perceiving and judging, and colleagues and clients with the same preferences are likely to be the easiest to like and understand. They will tend to have similar interests (because they share the same kinds of perceptions) and consider the same matters important (because they share the same kinds of judgment) (Myers, 1980).

On the other hand, it will be harder to understand and predict the behavior of colleagues and clients who differ on perception and judgment preferences. We are likely to take opposite stands on any issue with colleagues and clients who prefer different thinking processes (Myers, 1980). "The nurse-patient relationship is characterized by mutual growth of two individuals who 'dare' to discover love, growth and freedom together. The uniqueness of each or the two is valued, and differing values respected. Through dialogue, not monologue, the client's reality and worth are affirmed" (Stuart & Sundeen, 1991, p. 94).

If you would like to learn more about your preferences for perceiving and making decisions, as well as two other personality preferences, arrange with your school's counseling or guidance department to take the Myers-Briggs Type Indicator (MBTI). The aim of the MBTI is to identify, from self-reporting of easily-recognized reactions, the basic preferences of people in regard to perception and judgment (Myers & McCaulley,

1985). Learning about your own preferences will make you more aware of how your way of thinking influences the client-nurse helping relationship.

Affective

All clients and nurses have positive and negative feelings about the helping relationship; also, each has biases about the other. Both have different priorities for working on particular health concerns. The attitudes of both the client and the nurse will greatly affect whether they will work in harmony or discord; whether their respective knowledge will surface or submerge; and each will carry out the commitment of improving the client's health.

The major source of our value system is our culture. In America today, the culture is heterogeneous (with a variety of cultural groups in the American society), so that nurses and clients are likely to encounter different beliefs and values, particularly as the United States increasingly becomes home to people from all parts of the world. Modern medical and nursing practices become two of the external forces immigrants encounter (Leininger, 1978). This encounter with the American health care system is loaded with choices for immigrants to make in deciding how much of their culture's traditional medical practices they wish to maintain. Cultural patterns are one of the important means by which people adapt to recurrent change in their environments. Cultural patterns make life secure, a valuable factor in the emotional, mental, physical, and social health of a cultural group (Leininger, 1978).

Leininger believes that America has entered an era in which health care professionals are interested in and emphasize their clients' cultural and social values. In the late 1970s she predicted that "this new era will be dependent upon nursing and medical staff who have knowledge of sociocultural factors influencing patient behavior" (Leininger, 1978, p. 122). Obviously, this brings the responsibility for nurses to know the major cultural values of their own country. Her outline of the major American cultural values and how they influence thinking and action follows.

- **The cultural value of optimal health:** The marked emphasis given to optimal health for all Americans definitely contrasts with that of other societies where health is not the major concern and where little financial, social, and political effort may be given to health (Leininger, 1978, p. 128).
- **The cultural value of democracy:** The principles, policies, and norms of democracy are emphasized by social equality, representation by the people, and equal participation by anyone who wants to be heard or desires to participate in American affairs (Leininger, 1978, p. 129). For nurses, this cultural value carries the responsibility to provide all clients with equal time and consideration.

- **The cultural value of individualism:** Those religious beliefs which stress human rights and dignity buttress individualism (Leininger, 1978, p. 130). This emphasis contrasts with many cultures where it is the social group, and *not* the individual, that receives primary consideration.
- **Cultural values of achieving and doing:** Americans are urged to work hard, to keep busy, and to achieve in order to be successful. The cultural value of achievement keeps one moving and acting in order to convince others of one's motives and worth.

  In contrast, a number of cultures have learned to enjoy what they have. Moreover, they do not feel the urgency to be perpetually moving about and working feverishly for some goal or material object, or to produce something (Leininger, 1978, p. 131).
- **The cultural value of cleanliness:** Cleanliness, a dominant value in this culture, is closely related to optimal health. Leininger points out that there are few countries in the world that emphasize cleanliness as Americans do. Some other cultures are shocked by the way Americans order their lives around cleanliness. Often non-Americans are quite relaxed about being dirty, and may see a positive value in having some dirt on and around them.
- **The cultural value of time:** In our culture there is a perpetual emphasis placed on time and schedules. Time is precious. Time dictates where we will be during each hour of the day and night. In contrast, some cultures do not even have a time instrument, and people do not subject themselves to the slavery of clock-watching (Leininger, 1978, p. 132).

Think about the cultural values that influence you in your client-nurse helping relationships. What cultural values affect your clients?

Psychomotor

A client needs to know what skills the nurse has, and a nurse should find out about her client's ability to participate in his treatment plan. Both parties must come to an agreement about what their respective tasks will be in their effort to improve the client's health status.

CLIENT PRIVILEGES IN THE HELPING RELATIONSHIP

Far more than simple discourse between nurse and client, the professional interpersonal relationship is a purposeful dynamic interplay of energy, resources, and commitment to confronting human issues of meaning, self-realization, and personal growth in a variety of clinical settings (Arnold & Boggs, 1989).

As consumers of our health care services, clients have the right to:
- Expect a systematic and accurate investigation of their health concerns by a thorough and well-organized nurse

- Be informed about their health status and have all their questions answered so that they clearly understand what the nurse means
- Receive health care from a nurse, with current knowledge about their diagnosis, capable of providing safe and efficient care
- Feel confident they will be treated courteously and that the nurse will show genuine interest in them
- Trust that any issues of personal confidentiality will be respected
- Be informed about any plans of action to be carried out for their benefit
- Refuse or consent to nursing treatments without jeopardizing their relationship with the nurse
- Secure help conveniently and without hassles or roadblocks
- Receive consistent quality of care from all nurses

Features of the Client-Nurse Helping Relationship

The client-nurse relationship is a special helping relationship which is characterized by the following features:
- It is a **partnership** between the client and nurse. Both work together to improve the client's health status.
- It represents the nurse's **philosophy** about human nature and what motivates humans in health and illness. As nurses, we should know our beliefs and values and be able to articulate them clearly.
- It is **purposeful** and **productive.** Together, the client and nurse agree about the nature of the client's health problem, and they develop and implement a plan designed to reach agreed-upon objectives. Client and nurse together evaluate the outcomes and decide whether the desired and expected outcomes have been achieved.
- It can **preserve** the client's present level of health, and **protect** him from future threats to his health, because of the increased knowledge he gleans in the helping relationship.
- It can **palliate** the client's worries and fears through the nurse's reassurances, and ease his pain through soothing comfort measures.
- It can be a **psychic** or morale booster. Clients perk up from the positive attention and interest they receive from nurses.
- It can be **practical** when it offers efficacious, effective and efficient ways of handling health concerns.
- It is **portable** and takes place wherever and whenever a client and nurse come together.
- It has **phases.** There is a beginning (initiation), middle (maintenance), and end (termination) to each encounter between client and nurse.
- It should be **personally** tailored to the needs of each particular client.
- It is **platonic** and not passionate. Even though nurses may have strong caring feelings for their clients, it is expected that they can maintain adequate objectivity and perspective to provide therapeutic assistance.
- It is a **private** relationship in which clients may disclose intimate details about their lives. It is the nurse's responsibility to protect her clients' confidentiality.

- It can be a **powerful** relationship. Clients and nurses can develop attachments for each other, which makes their relationship special for each.

Pertinent Pointers to Guide You in the Client-Nurse Helping Relationship

This section offers some "dos" and "don'ts" for conducting yourself in the client-nurse helping relationship. Here are the "dos."

Do:

- Be **prepared** mentally, emotionally, and physically to assist your clients in resolving their health-care problems.
- Be **punctual** and **polite** in your manner of relating to clients.
- **Promote** clients' well-being, comfort and increased health status.
- Be **philanthropic** in your approach to clients by putting their needs and concerns first.
- Be **plucky** in planning and generating creative solutions to your clients' health concerns.
- Be **proficient** in the nursing skills required to safely and successfully care for your clients.
- **Praise** and encourage clients in their efforts to take better care of themselves.
- Be **patient** and understanding about clients' reactions to their particular health situations.
- **Persevere** in pursuing your pledge to help clients preserve their health.
    It is helpful to have in mind some of the "don'ts" as well as some of the "dos" about nurses' behavior in the helping relationship. Here are the "don'ts."

Do Not:

- **Patronize** clients.
- **Preach** at or **pressure** them to change.
- **Pigeonhole** clients with labels such as "good," "lazy," "uncooperative," which prevent you from seeing clients as they really are.
- **Procrastinate** following through on clients' reasonable requests.
- **Put down** clients by using medical jargon, or in any way making them feel inadequate or estranged.
- **Punish** clients for acts of omission or commission which have negatively affected their health.
- Reveal **prejudices** against the race, religion, or creed of clients.
- Be **pleasure-seeking** or trying to meet your own needs through the client-nurse relationship.
- **Pretend** or attempt to pull the wool over clients' eyes. It is their health

with which you are dealing and clients have the right to receive honest, forthright communication.

Being an Effective Nurse-Helper Requires Being Assertive and Responsible

As a nurse, it is your responsibility to ensure that a thorough assessment is made of your client's health concerns, that suitable nursing actions are chosen and implemented to help the client, and that an evaluation of the results is carried out. Assuming this leadership does not mean that you take over and do *for* or *to* your client. The quality of your nursing care is determined by the completeness of the interchange of knowledge, attitudes, and skills between you and your client.

To be most helpful to your client, make sure that you solicit his knowledge, become aware of his feelings and attitudes, and take into account his strengths and limitations for self-care. You must use this information in order to tailor your nursing care to suit your client. In addition, you need to be aware of how your knowledge, attitude and skills affect your ability to be helpful.

Effective nursing requires being assertive and responsible. Your goal is to help your clients achieve their best possible health status and do so in a way that allows expression of your professional competence. It is expected that you attempt to meet both these desired outcomes.

You must act responsibly to achieve your nursing goals. You need to collect pertinent information from your clients and make an accurate assessment upon which you will base your nursing care. The interpersonal communication behaviors in this book will help you develop your skills in these areas. The next chapter will show you how to make your problem-solving a mutual affair between you and your clients. Using this approach, you will be an assertive and responsible nurse-helper.

The following exercises will help you get to know yourself as a nurse-helper.

Practicing Helping

Exercise 1. The following questions have been designed to get you thinking about yourself as a nurse-helper. They are not easy questions, for they tap your basic beliefs and values about being a helper. To begin, answer the questions on your own. Later, get together with your classmates and discuss your responses. You will learn a lot from each other.
- What does health mean to you?
- What factors positively influence clients to take care of their health?
- Do you think health is a right or a privilege?
- To what extent do you think clients are responsible for the development of their health problems?
- What can you do, as a nurse, to increase the likelihood that your clients will take better care of themselves?

To be an effective helper it is important that you know how your feelings about being a helper influence how you relate to your clients.

• To what extent do you think clients are responsible for solving their own health care problems?
• With what degree of dependence (independence) in your clients are you comfortable?
• What is it you like most about helping clients?
• What is it you like least?

Nurses are expected to be proficient in carrying out a range of nursing treatments.

• How competent do you feel implementing the most essential nursing interventions in your clinical area?
• How would you rate your ability to teach clients how to take care of their own health?

Exercise 2. You have relationships with colleagues, friends, family members, and clients. How do your relationships with your clients differ from these? How are they the same? To help you answer this question, observe and make notes about the differences and similarities as you actually engage in these relationships. Once you have formulated your ideas, compare and contrast them with the views of your colleagues.

Exercise 3. What knowledge, attitudes, and skills in the nurse create and foster a therapeutic relationship? Think about your response on your own and then pool your ideas with your classmates.

Your responses to this question will help point out where your knowledge, attitudes, and skills are conducive to a helping relationship, and help you map out areas that need refinement to make you a better helper.

Exercise 4. American nurses will increasingly work with foreign-educated colleagues and immigrant clients; a number of social-psychological characteristics will affect how the foreign-educated and -born behave in the host country (Furnham & Bochner, 1986, p. 230). Review the following characteristics of host countries, and ask yourself to what extent these characteristics are present in your part of the United States.

• *Ethnocentrism:* the extent to which a country boosts its own identity and looks with contempt on outsiders. How do nurses and other health professionals show respect for people from other countries?
• *Territoriality:* the extent to which the host culture protects and defends its own territory. Do nurses encourage foreign-educated nurses to attend professional meetings, parties, or conferences? Does the hiring policy welcome and even encourage the hiring of foreign-educated nurses? Does the admission protocol have an open-door policy for clients from all cultures?
• *Shunning of dissimiliarity:* the extent to which a culture experiences differences from itself in terms of arousal and negative affect. Do American nurses give consideration and a fair trial to nursing procedures de-

veloped in other countries? Or do American nurses actively shun nursing ideas that haven't been developed in their own country? What reactions do nurses have to different food preferences, child-rearing practices, or relationships between the sexes in other cultures?

• *Competitiveness:* the extent to which a culture seeks out or feels competition from other cultures/groups. To what extent do American nurses and health profesionals acknowledge foreign methods or procedures as worthy, or show the ultimate compliment by adopting the innovation?

• *Search for control:* the extent to which a culture requires people to accept its belief and value systems that function to ensure predictability and control. Do American nurses allow clients to believe in and practice alternative health practices? What range and variation in dress and accent do nurse and health professionals permit?

Compare your responses with others in your class. Are you surprised by your responses?

REFERENCES

Arnold, E., & Boggs, K. (1989). *Interpersonal relationships: Professional communication skills for nurses.* Philadelphia: W.B. Saunders Company.

Congress for Nursing Practice, American Nurses' Association (1973). *Standards of nursing practice.* Kansas City, Mo.: The Association.

Furnham, A., & Bochner, S. (1986). *Culture shock: Psychological reactions to unfamiliar environments.* London: Routledge.

Jette, S.H. (1983). Interpersonal communication in nursing. In J.B. Lindberg, M.L. Hunter, & A.Z. Kruszewski (Eds.), *Introduction to person-centered nursing* (pp. 195-222). Philadelphia: J.B. Lippincott Company.

Lawrence, G. (1982). *People types and tiger stripes: A practical guide to learning styles* (2nd ed.). Gainesville, Fl.: Center for Application of Psychological Type, Inc.

Leininger, M. (1978). *Transcultural nursing: Concepts, theories, and practices.* New York: John Wiley & Sons.

Myers, I.B. (1980). *Gifts differing.* Palo Alto, Calif.: Consulting Psychologists Press, Inc.

Myers, I.B., & McCaully, M.H. (1985). *A guide to the development and use of the Myers-Briggs type indicator.* Palo Alto, Calif.: Consulting Psychologists Press.

Page, E.C. (1983). *Looking at type: A description of the preferences reported by the Myers-Briggs type indicator.* Gainesville, Fl.: Center for Application of Psychological Type, Inc.

Stuart, G.W. and Sundeen, S.J. (Eds.). (1991). *Principles and practice of psychiatric nursing* (4th ed.). St. Louis: Mosby–Year Book.

SUGGESTIONS FOR FURTHER READING

Avila, D., Combs, A.W., & Purkey, W.W. (Eds.) (1977). *The helping relationship sourcebook* (2nd ed.). Boston: Allyn & Bacon, Inc.

This book provides the beginning helper with an overview of the essential philosophical questions related to the helping process. For beginning nurses, the chapter by Carl Rogers, "The characteristics of a helping relationship", provides suggestions about formulating a helping relationship. Rogers makes a useful comparison between helpful and nonhelpful relationships.

Brammer, L.M. (1979). *The helping relationship: Process and skills* (2nd ed.). Englewood Cliffs, N.J.: Prentice-Hall, Inc.

Brammer's first three chapters are useful for student nurses wanting to read more about the helping relationship. In these chapters he describes helping and outlines characteristics of helpers and the skills needed to develop a helping relationship. He points out some of the problems encountered by helpers in various stages of the helping relationship.

Carkhuff, R.R., Pierce, R.M. & Cannon, J.R. (1980). *The art of helping IV* (4th ed.). Mass.: Human Resource Development Press Inc.

The essential skills needed by helpers are illustrated with cartoons, which drive the points home. Students can do a pre- and post-test of their helpfulness, and gauge how they are improving.

Combs, A.W., Avila, D.L., & Purkey, W.W. (1978). *Helping relationships: Basic concepts for the helping professions* (2nd ed.). Boston: Allyn & Bacon, Inc.

For the nurse who wants to read about the humanistic approach to helping, this book provides a comprehensive overview. The last chapter, "Being and becoming helpers", raises issues all helpers need to look at in themselves.

Cormier, W.H., & Cormier, L.S. (1979). *Interviewing strategies for helpers: A guide to assessment, treatment, and evaluation.* Monterey, Calif.: Brooks/Cole Publishing Company.

In the chapter, "Ingredients of an effective helping relationship", the authors have some excellent self-learning exercises for helpers. You can learn about your competence, power, and intimacy assessment. The whole chapter invites interaction by the reader.

Gazda, G.M., Walters, R.P., & Childers, W.C. (1975). *Human relations development: A manual for the health sciences.* Boston: Allyn & Bacon, Inc.

In the first chapter the authors have summarized a review of the literature to defend the importance of the need for facilitative human relations in the delivery of health care.

Hames, C.C., & Joseph, D.H. (1986). *Basic concepts of helping: A holistic approach* (2nd ed.). Norwalk, Conn.: Appleton-Century-Crofts.

A compact historical overview of helping through history; will be of interest to students.

Northouse, P.G., & Northouse, L.L. (1985). *Health communication: A handbook for health professionals.* Englewood Cliffs, N.J.: Prentice-Hall, Inc.

The beginning chapter, which provides a clear study of selected models of communication, including the strength and limitations of each, presents a good approach for nurses. Chapter 3, on communication in health care relationships, outlines a new way of considering some of the potential problem areas in the helping relationship.

Sundeen, S.J., Stuart, G.W., Rankin, E.A., & Cohen, S.A. (1989). *Nurse-client interaction: Implementing the nursing process* (4th ed.). St. Louis: Mosby–Year Book.

In Chapter 5, the authors blend, in a unique way, a number of significant concepts for the helping relationship. Students will delight in the selected concepts, including that of hope. The authors' detailed explanation of the stages of the course of the helping relationship is another strength.

Ujhely, G (1968). *Determinants of the nurse-patient relationship.* New York: Springer Publishing Company, Inc.

This is not a "how to" manual, but a readable overview about what the nurse and client bring to the helping relationship, and the importance of the context within which the helping relationship takes place.

CHAPTER 3

Mutual Problem-Solving in Nursing

"Equal opportunity and mutual respect are matters not only of law, but also of the human heart and spirit, and the latter are not always amenable to law."

Dwight D. Eisenhower

OBJECTIVES

This chapter will reaffirm your beliefs in the process of mutual problem-solving. The examples provided will illustrate some of the ways to validate each step of the problem-solving process with your clients. The exercises will give you a chance to practice mutual problem-solving so that it becomes a well-integrated and natural part of your approach. You will be introduced to making contracts with your clients.

WHAT IS THE DIFFERENCE BETWEEN PROBLEM-SOLVING AND MUTUAL PROBLEM-SOLVING IN NURSING?
Problem-Solving: The Nursing Process

It is generally agreed that there are eight steps to the problem-solving process in nursing (also called the nursing process):
1. Collection of data
2. Analysis of data
3. Formulation of nursing diagnoses
4. Prioritization of nursing diagnoses
5. Determination of desired and/or expected outcomes
6. Decision-making about nursing strategies to achieve outcomes
7. Implementation of nursing actions
8. Evaluation of outcomes
   The Standards of Nursing Practice (1973), developed by the Congress

34

for Nursing Practice of the American Nurses' Association, are stated according to this systematic approach to nursing practice: the assessment of the client's/patient's status, plan of nursing actions, implementation of the plan, and evaluation (p. 1).

The Mutual Problem-Solving Process in Nursing
Validation

Validation makes the difference between problem-solving *for* clients and mutual problem-solving *with* clients. Incorporating validation keeps us focused on the rights and obligations of clients to make their own decisions about their health.

The important activity of validation must be incorporated at each step of the problem-solving process in nursing. Validation is consciously seeking out our client's opinions and feelings at each phase of the nursing process. Validation means unearthing any questions or concerns he has about plans for his health care, and securing his understanding and willingness to proceed to the next step. Incorporating validation into our problem-solving stops us from forging ahead and *doing to* our clients. It ensures that we obtain complete agreement and commitment from our client about the nursing care plans being considered for his particular health problem.

A mutual problem-solving process in nursing looks like this:
1. Collection of data
2. Analysis of data
3. Validating your interpretation of data with the client
4. Identifying actual or potential problems with the client
5. Validating the nursing diagnoses with the client
6. Setting priorities for resolution of identified problems with the client
7. Determining expected and desired outcomes of nursing actions in collaboration with the client
8. Deciding on the nursing strategies to achieve these outcomes in collaboration with the client
9. Implementing nursing actions with assistance from the client
10. Encouraging client participation in carrying out nursing actions to meet the outcomes
11. Evaluating the outcomes of nursing care in consultation with the client

Including validation in the nursing process increases the number of steps but does not necessarily increase the time or energy required to carry out nursing care. Much of the checking can be done quickly and naturally while interacting with our clients. Ensuring that our clients understand and agree with each step of the nursing process increases the probability that they will do their part to comply with treatment. Clients who have a clear understanding of their health problems, and what they and their nurse can do about it, will expend less energy worrying and more energy doing something constructive. Clarity about their nursing diagnosis, and having a say in how best to handle it, gives clients a sense of control.

Validation invites the collaboration that is essential for successful client change (Risner, 1986). The trust developed from working together is likely to increase the accuracy and validity of the database, enriching the foundation for the rest of the nursing process. The trust growing out of mutuality provides the client with an "anchor," giving him the support he needs to risk changing health behaviors. Collaboration ensures the benefits of two heads working on a health problem; this is essential because nursing cannot exist in a vacuum, striving for perfection without including full participation of the client (Risner, 1986, p. 161).

Many of today's health care consumers are speaking up, asking questions, seeking second opinions, demanding alternative health care options, and forming their own self-help groups to take action. This assertiveness and independence reflects the true meaning of the label "client," designating those who claim the rights and privileges of partnership in health care (Lindberg, Hunter, & Kruszewski, 1983). "A client is a person who has contracted for services from another who is qualified to provide these services. There is an assumption that this kind of relationship is a negotiated partnership and that the client is capable of taking the information provided and utilizing it in some fashion or other" (Lindberg, Hunter, & Kruszewski, 1983, p. 8).

Not all health care consumers are this self-protective. Some do what health care professionals tell them, living out the definition of the label "patient": ". . . an individual awaiting or under medical care or treatment; the recipient of various person services" (Lindberg, Hunter, & Kruszewski, 1983, p. 8). The passivity of this stance creates an inequitable relationship between nurses and people. As nurses, we can help reverse this apathy and listlessness by encouraging our clients to be partners in their health care (Lindberg, Hunter, & Kruszewski, 1983, p. 9). This means appreciating the worth of our clients and calling on their strengths. We can transform our nursing care into a mutual problem-solving process when we invite, even request, the full participation of our partners—the clients.

Earlier in this century patients were more satisfied with a system of illness care that focused on disease eradication (Lindberg, Hunter, & Kruszewski, 1983, p. 134). As the influence of science and technology on health care swelled, discontent emerged along with resentment of the chauvinism of all-knowing health care professionals. People began demanding more say in their health care and requesting more individualized care. Evidence of this movement materialized in 1972, with the publication of the Patient's Bill of Rights (presented by the American Hospital Association). This document describes the expectations for respect, knowledge, privacy and confidentiality, and access to any information essential for adequate treatment. Pelletier (1979) warned of the need to focus on the individual's responsibility for health care, as well as his rights (Pelletier, 1979, p. 65). For nurses, it is important to emphasize what clients can do to take care of themselves, as well as to safeguard their right to quality, informed care.

The following statements from the Standards of Nursing Practice (1973) demonstrate the support of the American Nurses' Association for a mutual problem-solving approach with clients:

Standard V. Nursing actions provide for client/patient participation in health promotion, maintenance and restoration.

This standard demands that clients/patients and family are kept informed about current health status, changes in health status, total health care plan, nursing care plan, roles of health care personnel, and health care resources. Clients/patients and family must be provided with the information needed to make decisions and choices about: promoting, maintaining and restoring health; seeking and utilizing appropriate health care personnel; and maintaining and using health care resources.

Standard VII. The client's/patient's progress or lack of progress toward goal achievement is determined by the client/patient and the nurse.

The client is an essential part of the comprehensive and intelligent determination of nursing's impact upon the health status of the client/patient. The client/patient evaluates nursing actions and goal achievment.

Incorporating Validation into the Nursing Process

The following example will illustrate some suggested methods for ensuring maximum client participation in a mutual problem-solving approach.

Validating the Nurse's Interpretation of the Data Collected with the Client

From the time a client enters our nursing care we start asking him questions about his health problem. As we receive information about his situation from the answers he gives us, the way he answers our questions, and objective data from laboratory tests and physical assessment, we start to piece together a meaningful picture. That picture is our interpretation of the data; it starts off fuzzy and develops into a clear explanation of our client's health problem(s).

Nurses are not the only ones who crave a clear picture of what is going on—the client is usually eager to know about his situation. Put yourself in the following clinical nursing situation in which your client seeks information from you.

Mrs. Woods is a 46-year-old who was admitted to your medical unit a week ago upon discovering that her adult-onset diabetes is out of control.

She has been on oral hypoglycemic agents for the past 2 years. Her admission blood sugar was 350 mg per 100 ml.

While talking with Mrs. Woods you learn that she has little knowledge about the special care she must take as a diabetic to ensure that her nutritional intake is satisfactory, that her skin care is thorough, and that she checks her urine daily for sugar. You learn that she has been given verbal and nonverbal messages from her parents and husband that she must be a perfect wife and homemaker. Her sisters are all perfectly healthy women and her husband is a fitness fanatic who tells her that he will not tolerate any sickness. When the symptoms of hyperglycemia were surfacing, Mrs. Woods tried to ignore them and pretend that nothing was wrong. It was at the insistence of her neighbor that she conceded to see her family doctor about her increased thirst and appetite and her diminished strength and weight loss.

> **Mrs. Woods:** "I can't wait to get home again. I can't stay in here. My husband is complaining that things are getting out of hand at home while I 'lie around the hospital having all these tests done.' Lots of people have diabetes and I'm sure I'll be fine. When do you think I can go home? My husband wants me home in tiptop condition."

At this point you want to make Mrs. Woods aware of your assessment that she has very little knowledge about how to safely look after her diabetic condition, and to ensure that she avoids the many possible complications of diabetes. Your hunch is that she has never really learned much about diabetes because she wishes to pretend that she does not have a chronic illness, in an effort to live up to her parents' and husband's expectations. You sense that she may mistakenly assume that she may not be able to live a completely active and full life as a diabetic.

You validate this interpretation of the information with the following statement:

> "Mrs. Woods, I can see that you are really eager to leave the hospital and get home. However, I have some concerns about your heading home without learning more about taking care of yourself and your diabetes. You can feel and look like a healthy and vital woman when you know some of the ways to manage your diabetes. From what you've told me I know it's important for you and your husband that you're healthy. To keep that way, I think you need to accept that diabetes won't stop you from doing anything you want, if you know how to take care of yourself. What do you think?"

This validation respectfully lets your client know your thoughts about her health situation. Your ending question allows Mrs. Woods to agree, disagree, or ask questions about your interpretation of her health care situation.

Identifying Actual or Potential Problems with the Client

When Mrs. Woods has either agreed with or amended your interpretation of her situation, you can then formulate and validate the nursing diagnoses.

Mrs. Woods may say something like:

"What else is there to learn? I've been taught to give my own insulin and I can't just sit around here when I'm needed at home."

Her response provides you with an opening to inform her about the potential problems diabetics need to avoid. You could respond with:

"You have skillfully mastered taking your insulin, Mrs. Woods; however, there is a lot to learn in addition to that. All diabetics need to understand the signs and symptoms of low blood sugar and have a plan for emergencies. Because all diabetics can suffer from poor circulation, you would benefit from learning about special techniques for skin care. How to regulate your calories to adjust to your changing levels of energy is also essential to understand. Learning how to manage your day-to-day activities will make you feel as normal as everyone else."

This identification of some of the potential problems for diabetics would alert Mrs. Woods to some of the special considerations she has to make. Worded this way, your response engenders hope that she can live normally.

She might respond with:

"Oh. I thought all I had to do was give myself this insulin every day and I'd be okay. I guess there's more to it. My husband wants me to be healthy, and you've got to be healthy to keep up with him, so I'd better learn these things you're talking about."

Validating the Nursing Diagnoses with the Client

Mrs. Woods has acknowledged that she needs to learn how to take care of herself to prevent problems. Your next step as the nurse is to validate the nursing diagnoses with her. You might do that by saying:

"The three main areas to learn about are: adjusting your caloric intake to match your activity level; taking special precautions with your skin care—especially your feet; and getting a plan to cope with low blood sugar, should that occur. Does that pretty well cover it from your point of view?"

Your list of problem areas has been checked out with Mrs. Woods to see if she has any additions. She might respond with:

"That sounds like more than enough to learn before I leave here. The thing that boggles my mind is the bit about the skin care. I've always had good skin and I can't imagine having any problems with it."

Setting Priorities for Resolution of Identified Client Problems with the Client

Unless there is a life-threatening problem that should be treated first, there is some leeway in determining which problem to begin working on. The client may have preferences, or the amount of time available may determine where to start. It may be that by initially working on one problem, the other problems will clear up or diminish. For example, in this situation it is highly likely that Mrs. Woods will grow closer to accepting her diabetes when she learns to prevent potential problems. Your next step is to decide with Mrs. Woods what potential problem to work on first.

Mrs. Woods has indicated an interest in skin care. That may be a place to begin but you need to check it out with her. You suggest:

"Since you brought up the question of skin care, you may wish to begin there. The three areas are equally important and we can cover all three in any order you like."
"Well, I am most curious about the skin part," Mrs. Woods says.
"Well, let's start there then," you concur.

This validation has given Mrs. Woods some say in the order of handling her concerns and issues.

Determining Expected and Desired Outcomes of Nursing Actions in Collaboration with the Client

You and your client are aiming at outcomes. It is important for the nurse and client each to reveal their goals for nursing care. If nurses do not consult clients, it could happen that each will aim in different directions. Making the end results explicit provides you both with a benchmark for knowing when you have accomplished your goals.

You are at the point of clarifying and agreeing on the expectations for nursing care with Mrs. Woods. To begin this negotiation you might start off with a suggestion that Mrs. Woods can alter:

"We both need to have some idea of where we are headed, Mrs. Woods, so that we'll know when we've completed our task. In terms of the skin care and management of low blood sugar I would expect you to be able to map out your strategies for prevention of skin breakdown and low blood sugar, and what to do if either occurs. And in the area of caloric adjustment it's my hope that you'll soon be able to figure out your daily caloric balance so that you have the energy you need to live an active life. That sounds like a tall order but we can get started while you are in the hospital, and when you are discharged you can follow up at the diabetic clinic if you like. Those are my expectations of where we could head. I'd like to hear what you think."

These suggestions make it clear what you want Mrs. Woods to accomplish. Now it is her turn to indicate her goals.

Mrs. Woods: "It does seem like a lot to learn, but I guess I don't have much choice. I felt pretty sick before I came into the hospital and I don't really want to feel like that again. I don't think either my husband or I can take going through that. What you are saying makes sense. I'll give it a try."

You: "We can start with those goals. I think when you accomplish them you are going to feel like a new person. I am willing to wager that you'll feel more in control and not so strange about taking insulin and being a diabetic. In time everything will be more natural for you."

This reply provides Mrs. Woods with another good reason for learning about her condition; it introduces another desired outcome.

Deciding on the Nursing Strategies to Achieve These Outcomes in Collaboration with the Client

Now that you and Mrs. Woods have come to an agreement about where you are headed, you have to work out how you will get there. As nurses we have access to knowledge, people, and material resources to help our clients achieve their expected and desired outcomes. Clients bring their personal preferences, cost and time limitations, their own suggestions about the best treatment methods, and a willingness to learn. In this particular situation Mrs. Woods knows very little about diabetes and would most likely appreciate your input about the best way to improve her knowledge. You offer the following suggestion:

"You indicated you would like to start off with the skin care precautions. We have an excellent slide-tape show on the unit that has clear pictures and many examples of how to ensure that your skin doesn't break down. Or we have some pamphlets on skin care. And I'd be glad to go over any questions you have about it. Which method would help you to learn best?"

Mrs. Woods: "Gee, I don't know. It's been so long since I've been to school. I think I'd better see the tapes and read the flyers. And I want to talk to you about it afterwards, too."

You: "I'll get you the flyers when we have finished talking. The slide-tape show is set up in the resource room and I'll show you how to work it. We can talk when I don't have meds to give and you don't have visitors to entertain! How does that sound?"

Mrs. Woods: "Sounds fine."

Now that you have checked out this plan with your client you can continue.

You: "I need your opinions on the other two areas. We have a nutritionist who comes to the unit; she sees clients on an individual basis to go over their needs for calories and their desire for exercise, and helps them work out their menu planning so that it becomes second nature. She also has a class once a week to go over any questions that all the diabetics in the hospital might have. Would you like to see her individually or attend the class?"

Mrs. Woods: "She sounds like the expert, so I'd better see her. But I don't want to go to the group. I hate groups . . . I just clam up in them and I'm scared to open my mouth so I don't get anything out of them. I'd prefer to see her alone."

You: "Fine. I'll ask Mrs. Neufield, the dietitian, to see you as soon as possible about your menu planning. The only thing left to arrange for is the preparation for any diabetic emergencies. Since you don't wish to join the diabetic group how would you feel about talking to just one other diabetic client about how she manages?"

Mrs. Woods: "I'm not sure . . . I don't think so . . . I don't want everybody to know about my problems. No. I think I'd rather just talk to you about that."

You: "I'd be glad to teach you the signs and symptoms to watch for and what to do if you need help in a hurry. If you reconsider later and want to talk to another diabetic client, I'd be glad to arrange it."

Although the nurse in this negotiation has done most of the initial suggesting, Mrs. Woods has had plenty of opportunity to indicate her desires because they have been solicited and respected by the nurse. If clients are pushed or given ultimatums about how to take care of their health problems, they are less likely to really become interested in the process and follow-through.

Implementing Nursing Actions with Assistance from the Client; and Encouraging Client Participation in Carrying Out Nursing Actions to Meet the Outcomes

In Mrs. Woods' situation, your main focus would be on encouraging her participation in the various forms of learning how to manage her diabetes. One way to show your interest in her progress is to ask her open-ended questions that invite her to reveal how she is progressing. For example:

"How did you find the slide-tape show on skin care for diabetics?"

"What was useful for you in the pamphlet on skin care for diabetics that you read?"

"What questions do you have about skin care, either from the slide-tape show or the phamplets, that we might be able to discuss together?"

"What did you learn from the nutritionist about calorie adjustments?"

Questions like these would show your interest in her endeavors to learn about diabetes, and might also indicate where she needs encouragement or prompting to do more work. Finding out about clients' progress gives us an opportunity to offer them praise as well.

Evaluating the Outcomes of Nursing Care in Consultation with the Client

At this point you and your client check to see if your mutually agreed upon outcomes have been met.

After Mrs. Woods has had a chance to view the slide-tape show, read the manual, consult with the dietitian, and talk things over with you, it is time to evaluate the outcomes. This step need not be threatening to your client. Rather, it can be incorporated into your usual contact periods. In a situation where the client has carried out many of the activities in the care plan, it might even be appropriate to have a "test day" to check out his or her knowledge. With Mrs. Woods you decide to use humor to make the evaluation more fun.

You: "Well, Mrs. Woods! It's the day of reckoning! Are you ready for a quiz on all you've learned about diabetes?"

Mrs. Woods: "Well, if I don't know more than when I came in here, then something's wrong! I almost feel like I've been in school instead of the hospital!"

You: "You have been working hard, so I'd like us to review what you've been learning. The first thing we agreed on was that you would be able to map out strategies for the prevention of skin breakdown. Can you tell me how you're going to prevent any damage to your skin?"

Mrs. Woods: "I've learned a lot. First of all, out with my tight shoes! They *are* fashionable, but over time they may pinch my circulation. I'm going to chuck my knee-highs too. I've learned they can be like a vise on my calves, cutting off circulation. There was a good picture on how to cut your toe nails straight across. Thank goodness I already do that all right. And I know enough now to pat dry with the towel instead of making sandpaper out of my skin by rubbing it off with the towel! How's that?"

You: "You've really learned a lot and it sounds like you are going to make a lot of changes to protect your skin. The only two things I can think to add are making sure you are warm enough and using hand and body lotion to prevent your skin from drying. Even the motion of rubbing it in will improve your circulation. How about preventing low blood sugar; what have you learned about that?"

Mrs. Woods: "I had no idea this was so serious. Now I know what to watch for: hunger, feeling faint, getting edgy, and shaking. The part that scares me is that it can get bad enough that I can have a 'fit.' Now I understand why it's so important to check my urine every day. That way I'll pick up on things before they go completely out of whack. You've seen me check my urine four times a day so you know I can do that. And the dietitian went over with me how to adjust my diet when I exercise more, or when I'm less active."

You: "It sounds like you will take care to prevent your blood sugar from going down. The importance of it has made an impression on you. Did you learn about carrying some sugar with you?"

Mrs. Woods: "Oh yes, I forgot! And I'm going to get a card for my wallet about being a diabetic, and I'd like to wear one of those medic-alert bracelets in case I get in trouble. Then anyone who finds me will know to give me sugar. I've even got my hard candy on me now, see? I know to take it if I feel weak. The dietitian said my speech might get a little slurred if my blood sugar gets too low. So, I'll be on the lookout for that too."

You: "I am positively impressed with how much you have learned. With this knowledge you'll be able to live an active, normal life because you will know how to protect yourself. And I've seen your daily menu plans that you have prepared the last couple of days. It's clear you understand all about the carbohydrate substitutions and how to adjust your intake for periods when your activity is greater. You've accomplished a lot in the past few days."

Mrs. Woods: "Yes, even though I was too scared to face that I had diabetes at first, now I think I can lick it. It's a lot more complicated than I thought at first, but even in the last 3 days I felt more like I know what I'm doing when I'm testing my urine and doing my diet planning. There's hope!"

You: "What you're saying tells me that you are starting to feel more comfortable with being a diabetic. I'm happy that your confidence is growing. Is there any other area of your diabetes that you'd like to cover before you are discharged?"

Mrs. Woods: "Right now I can't think of anything. When I get home I'm sure that I'll have lots of questions as I get into my daily routine. I've decided to keep regular appointments at the diabetic clinic just to have someone to ask questions. You never know— someday I may even join the diabetic self-help group!"

To do this evaluation you and Mrs. Woods reviewed the expected outcomes that you had agreed on earlier. In this situation Mrs. Woods had met most expectations, and you were able to add points she had not included. Mrs. Woods is almost ready for discharge because she has accomplished the goals you set out.

One aspect of Mrs. Wood's health and well-being that hasn't been discussed is how her family can help her continue to comply with the self-care advances she has accomplished. The support and understanding of her husband and her parents will likely enhance her health. The family context is where health and illness are learned (Friedman, 1986) and fostered, so it is essential to include Mrs. Wood's family in discharge plans.

Mrs. Wood's illness has undoubtedly affected her husband in a number of ways. He may need help adjusting to the idea that his wife has a chronic illness, and encouragement to appreciate that a wife with less than perfect health can be productive and happily share life with him. In practical terms, he requires basic understanding of the safety measures Mrs. Woods has just learned. At this point a preparation-for-discharge interview with Mr. and Mrs. Woods could be set up, with agreement of all.

Benefits of Mutuality That Go Beyond the Client-Nurse Dyad

March (1990) believes that the benefits of the collaborative client-nurse relationship (which she terms *therapeutic reciprocity*) go beyond any isolated meeting and contribute to growth and development for both clients and nurses. The shared meanings about the client's experience are a natural precursor to the shared control and responsibility for the outcomes of their relationship. They gain trust in each other as human beings, and in their own ability to relate effectively in the helping relationship (March, 1990, p. 55). This discovery, although of primary value for the health care context, enhances their views of humans in general.

Matheis-Kraft, George, Olinger, & York (1990) claim that clients who take more active roles in their treatments recover faster. This benefits hospitals, which are struggling to contain costs of health care. Matheis-Kraft et al. reported how one American hospital instituted patient-driven health care. The goal of the hospital's patient-centered approach is to create a caring, dignified, and empowering environment in which their clients truly direct the course of their care and call on their inner resources to speed the healing process (Matheis-Kraft, George, Olinger, & York, 1990, p. 128). The staff promotes client realization of how their own physical, mental, and spiritual resources can promote healing.

In addition to the endorsement by clients and their families, nurses working in an environment with this philosophy active reported a number of spinoffs that have boosted their morale:

- Opportunity to bring more nurturing and caring into their profession
- Enjoyment of expanded autonomy and authority, allowing them to make a real difference

- A more equal relationship with physicians, who listen to their recommendations and even seek their counsel
- Satisfaction of being client advocates as they were educated (Matheis-Kraft, George, Olinger, & York, 1990, p. 128)

Schwertel-Kyle & Pitzer (1990) describe their implementation of Orem's self-care model for nursing in a critical nursing care unit as a way of providing optimal care to clients within concise time frames. Originally spurred by the financial restraints of prospective payment systems (decreased length of hospital stay, increased acuity, and decreased care-giving resources resulting from set reimbursement rates), the plan enhanced clients' self-confidence and feelings of accomplishment. The transformation from passive, dependent patient to active partner is one way for America's nursing clients to start taking the responsibility for their health care, in addition to securing their health-care rights.

Some Pointers about How to Make Your Clinical Problem-Solving a Mutual Affair

1. Explore what you believe about the issue of clients having an active part in their health care. The extent to which you uphold clients' responsibility for their health will mirror how you involve them in the nursing process.
2. Practice revealing your opinions to clients. Increase your confidence in telling clients about your assessment in their particular situation.
3. Avoid giving nursing care without checking with your client to see where he would like to start. Do not assume you know best because you are the nurse. Clients usually have personal preferences for where to start working on their health care problems. While you might go from easiest to most difficult, your client may want to work on the most complex problem first.
4. Do not negotiate the nursing strategy if there is in fact no choice for the client. Occasionally the philosophy of the institution in which you work, technical policies, time, and/or staff shortages dictate the prioritization and methodology. Most clients resent being given the false impression that they have some choice.
5. Before just about everything you do for your client, ask yourself: Could my client be doing this (turning, transferring, making a telephone call, speaking to a relative, making a bed, changing a dressing) for himself? By doing *for* our clients we rob them of the opportunity to discover their own power to take care of themselves. Every time we provide clients with the wherewithal (information, equipment, contacts) to do something for themselves, we save ourselves time and energy, two precious commodities in this time of restraint on health dollars.
6. Remember to evaluate with your clients. If you have been successful in collaborating through all the steps of the nursing process, then continue your good performance through this last phase. The only way to know if your clients are satisfied with the outcomes of your nursing care is to ask for, and listen to, their opinions.

7. Keep in mind that validating is an assertive act. We are not effective when we hesitate to express our points of view or shy away from seeking those of our clients. Validation does not mean commanding or coercing clients. Mutual problem-solving is a two-way street; open communication is exchanged between clients and nurses.

Making a Contract with Your Client

Once you have mastered the skills of validation and mutual problem-solving, you will have the basic ingredients for making a contract with your clients. This agreement involves formalizing many of the steps you already carry out in your nursing practice.

A contract is an agreement between you and your client outlining what activities and responsibilities each of you will be accountable for. The contract is often a motivator for learning for both client and staff (Rankin, 1990, p. 183). Good client contracts are realistic, measurable, dated, positive, and rewardable (Herje, 1980). In a formal contract both parties would spell out the availability, amount of time, skills, commitment, and area of responsibility they will contribute to the improved health status of the client. This negotiation can usually be covered in a verbal agreement. In some situations you may wish to make a written, signed agreement.

Under the terms of a contract both parties must fulfill their complementary obligations. The nurse has the right to make her client aware if he has not carried out those tasks to which he agreed, and the client can point out to the nurse if she has reneged on her part of the bargain. And conversely, they are both eligible for praise when they have successfully accomplished their respective tasks.

When the nurse and client have each done their part to fulfill the activities agreed on, then they evaluate the effectiveness of their efforts and determine if their contract is completed. A contract provides standards for evaluation because the expected outcomes are clearly spelled out (Rankin, 1990). If both parties are satisfied with the results, then termi-

---

ELEMENTS OF A CLIENT-NURSE CONTRACT

Here is a list of components of a client-nurse contract for you to adapt to your workplace (adapted from Stuart & Sundeen, 1991, p. 104):
- Names of client and nurse
- Purpose of the client-nurse relationship
- Roles of client and nurse
- Responsibilities of client and nurse
- Expectations of client and nurse
- Specific details such as meeting times and structure for confidentiality
- Conditions for termination

nation will occur. If the client wants more treatment, he must negotiate with the nurse, who may or may not be willing to continue. Or it may be the nurse who wants the client to do more for himself or to reach a higher level of health. If so, she must entice the client to pursue further treatment and make clear her part in the extended contract.

Herje (1980) argued that one benefit of working out a contract with clients is that they become activists, who choose the options they can realistically follow, rather than passive victims of the health care system. As clients get more assertive about taking an active part in their health care planning, nurses will be forced to respond by renegotiating the terms of their mutual commitment. As we nurses become more vocal about our contribution to health care, we become more accountable. Whether for legal, ethical, or philosophical reasons, we are likely to become much more explicit about the terms of contracts with our clients in the years to come.

PRACTICING THE SKILL OF MUTUAL PROBLEM-SOLVING

Exercise 1. For this exercise work in threes. One will roleplay a client, one the nurse, and the third will be the observer who gives feedback. The purpose of this exercise is to give you an opportunity to practice mutual problem-solving and to receive feedback on your performance.

The client will approach the nurse with a specific problem that the nurse will help the client begin solving using the principles of mutuality.

After 12 to 15 minutes of discussion, debrief the nurse on how effective she is in making her relationship with the client a mutual problem-solving affair. The following questions can be used as guidelines for debriefing:

As the nurse, did you:
- Allow your client to provide you as much information as possible about his health problem(s)
- Show interest in your client's assessment of his situation
- Check out your analysis and nursing diagnosis(es) with your client
- Find out your client's reactions to his health problems
- Discover what goals your client has for treatment
- Discuss your hopes and expectations for his care
- Elicit your client's opinions of all possible nursing actions
- Work out how your client could be more actively involved in implementing his treatments
- Assess together how effective the treatment plans had been?

Review the 11 steps of a mutual nursing process to see where you were successful and where you could improve. What made it possible for you to validate in some instances but not in others? Compare your experiences with those of your colleagues.

As the client and the observer:
1. How well did the nurse follow the steps of mutual problem-solving?
2. What suggestions for improving her ability to incorporate validation into her nursing process would you make?

In 12 to 15 minutes the nurse and client may not get through all the phases of the nursing process. Review how mutual the problem-solving process was for the stage that was reached.

Switch roles so that you each have a chance to roleplay all roles.

Exercise 2. For each of the following client situations describe what you would say to these clients to encourage them to take a more active part in their health care:
1. Mr. Bane is a 33-year-old newly diagnosed epileptic. He has to take medication every 4 hours.
2. Mrs. McNeil is a 63-year-old client with arthritis. She has been urged by her physician to do wrist and finger range of movement exercises 3 times a day.
3. Johnnie is a 17-year-old client who has been advised to use specially prepared soap for his facial acne.
4. Beth is a tense young client who has been urged to do daily muscle relaxation exercises that the physiotherapist taught her.
5. Mr. Jameson has a high cholesterol level. He has been taught how to reduce the cholesterol in his diet. He selects his own menu daily.

Compare your strategies for approaching each client situation with the suggestions of your colleagues.

Exercise 3. For each of the following case studies write down how you would discuss the problem that your client has broken the agreement mutually reached about what actions he would take to improve his health status. Write out specifically what you would say when you approach the topic with your client.
1. Miss Marson is a 19-year-old admitted for investigation of severe, debilitating headaches. She has agreed not to consume any of her own over-the-counter drugs to alleviate her pain while tests are being done to discover the source of her headaches. On your night rounds you find Miss Marson in the washroom swallowing one extra strength pain reliever tablet and about to take another
2. Mrs. Dodds is a 22-year-old client admitted for investigation of severe and rapid weight loss. She has agreed to stick to a bland diet while the reasons for her weight loss are being unearthed. On the evening shift you discover her eating spicy chili her visitor brought her from the local deli.
3. Mr. Jones is a 45-year-old who is five hours postoperative. Preoperatively he agreed to do his deep breathing and coughing after surgery, yet now he has been adamant that he has no intention of letting you support his incision so that he can cough. He only wants to sleep peacefully.
4. You are completing a health history on a client who has had chest pain in the past few weeks. She has agreed to bring you the pertinent information about her family's cardiac health history for her appointment today. She comes without the information, telling you that she

was too busy with her friends this week to get the information from her aunt.

After you have done this exercise on your own, compare your responses with those of your colleagues in your class. Be aware of the many ways to assertively inform your clients that they are not completing part of the nursing care plan to which they agreed.

Exercise 4. In the following situation you and your client disagree about the priority of the client's health problem. Think about how you would assertively handle such a situation and be prepared to discuss your suggested strategies with your colleagues in your class.

Mrs. Boyd is a 30-year-old admitted for a cholecystectomy. She is 2 months postpartum and is eager to continue breast feeding even though she is about to undergo surgery. You are concerned about her physical health because Mrs. Boyd is lethargic and jaundiced and has dry, itchy skin and severe abdominal pain. She wishes to have her baby brought in to be nursed at his regular feeding periods. You would prefer that she get as much rest as possible and start her baby on formula feedings.

Mrs. Boyd feels strongly that breast feeding is essential to the health of her baby. She acknowledges that it may be difficult to continue breast feeding at this time but she fears if she stops she will not be able to restart, and then her baby would suffer. In addition, breast feeding is a special part of being a nurturing mother for Mrs. Boyd, and she does not want to miss the experience.

Compare your strategy for working out this difference in priorities with Mrs. Boyd to the suggestions of your colleagues.

Exercise 5. The next time you are on the nursing unit where you are doing your clinical course, attempt to practice a mutual problem-solving approach with your assigned clients. Use the following questions to evaluate your ability to validate with your clients:

Assessment phase
- Do you allow clients the space to tell you what they know and believe about their health concerns?
- In what ways are your views about health congruent with your clients', and where are they divergent?
- What client knowledge gaps surfaced, allowing you to teach?
- What have you learned about your clients' health beliefs, health care habits, and problem-solving ability?

Validating the Nursing Diagnosis with Your Clients
- Do you determine what your clients think their problem is, and what they think might be causing it?
- Do you inform clients about your assessment of their health problem?
- Do you and your clients agree on the assessment?

- How do you handle the situation when your views are disparate?
- Do you explore how your clients feel about their nursing diagnosis(es)?
- How comfortable are you with sharing your views about the nursing diagnosis(es) with your clients?

Determining Desired Outcomes for Your Clients

- Are you and your clients congruent about the desired outcomes?
- Are you realistic in your hopes and expectations for your clients' health?
- Are you and your clients able to agree on mutually acceptable outcomes?

Choosing Nursing Strategies to Help Your Clients Achieve Their Expected and Desired Outcomes

- Do you take into account how your clients feel about the options?
- Do you take into account your clients' personal and cultural preferences, schedules, finances, and abilities?
- Are you able to inform your clients about the efficacy of the various options?
- Are you willing to express your opinions about the various treatment choices?

Implementing a Plan of Action to Help Meet Your Clients' Needs

- How much consideration do you give to your clients' ability to carry out the plan themselves?
- Do you do for your clients when they could be doing for themselves? Or, conversely, do you expect too much from your clients without adequately training them?
- Do you take the opportunity to find out how your clients feel about carrying out the plan?
- Do you make certain your clients are ready and willing to continue with the plan?
- Do you make clear what your role, and that of your clients, is?

Evaluating the Outcomes Together

- How extensively do you ask your clients their opinions and feelings about the outcomes of treatment to date?
- To what extent do you share your views about progress with your clients?
- How do you handle situations when you and your clients disagree (they are pleased with the outcomes and you wish to persevere for greater excellence or vice versa)?

• How well do you prepare your clients for termination?

Answering the questions that are posed above will crystallize your awareness of how you may already be encouraging mutual problem-solving with your clients, and stimulate your anticipation of where you can facilitate even more interchange.

Exercise 6

The next time you are a client (of a lawyer, a nurse, a pastor, priest, or rabbi, a physician, a dentist) make note of how much this professional engages you in mutual problem-solving. Notice exactly what the professional does to make you feel included in the planning.

• In what ways does your professional make you feel your opinions are important?
• In what ways could your professional include you more in the problem-solving process?
• How do your feelings differ when you are included and when your professional takes over and does not consult you?

Compare your experiences with those of your classmates. What has this exercise taught you about mutual problem-solving?

REFERENCES

Congress for Nursing Practice, American Nurses' Association, (1973). Standards for nursing practice. Kansas City, Mo.: The Association.

Friedman, M.M. (1986). Family nursing: Theory and assessment (2nd ed.). Norwalk, Conn.: Appleton-Century-Crofts.

Herje, P.A. (1980). Hows and whys of patient contracting. Nurse Educator, Jan-Feb, pp. 30-34.

Lindberg, J.B., Hunter, M.L., & Kruszewski, A.Z. (1983). Introduction to person-centered nursing. Philadelphia: J.B. Lippincott Company.

March, P. (1990). Therapeutic reciprocity: A caring phenomenon. Advances in Nursing Science, 13(1)0, 49-59.

Matheis-Kraft, C., George, S., Olinger, M.J., & York, L. (1990). Patient-driven healthcare works! Nursing Management, 21(9), 124-128.

Orem, D.E. (1980). Nursing: Concepts of practice (2nd ed.). New York: McGraw-Hill Book Company.

Pelletier, K.R. (1979). Holistic medicine: From stress to optimum health. New York: Delacorte Press/Seymour Lawrence.

Rankin, S.H., & Stallings, K.D. (1990). Patient education: Issues, principles, and practices (2nd ed.). Philadelphia: J.B. Lippincott Company.

Risner, P.B. (1986). Diagnosis: Diagnostic statements. In J.W. Griffith-Kenny and P.J. Christensen, (Eds.), Nursing process: Application of theories, frameworks, and models (pp. 151-158). St. Louis: Mosby–Year Book.

Schwertel-Kyle, B.A., & Pitzer, S.A. (1990). A self-care approach to today's challenges. Nursing Management, 21(3), 37-39.

Stuart, G.W., Sundeen, S.J. (1991). Principles and practice of psychiatric nursing (4th ed.). St. Louis: Mosby–Year Book.

SUGGESTIONS FOR FURTHER READING

Bailey, J.T. & Claus, K.E. (1975). Decision making in nursing: Tools for change. Saint Louis: Mosby–Year Book.

This book goes into great depth to describe all the variables that influence decisions nurses make, many of which are client related. Models of decision making are demonstrated to show readers how to apply a systematic policy.

Bower, F.L. (1982). The process of planning nursing care: Nursing practice models (3rd ed.). St. Louis: Mosby–Year Book.

What this book offers that is different from other texts on the nursing process is how to use a model of nursing practice when going through the steps of the nursing process. Some attention is given to the step of validation.

Carpenito, L.J. (ed.) (1987). Nursing diagnosis: Application to practice (2nd ed.). Philadelphia: J.B. Lippincott Company.

For nurses becoming familiar with nursing diagnoses this text is an excellent resource. The first four chapters provide a carefully written introduction demonstrating the relationship between nursing diagnoses and the nursing process. The remainder of the text contains a well-presented illustration of employing nursing diagnoses in clinical practice.

Gordon, M. (1987). Nursing diagnosis: Process and application (2nd ed.) New York: McGraw-Hill Book Company.

For nurses more familiar with the concept of nursing diagnosis in clinical practice, Gordon's text provides a theoretical exposition of nursing including: the thinking processes involved by the clinical nurse; ways of making accurate nursing diagnostic statements; and the implications of introducing nursing diagnoses into the health care system.

Griffith, J.W., & Christensen, P.J. (1986). Nursing process: Application of theories, frameworks and models (2nd ed.). St. Louis: Mosby–Year Book.

This is a very practical textbook on the problem-solving process in nursing. The authors include an overview of selected theoretical approaches so that nurse readers can learn how to use a nursing model to complete the nursing process. Students find this text very helpful.

La Monica, E.L. (1985). The humanistic nursing process. Monterey, Calif. Wadsworth Health Sciences Division.

This well-organized text will familiarize you with the nursing process. Each section of the book covers a phase of the problem-solving process in nursing.

Marriner, A. (1979). The nursing process. St. Louis: Mosby–Year Book.

This text provides a clear understanding of the nursing process for beginning student nurses. The implementation stage is extensively covered with detailed examples. Validation and the role of clients in planning care are given some attention.

O'Banion, D.R., & Whaley, D.L. (1981). Behavior contracting: Arranging contingencies of reinforcement. New York: Springer Publishing Company.

This text is for the student with a knowledge of principles of behavior modification. It is an excellent overview on contracting in general, describing theoretical assumptions and how to set up a contract.

Sackett, D.L., & Haynes, R.B. (Eds.) (1976). Compliance with therapeutic regimens. Baltimore: The Johns Hopkins University Press.

This text provides an excellent overview of factors related to compliance. Chapter 3, "A critical review of the determinants of compliance", informs nurse readers of how factors in their relationship with clients affect adherence to treatment. Becker's Health Belief Model, described in Chapter 4, gives nurses a framework for understanding what motivates clients to take care of their health. These ideas could have an effect on how you carry out mutual problem-solving with your clients.

Smith, J.A. (1981). The idea of health: A philosophical inquiry. Advances In Nursing Science, 3(3), pp. 43-50.

This article clarifies the concept of health and provides an overview of four different models of health. It is important for nurses to know from which model we operate, and how our clients view health, so that we articulate our views about health to clients and are open to clients' ways of thinking.

Steckal, S.B. (1982). Patient contracting. Norwalk, Conn. Appleton-Century-Crofts.

This is a dynamically written book about writing behavior contracts with patients. It provides readers with theoretical background and practical guidelines. A prominent theme throughout the book is how we as nurses are responsible for how we influence our clients.

Vaughan-Wrobel, B.C., & Henderson, B.S. (1982). The problem-oriented system in nursing: A workbook. St. Louis: Mosby–Year Book.

This book helps beginning nurses to chart their nursing notes using a problem-solving format. This practical text will help students become familiar with the nursing process.

Wu, R. (1973). Behavior and illness. Englewood Cliffs, N.J.: Prentice-Hall, Inc.

This readable book offers nurses an excellent overview of illness and health. This book has an excellent summary of the various models of illness which will help you articulate your views.

Yura, H., & Walsh, M.B. (1983). The nursing process: Assessing, planning, implementing, evaluating (4th ed.). Norwalk, Conn.: Appleton-Century-Crofts.

This classic book provides readers with a history of the nursing process. It goes into depth on the components of the nursing process and demonstrates application to individuals, families, and the community.

CHAPTER 4

Warmth

"I love thee for a heart that's kind—
not for the knowledge in thy mind."

W.H. Davies

OBJECTIVES

After studying this chapter you will be able to describe a variety of ways in which warmth is displayed, and to articulate the importance of warmth in human interactions. You will be encouraged to practice augmenting your warmth in day-to-day encounters with clients and colleagues.

THE BENEFITS OF WARMTH FOR YOUR CLIENTS AND COLLEAGUES

Warmth is the glue in the bonding between people and the magnetism that draws us to a closer intimacy with others. It is a special ingredient, even a catalyst, in our human relationships. Warmth in people makes us feel welcomed, relaxed, and joyful.

Warmth has been identified as an essential attribute in psychotherapists. Studies have demonstrated that the therapist's warmth, along with empathy and genuineness, accounted for client improvement (Truax, 1963; 1966), and led to more open, full relationships for clients in and out of therapy (Shapiro, Krauss & Truax, 1969).

Most of you will not be psychotherapists. However, your expression of warmth to your clients will make them feel welcomed and unjudged. These positive emotions will foster feelings of well-being and likely promote healing. Clients who sense your warmth are more likely to engage in dialogue with you and provide you information about their health condition. This communication helps you to make a nursing diagnosis, determine expected outcomes, work out a nursing care plan, and mutually evaluate the progress of nursing care.

Exchanging warmth with colleagues makes the workplace a more pleasant environment. Warmth enhances closeness, which has social and work-related benefits. Extending our warmth makes us more approachable by colleagues. Increased communication between colleagues ensures that important messages about clients or unit policies and procedures will be transmitted.

Although we often refer to others as warm, it is a human quality difficult to pin down and say, "Yes, that's it! That's warmth." It is one of the most difficult interpersonal communication behaviors to learn. Warmth involves not only attitudinal and psychomotor behavior but also a total way of offering oneself to another person. Showing warmth to others means conveying that you like to be with them and accept them as they are. In this sense warmth is a way of showing respect to clients and colleagues (Egan, 1977).

Warmth is not communicated in isolation; it enhances and is enhanced by other facilitative communication behaviors you will learn about in later chapters (such as respect, genuineness, and empathy). By itself warmth is not sufficient for building an effective helping relationship, developing mutual respect, or problem-solving; but warmth enhances these processes (Gazda, Asbury, Balzer, Childers & Walters, 1984).

Knapp cautioned that "nonverbal communication should not be studied in an isolated unit, but as an inseparable part of the total communication process. Nonverbal communication may serve to repeat, contradict, substitute, complement, accent, or regulate verbal communication" (1980, p. 21). Levine and Adelman reported a study done in the United States wherein it was discerned that 93% of the message was transmitted by the tone of the voice and facial expression, and only 7% by the words (1982, p. 43). It is possible that we tune into the nonverbal expression of emotions and attitudes more than the verbal. Because expression of warmth is predominantly nonverbal, it is wise to heed these findings.

How to Display Warmth to Your Clients and Colleagues

Warmth is displayed mostly nonverbally (Knapp, 1978; Gerrard, Boniface & Love, 1980). Subtle facial and body signs, as well as gestures (small movements of a hand, brow or eye), convey our inner relaxation and attentiveness to another person.

The specific features of warmth will be described, beginning with the face and then the rest of the body.

FACE	HOW WARMTH IS DISPLAYED
Forehead	Muscles are relaxed and forehead is smooth; no furrowing of the brow
Eyes	Comfortable eye contact is maintained; dilated pupils; natural eye movements where gaze is neither fixed nor shifting and darting
Mouth	Loose and relaxed as opposed to tight or pierced; absence of gestures like biting lip or a stiff or forced smile; jaw is relaxed and mobile, not clenched; smile is appropriate

Expres-sion	Features of the face move in a relaxed, fluid-like way; worried, distracted, or fretful looks are absent; shows interest and attentiveness

There is a lot that you do with your face to convey warmth. When you are talking to another person attention is largely focused on the face, so it is important to know how to make facial expressions that maximize your warmth.

Knapp (1980) calls the face a multimessage system that can communicate information regarding our personalities, interests, and responsiveness during interaction, as well as our emotional states. The face is a conversational regulator, opening and closing communication channels (Knapp, 1980, p. 178). The context, including the relationship, determine the meaning of our facial expressions (Levine & Adelman, 1982). Also, the degree of facial expressiveness varies among individuals and cultures (Levine & Adelman, 1982, p. 45). In relationships with clients and colleagues, it is wise to remember that when people from other cultures do not express emotions (such as warmth) openly, it does not mean that they do not experience these emotions; rather it might mean the amount of nonverbal expressiveness is culturally contained (Levine & Adelman, 1982, p. 45-46).

Americans express themselves facially in varying degrees. People from certain ethnic backgrounds in the United States may use their hands, bodies, and faces more than others. There are a variety of ways to express warmth, and, in contrast, it is usually considered negative or suspicious to have a "poker face" or "deadpan" facial expression (Levine & Adelman, 1982, p. 46).

We learn that there are culturally prescribed rules for displaying our warmth, related to factors such as the need, occupation, status or role position, and sex of both people involved. Situational variables such as the appropriateness of the place, nature of the event, and number of people around will also affect our expression of warmth (Knapp, 1980, p. 164).

"Eye contact is important because insufficient or excessive eye contact may create communication barriers. It is important in relationships because it serves to show intimacy, attention and influence" (Levine & Adelman, 1982, p. 46). There are no specific rules governing eye behavior except that it is considered rude to stare, especially at strangers. "In a conversation, too little eye contact may be seen negatively because it conveys lack of interest, inattention, or even mistrust."

Posture is the other place from which your warmth emanates. Movements or ways of holding yourself that encourage communication, interest, and pleasure in being with the other person constitute warmth.

POSTURE	**HOW WARMTH IS DISPLAYED**
Body position	Facing client squarely; shoulders are parallel to client's shoulders

Head position	Sitting or standing at same level as client; nods head periodically to show interest and attentiveness
Shoulders	Level and mobile; not hunched and tense
Arms	Loose and able to move smoothly; or holding stiffly onto a chair or the wall
Hands	Natural gesturing; not clenched or grasping a clipboard or chart; held in what seems to be a comfortable position; no agitated mannerisms like tapping pen or playing with an object
Chest	Breathing is at an even pace, not noticeably shallow or jarred; chest is open and neither slouched nor extended too far forward in feigned attentiveness; leaning slightly forward
Legs	Whether crossed or uncrossed, legs are in what seems to be a comfortable and natural arrangement for the speaker; when standing knees are flexed and not locked
Feet	Not fidgeting, tapping, or kicking

Knapp reports that warmth indicators include a shift of posture toward the other person, a smile, direct eye contact, and still hands (Knapp, 1980, p. 155). In Knapp's study, gestures such as looking around the room, slumping, drumming fingers, and not smiling detracted from warmth. In a dialogue situation, the positive warmth cues coupled with verbal reinforcers such as "mm-hmm" were effective for increasing verbal output for the interviewee (whereas the verbal cue alone was insufficient). This finding has implications for nursing, where so much client information is gleaned through interviewing.

Purtilo points out that in addition to whole-body posturing and positioning, gestures involving the extremeties—even one finger—can suggest the meaning of a message (Purtilo, 1990, p. 142). Think about how the following gestures would affect your message of warmth: shrugging your shoulders, folding your arms over your chest, rolling your thumb, shuffling your foot, or silently clenching your fist. Even if other parts of your body were focused on conveying warmth, these partial gestures might minimize or wipe out the message of warmth you were trying to send.

Another point to register about gestures in relation to warmth is that not all gestures embody universal meaning; the interpretation of a wink or a hand gesture may not be received in the same mood of warmth in which it was delivered (Levine & Adelman, 1982, p. 44). For example, our OK sign (circle made with thumb and forefinger) is a symbol for money in Japan, and the same gesture is obscene in some Latin American countries.

The spatial distance or closeness we create between us and our clients and colleagues can affect the warmth received. For Americans, distance in social conversation is about an arm's length to 4 feet (Levine & Adelman, 1982, p. 47). In our exuberance to display warmth we may invade this unseen but well-defined circumference in an attempt to get closer. Not all clients or colleagues will feel comforted by this gesture. Some may feel intruded upon, and others may feel threatened and act defensively.

Touching is another way to affectionately transmit warmth. From the briefest touch on the shoulder to an embracing hug or extended hand, you can convey warmth to others. The warmth in the touch is augmented when you are truly comfortable with the act of touching. Being overly tentative emphasizes your uncertainty and embarrassment rather than your warmth. Being overly jocular or possessive in your touching may engulf and dissolve your warmth. When touching, it is important to be sincere so the warmth intended reaches the other person.

Knapp (1980) consistently reminds us of the context of any interpersonal situation and how the variables affect the meaning attached to nonverbal gestures. In terms of touch, the number of factors influencing the intended message are many; meanings vary according to: the part of the body being touched, how long the touch lasts, the strength of the touch, and the method and frequency (Knapp, 1980, p. 158). Touch also means different things in different environments and with varying age groups, sexes, and stage of a relationship. The silent language of nonverbal behavior is much louder than it first appears (Levine & Adelman, 1982).

Warmth can be conveyed verbally as well as nonverbally. The volume of the voice is related to warmth. Softer, modulated tones convey warmth more than loud, aggressive tones that are vexatious to the ears. A pitch that seems comfortable for the speaker transmits warmth more than an unnatural pitch, which may seem to be out of the speaker's range. The pacing of your words is also important. Pressured, stilted, or stoic speech detracts from the warmth that can be conveyed through rhythmic speech, whose pacing is in keeping with the speaker's natural breathing. The actual words you speak have the power to extend warmth to others. Loving, soft words are warmer than harsh, thoughtless words: "So, you've never exercised before and now you think you'll become a 'super-jock' and take up jogging," is cold and judgmental compared with "You'd like to improve your fitness level so you're taking a new lease on life and learning to jog."

As you may have noticed, many of the features of warmth are those of a relaxed person. In addition to being relaxed, it is only possible to convey warmth when you have a genuine interest in the other person and a wish to convey that welcomeness and pleasure to him. A desire to be warm is based on the belief that each person you encounter is worthy of receiving the acceptance and comfort that your warmth generates.

Gazda, Asbury, Balzer, Childers, & Walters (1984) maintain that when you display high-level warmth you are completely and intensely attentive to the interaction between you and your clients or colleagues, making them feel accepted and important. The opposite—cold behavior—is when you convey disapproval or disinterest.

Extending and Withdrawing Warmth

Any time you wish to get closer to one of your clients or colleagues, or give the message that you really care, calls for the expression of your warmth. There are degrees of warmth. An attitude of, "I like that client (colleague); I feel warmly toward him with all his strengths and weaknesses," is warmer than, "I don't feel any revulsion for my client (colleague)." The warmth you express should be congruent with your genuine feelings. Your expression of warmth to your colleague whom you would like to date will likely be more open and intense than the warmth you might express to a client in your care.

Some factors that make it possible to convey warmth are the physical ability to control the facial, postural, tactile, and verbal features of warmth, and the ability to overcome any of the cognitive or affective influences mediating against warmth. What are some of these factors working against the expression of warmth? Any thoughts or feelings that distract the nurse's attention from the other person block the expression of warmth. Being rushed, overcome with strong emotions, shocked, or judgmental about the other's behavior are distractions that divert the nurse's attentions toward her own problems. When feeling hurried, the nurse's concern is for herself and her expression of enjoyment in the other person diminishes or disappears.

There may be occasions when what we feel conflicts with the expression of warmth. It is only natural to withdraw our warmth when we have feelings of anger toward another. When we feel hurt, bitter, irritated, or enraged with a client or colleague it would be insincere to try to convey warmth. At times we may feel insecure or ill-confident about whether we will be received or rejected by another person. Then, we might hide behind crisp attentiveness until we feel safe enough to allow our warmth to surface.

There may be occasions when we withhold our warmth for fear of being too warm, such as when we have romantic feelings for a client or an unavailable colleague (or vice versa). It is likely that we all have encountered someone who has treated us coldly, with disdain, or even mistreated us with rudeness or contempt. It would be difficult for most of us to be freely warm with those who have treated us in this way. When we want to protect ourselves from perceived or actual uncaring or disinterest, we may withdraw our warmth or refrain from offering it.

It is assertive to express your warmth to clients and colleagues when you wish to. It is unassertive to withhold the warmth you feel. In contrast, it is aggressive to exude a warmth beyond the measure of your feelings. When you sincerely convey the warmth you feel you bring to life the assertive position: "I like myself; I like you." This warmth is nonpossessive and allows the other person room to be himself.

The following exercises will make you aware of your warmth and give you pointers on how to convey your warmth when you wish to.

PRACTICING WARMTH

Exercise 1. Before you start trying to observe or change your own warmth behavior, take a few days to observe the warmth emanated by colleagues and friends. Keep some notes of what you notice and your reactions. What did you notice about:

• Facial expressions
• Posturing
• Verbal expression
• Touching

What felt good to be receiving? What warmth behaviors would you like to emulate?

Compare your observations with those of your classmates. What did you learn from each other about the communication behavior of warmth?

Exercise 2. For a few days, focus on your delivery of warmth. What is it you do to show your loved ones that you care? How is this expression different from your display of warmth to co-workers and clients? What is the same? Would you like to display more affection for others than you do? Make note of what you could change to be warmer. Find a partner in the class and exchange notes on the self-observations you have made.

Exercise 3. Find a full-length mirror and really take a good look at yourself. Make a statement about the warmth your image projects. Does the set of your face convey warmth? Why? Why not? Note how you are holding your facial muscles. Do your eyes twinkle or are they cold? Are your lips softly mobile or tightened? Now, change your expression to make it warmer. Note what you do. How does it feel to soften your facial expression? Recall that feeling, for you need that memory to call on when you want to convey warmth to another person (and you don't have your mirror handy!).

Next, turn away from the mirror and attempt to recapture that same warm facial expression. Then turn to check in the mirror. Have you got it? Or does your head need tilting, your smile broadening, or your eyes crinkling?

If you want to convey warmth, you need to practise these nonverbal gestures so that you will feel confident you are sending out the warmth you want your client or colleague to receive.

Exercise 4. Now stand up in front of the full-length mirror and look at how you are holding your body in space. Do your slouched shoulders suggest that you are lackadaisical, conveying disinterest? Are you hunching your shoulders so much to compensate for poor posture that you look frozen? What are you doing with your hands? Are they on your hips in defiance? Are you twisting them nervously in front of you, or are they comfortably placed? Look at your lower body. Are your knees stiffly locked or in a relaxed stance?

What are you learning about the warmth you convey through your facial expression and posturing?

Exercise 5. In front of the mirror, try out a few gestures that you commonly display in your roles as spouse, student, teammate, nurse, and so on. Examine in the mirror what looks comfortable and natural for you.

Exercise 6. Now try shaking hands with your image. Where do your eyes focus? Do you smile when you look at your image? How does it feel to be receiving a handshake from you? Does it feel warm? What would make it warmer? Try it and see! Does your handshake look assertive?

Exercise 7. Try sitting and keep your eyes on your image in the mirror. What are your reactions to your posture in the chair? Is your slouch disengaging? Is your military posture stiff and cold? Or is your position nicely aligned and at ease? What are your feet doing? Are your toes tucked under the chair ready to pounce, or placed in a natural line? Try some different positions and judge which look most relaxed and warm to you.

Exercise 8. Talk to yourself out loud. How does your voice sound? Is it soft and warm? Try a different tone. Which one sounds warmer to you? You can also record your voice and listen to it.

Exercise 9. In the classroom find a partner with whom to work. Engage in a conversation with each other. The conversation can be about any topic you wish (such as a summer holiday or a movie). In addition to talking and listening to each other, observe what you like about each other's expression of warmth.

After an exchange of 4 minutes, give each other feedback on how you expressed your warmth. If there is just *one* way in which you think your partner could change in order to be warmer, and if your partner would like to hear your idea, then make your suggestion. If a change is suggested to you, think about it and if you judge that it could make you come across as a warmer person, then act on it.

Exercise 10. Assessing Your Warmth Skills (see legend under Figure 4-1.).* This exercise will help you develop skills in assessing warmth and provide you with feedback on your own warmth skills.

For this exercise work in groups of four. During the week each group member is to make a 10-minute videotape of herself interviewing a client. (If clients are not available, group members can interview each other about a topic of personal significance to the interviewee.)

Each small group meets by itself to view the videotapes. As the first group member shows her videotape to the group, all the group members should use the Warmth Content Analysis Sheet (see Figure 4-1) to check off the warmth behaviors they see the interviewer demonstrating.

Instructions for the Warmth Content Analysis Sheet

Each time you observe the interviewer demonstrate one of the warmth behaviors listed below during a 1-minute interval, place a check mark in the appropriate column. For example, if during the first minute the interviewer smiles, has a warm voice tone, and leans slightly forward, place a check in the 1-minute column beside the appropriate rows. If the inter-

Name of Person Rated: _____ **Name of Rater:** _____

1-Minute Intervals

Interviewer's behavior	1	2	3	4	5	6	7	8	9	10	Total
1. Maintains eye contact											
2. Faces interviewee "squarely"											
3. Leans forward slightly											
4. Open posture: arms											
5. Open posture: legs											
6. Relaxed posture											
7. Nods heads to show interest											
8. Smiles											
9. Jokes											
10. Warm voice tone											
11. Face shows interest, attentiveness											
12. Speech content shows interest											

WARMTH RATING SCALE

Instructions: Place a check mark (✔) in the box beside the rating that indicates how warm you felt the interviewer's behavior was.

4.0 ☐ Very good response: very warm
3.5 ☐
3.0 ☐ Good response: warm
2.5 ☐
2.0 ☐ Poor response: cool
1.5 ☐
1.0 ☐ Very poor response: cold

Figure 4-1 Warmth Content Analysis Sheet (*The exercise on Assessing Your Warmth Skills and the Warmth Content Analysis Sheet are taken from Gerrard[B., Boniface, W., & Love, B., *Interpersonal Skills for Health Professionals*. Reston, Va.: Reston Publishing Company, 1980, pp. 124-127.)

viewer engages in a behavior more than once during a 1-minute interval, you still give it only one check mark. During each interval you are only checking off whether a behavior occurs—how often it occurs doesn't matter. When one minute is up, move to the next "minute" column and check off any behaviors that occur during that minute interval. During each 1-

minute interval you will be making a separate set of ratings. When the interview is over (or when ten minutes is up), add up your check marks in each row and write the total in the last column.

At the end of the 10-minute interview, after each group member has totaled her scores for her Warmth Content Analysis Sheet, each group member should use the Warmth Rating Scale (see Figure 4-1) to rate overall how warm she felt the interviewer's behavior was.

Note that these two scales measure different aspects of warmth. The content analysis sheet provides information on specific behaviors that occurred during the interview. The rating scale provides an overall assessment of the quality of warmth provided by the interviewer.

When the ratings are complete, each group member should give the interviewer feedback on her warmth scores; this feedback includes the overall warmth rating and the specific behaviors used to communicate warmth. As each group member completes her feedback, she should finish by telling the interviewer the one thing the interviewer did best to show warmth to the interviewee.

Repeat the above steps with each group member until everyone has had a turn receiving feedback on her videotape.

Exercise 11. Making Your Warmth Assessment and Care Plan. At this point you have a lot of information about your warmth ability. List those areas where your warmth is strong and in keeping with how you wish to be. You might write something like this:

'Facial and body expression of warmth to others adequate when feeling inwardly calm, respected by the other person, and caught up in my work.'

There may be situations when the expression of your warmth is less than you would like. You might write something like this:

'Diminished expression of facial warmth in situations when I'm expecting criticism.'
'Absence of facial warmth (to the point of coldness) and absence of postural warmth (to the point of rigidity) when encountering an angry client, because of fear of disapproval or dislike.'

Pinpointing the areas of concern helps you to realize how specific and isolated the occasions for improvement are, and it directs you to develop a plan for improving.

Exercise 12. Ways to Evaluate Improvements in Your Expression of Warmth. One of the most important barometers of your warmth gauge is your inner feelings. Are you feeling more relaxed and caring with clients and colleagues? Do you feel like you are expressing more affection and engaging more fully with others? Are your expressions of affection flowing more freely?

For an external evaluation you can monitor the verbal and nonverbal feedback you get from your client. Does your client talk more, look at you more, ask questions of you, shift to a relaxing position in the chair, and indicate that he feels cared for by you?

You might wish to receive even more specifically detailed feedback about your warmth ability. One way to secure these comments is to ask a colleague to watch your interactions with clients and colleagues and to let you know those ways in which your warmth is conveyed and where you might augment it.

REFERENCES

Egan, G. (1977). *You and me: The skills of communicating and relating to others.* Monterey, Calif.: Brooks/Cole Publishing Company.

Gazda, G.M., Asbury, F.R., Balzer, F.J., Childers, W.C., & Walters, R.P. (1984). *Human relations development: A manual for educators* (3rd ed.). Boston: Allyn and Bacon, Inc.

Gerrard, B.A., Boniface, W.J., & Love, B.H. (1980). *Interpersonal skills for health professionals.* Reston, Va.: Reston Publishing Company, Inc.

Knapp, M.L. (1978). *Nonverbal communication in human interaction* (2nd ed.). N.Y.: Holt, Rinehart & Winston.

Knapp, M.C. (1980). *Essentials of nonverbal communication.* New York: Holt, Rinehart & Winston.

Levine, D.R., & Adelman, M.B. (1982). *Beyond language: Intercultural communication for English as a second language.* Englewood Cliffs, N.J.: Prentice-Hall Regents.

Purtilo, R. (1990). *Health professional and patient interaction* (4th ed.). Philadelphia: W.B. Saunders Company, Harcourt Brace Jovanovich, Inc.

Shapiro, J.G., Krauss, H.H., & Truax, C.B. (1969). Therapeutic conditions and disclosure beyond the therapeutic encounter. *Journal of Counselling Psychology, 16*(4), pp. 290-294.

Truax, C.B. (1963). Effective ingredients in psychotherapy: An approach to unravelling the patient-therapist interaction. *Journal of Counselling Psychology, 10*, pp. 256-263.

Truax, C.B., Wargo, D.G., Frank, J.D., Imber, S.D., Battle, C.C., Hoehn-Saric, R., Nash, E.H., & Stone, A.R. (1966). Therapist empathy, genuineness, and warmth and patient therapeutic outcome. *Journal of Counselling Psychology, 30*, pp. 395-401.

SUGGESTIONS FOR FURTHER READING

Ekman, P., & Friesen, W.V. (1975). *Unmasking the face: A guide to recognizing emotions from facial clues.* Englewood Cliffs, N.J.: Prentice-Hall, Inc.

For the nurse reader who wants to learn more about nonverbal expression of feelings as they are displayed in the face, this book is creative and informative. The excellent photographs and explanations point out how all the emotions are represented in different parts of the face. This book is useful for the nurse who wants to be able to discriminate fine emotions on the faces of clients and colleagues.

Gazda, G.M., Walters, R.P., & Childers, W.C. (1975). *Human relations development.* Boston: Allyn & Bacon, Inc.

Chapter 10 provides a thorough overview of the nonverbal warmth behaviours. There are some creative individual and group exercises to augment your verbal and nonverbal expressions of warmth. Appendix D contains a scale for rating your warmth.

Schulman, E.D. (1978). *Intervention in human services* (2nd ed.). Saint Louis: Mosby—Year Book.

Chapter 8 describes extensively the skills of empathy, genuineness, and nonpossessive warmth via definitions, examples, rating scales, exercises, rating sheets, sample score sheets, discussion of nonverbal cues, and methods for self-evaluation. This is a helpful and complete chapter for nurses to assess their facilitative communication skills.

Vanier, J. (1970). *Tears of silence.* Toronto: The Alger Press Ltd.

This is a touching book of poetry which grabs readers in its plea to remember how important an influence we all have on each other—how even a look can generate hope and make another feel worthwhile. It's a "refresher" for nurses.

CHAPTER 5

Respect

*"We owe respect to the living;
to the dead we owe only the truth."*

Voltaire

OBJECTIVES

Respect is an essential building block in the foundation of a successful relationship between people. By the end of this chapter you will be able to explain the meaning of respect and to articulate the importance of demonstrating respect to others. You will increase your ability to show respect to your clients and colleagues in a consistent and reliable fashion.

THE BENEFITS OF RESPECT

When we show respect to our clients and colleagues we are sending them the message: "I value you. You are important to me." Together, warmth and respect form what Rogers (1961) and his successors called unconditional positive regard. When helpers demonstrate they care in a nonpossessive way, they transmit unconditional positive regard. It means accepting others for what they are, not on the condition that they behave in a certain way or possess special characteristics.

Receiving respect makes people feel important, cared for, and worthwhile. These examples illustrate such reactions. Your co-worker tells you: "I love going to my new physician. Besides being a good clinician, she makes me feel so important. She's on time for my appointments, her receptionist remembers my name, and any requests I have are followed up." Your neighbor tells you about her recent experience with the nursing staff on the unit where her husband is hospitalized: "The nurses are busy, of course, but they seem to have time to say 'hello' and pause for a few minutes to tell me something new about Jack. They never seem too busy for the little touches that make you feel so special. Not like unit M.H.

where they scowl if you ask for something or give you the impression that they don't have time for you."

In contrast, when people do not receive respect, they feel hurt and ignored. For example, a middle-aged woman talks about the ward clerk on a busy hospital unit: "She didn't even have the courtesy to raise her head to speak to me when I asked her where Dad's room was. I might as well not have been there." A nurse reports her frustration at the disrespect she encountered: "Boy, I'm glad I don't work there! When I came down to borrow some syringes the two nurses ignored me and kept on talking! They didn't even register that I was in a hurry and needed the stuff quickly." When people feel that they are not being treated with respect they feel angry and rejected.

There is a positive correlation between respect, warmth, empathy, and successful treatment outcomes in psychotherapy clients. Indirect evidence supports the notion that respect, in terms of access to desired physician, provision of convenient clinics, and reduced waiting times for appointments, has a beneficial influence on client compliance with therapeutic regimen (Haynes, 1976).

Showing Respect to Your Clients

Respect is communicated principally by the ways helpers orient themselves toward, and work with, clients. Although respect starts as an attitude, this mental outlook needs to be translated into behavior in order to demonstrate respect (Egan, 1986, p.60). The behavior that demonstrates respect is **acknowledgment.**

Acknowledging Your Client

It is not good enough to feel respect for your clients. They will only receive the message that you think they are important and worthwhile if you deliver it clearly and directly. The following list provides you with some concrete actions you can take to show respect to your clients.

- Look at your client
- Give your undivided attention
- Maintain eye contact
- Smile if appropriate
- Move toward the person
- Determine how he likes to be addressed
- Call him by name and introduce yourself
- Make contact with a handshake or gentle touching

Showing respect involves using verbal and nonverbal skills. Just looking right at our clients or colleagues as they speak shows attention; but the quality of our facial expressions reveals whether or not we are interested in what our clients or co-workers are saying (Knapp, 1980).

In the United States, introductions are accompanied by a firm, brief handshake. This custom may not be the same for all countries from which our clients or colleagues come. In some cultures handshaking is prolonged, and taking our hands away too quickly could be misinterpreted as rejection (Levine & Adelman, 1982, p. 4).

After the opening acknowledgements are made, there is usually a period of "small talk" during which impersonal and trivial subjects (such as the weather) are discussed to break the ice. Some cultures prolong this period of discussion, but North Americans usually keep this "warm up" brief, because our dominant cultural value of time makes us slaves to schedules (Leininger, 1978, p. 132).

Establishing the Nature of the Contact

After you have acknowledged your client, there are several things you can do to convey respect at the outset of a new or on-going client-nurse encounter.

For a first-time contact:
- Make it clear who you are and what your role is in the agency
- Ask what he needs or wants
- Be clear about how you can be of help
- Indicate how you will protect your client's confidentiality

For an on-going relationship:
- Ensure that he recalls who you are and your role in the agency
- Determine his needs at this point
- Indicate you recall details about him and his situation
- Review the issue of confidentiality
- Refrain from "gossiping" about other clients
- Suggest a referral where appropriate so that he will receive the required assistance

As nurses we must remember that the most intensely private and personal moments of clients' lives are revealed in hospital settings. At the outset of a client-nurse relationship, we have a duty to tell clients of others with whom we are likely to share the information they tell us, so that they understand the parameters of confidentiality in the agency. Some private information may need to be shared with other members of the health care team so that it is utilized in developing the treatment plan. We are obliged to diligently protect the confidences of our clients unless required to reveal them by law, or unless our clients give us permission to share these details (Calfee, 1989, p. 23). Merely releasing the status of a client's condition to the news media or general public does not create liability exposure, but disclosing more detailed information or a photograph without the client's consent should be avoided. In health care facilities where there is public stigma, such as a psychiatric or drug abuse treatment center, even releasing a client's name would be an automatic invasion of privacy (Calfee, 1989, p. 23).

Although the following ethical guidelines for confidentiality were written for psychiatric nurse specialists, these principles are applicable guides in any situation where nurses are striving to respect clients by protecting their confidentiality (Colorado Society of Clinical Specialists in Psychiatric Nursing, 1990):

1. Keep all client records secure
2. Consider carefully the content to be entered into the record
3. Release information only with written consent and full discussion of the information to be shared, except when release is required by law
4. Use professional judgment deliberately regarding confidentiality when the client is a danger to self or others
5. Use professional judgment deliberately when deciding how to maintain the confidentiality of a minor. The rights of the parent/guardian must also be considered deliberately;
6. Disguise clinical material when used professionally for teaching and writing
7. Maintain confidentiality in consultation and peer review situations
8. Maintain anonymity of research subjects
9. Safeguard the confidentiality of the student in teaching/learning situations (p. 43)

Establishing a Comfortable Climate

The following list describes the steps necessary to establish a comfortable environment for the patient.

- Indicate at the beginning how much time you have so that your client can gauge his discussion and prepare for your leaving.
- Arrange to meet at another time if the allotted period is too brief for the content to be discussed.
- Ensure privacy before engaging in a discussion of confidential matters.
- Ensure that phones or other people do not interfere with your giving undivided attention to your client.
- Arrange the room so that no barrier, such as a desk, separates you and your client, and avoid standing over a person in a wheelchair.
- Ensure that the environment is comfortable by making space for your client, having a place for his coat and personal belongings, and adjusting room temperature and lighting.
- Take care to be on time for appointments and try to avoid inconveniencing a client by switching appointments.
- If you are late or have to change an appointment time, explain the reason to your client so he understands it is not a put-down or a disrespectful gesture.

Promptness for appointments is important to Americans, and we consider it dependable to keep scheduled appointments. For Americans time is tangible, as is reflected by these phrases: "gain time," "spend time," "waste time," "save time," or "kill time" (Levine & Adelman, 1982). Because clients from other cultures may proceed at a different pace than

Americans, and have different ways of perceiving, regulating, and dividing time, we may have to be creative about negotiating the time customs around appointments. Clients from cultures with different values about time might have to learn about cancelling and rescheduling appointments.

An aspect of mutuality is a sense of equality in the partnership. One nonverbal way to achieve an egalitarian relationship with clients is to arrange the seating so you are both at the same height. "Authority can be communicated by the height from which one person interacts with another. If one stands while the other sits, the former has subconsciously placed himself or herself in a position of authority. . . . Height is unwittingly used to project a submissive role onto a patient when he or she is confined to a bed, a treatment table or a wheelchair" (Purtilo, 1990, p. 141).

The concept of privacy is different for every culture. People in the United States tend to achieve privacy by physically separating themselves from others. In countries where space is more limited, people achieve privacy by simply withdrawing (Levine & Adelman, 1982). American clients will feel most comfortable discussing aspects of their personal health history in a private space, far from the earshot of other clients and hospital personnel. Pulling the curtain around a bed protects visual privacy, but anyone in the vicinity can hear the whole conversation (whether trying to listen in or not). Clients or colleagues from other cultures that don't prize privacy as we do may find our efforts to secure this seclusion unproductive. It's a critical and sensitive cultural value that surfaces again and again in the life of a health care consumer, and warrants nurses' consideration at each relevant moment in the client-nurse relationship. Until some clients become assertive enough to ask for privacy, nurses may have to teach them their rights.

Terminating Contact

How the nurse ends her discussion with the client is just as important as the other phases of the discussion. Below are some guidelines for terminating the contact.

- If you have to leave early, prepare your client in advance
- Summarize what you have discussed
- Follow through with what you said you would do
- Make notes of any points you want to remember for future contact

For On-Going Relationships:

- Several visits before termination prepare your client for discharge
- Allow time and space for him to talk about his feelings of termination

- Express your thoughts and feelings about termination as a way of showing that you care
- If you are going to be away for a limited period of time, make arrangements for client coverage and be sure to check with your client these arrangements are suitable

To maintain cost-effectiveness in American hospitals, clients are being discharged earlier and their length of stay is decreasing (Riley, 1989). This limits the time for discharge planning, and the transition period from hospital to home is briefer and possibly not as smooth for clients (Riley, 1989, p. 64). Riley described the implementation of the Patient Call-Back System in an American hospital, whereby the primary nurses telephoned clients at home within 24 hours of discharge. This nursing follow-up facilitates early identification of any post-discharge problems and early problem-solving. Such respectfulness makes clients feel cared for, instead of shunned as they might with briefer hospitalizations. Riley reported that call-backs allowed clients the chance both to express their feedback about their satisfaction level regarding their treatment, and to secure any necessary post-discharge information such as a referral, encouragement, or support (Riley, 1989, p. 66).

Egan (1986) suggested additional ways we can show respect to our clients. Demonstrating willingness to work with our clients by being available and interested in their health care problems is respectful. Accommodating the uniqueness and individuality of each client is another way. Adopting the mutual problem-solving approach is respectful because it shows good faith in our client's desire to use his own resources to take care of his health.

You can apply many of the above suggestions for showing respect to your colleagues. Being courteous, attentive, and mindful of the unique contribution each colleague makes to the total health care team approach—all are ways of conveying respect to colleagues.

Leininger continues to remind nurses that individuals from different cultures perceive and classify their health problems in specific ways, and have certain expectations about the way they should be helped, just as Americans do. If we become ethnocentric—that is, convinced that our ways are the right ways and that we have the knowledge that others need—we will violate all rules of respectfulness (1978, pp. 116, 149). "We need to respect, protect, and defend the cultural variabilities as important to our full American way of life. But, most important, we need to develop ways to be flexible in our thinking, and practices to accomodate different cultural or minority group needs and goals" (Leininger, 1978, p. 152).

Being respectful embodies assertiveness. When we show respect we are granting the other person's right to be treated with dignity and consideration, while at the same time not ignoring our own needs to manage our time effectively and carry out the role for which we are qualified. Being respectful means acknowledging the other's needs to be: attended to, understood, and helped within the limits of the nurse's abilities and time.

It is important that we, as nurses, understand the effect we can have on people in every single encounter. Being respectful means showing our finely-tuned sensitivity to others with the full realization that we can affect their well-being. As nurses, we need to be aware of the power we have to make our clients and colleagues feel cared for, and, more importantly, to use that power consistently and with good intent.

One factor that facilitates nurses showing respect is a strong value that others have the right to be treated with regard for their feelings of worth. Nurses with less well-integrated values of human dignity might be less consistent in demonstrating their respect. If you find you are inconsistent in demonstrating respect, examine which of your values conflicts with being respectful in those situations. What is more powerful in influencing your behavior than your desire to be respectful?

PRACTICING RESPECT

Exercise 1. Find a partner with whom to work. For the first part of this exercise one of you will talk and the other will listen, and then you will switch roles. When the speaker is talking, the task of the listener is to be blatantly disrespectful. For example, when you first come together, do not acknowledge the other person; give limited attention to her concerns and demonstrate rude behavior such as reading, looking at your mail, forgetting her name, or terminating abruptly. After 4 minutes, stop talking and debrief.

As the speaker:

How did it feel to receive disrespectful communication?

As the listener:

How did it feel to be disrespectful?

Share these feelings with each other as a way of learning about the negative effects of disrespect. Now switch roles so that each of you feels what it is like to give and receive disrespect.

Exercise 2. For this exercise work in pairs, with one being the speaker and one the listener. This time the listener is to show as much respect as possible throughout the interview, by exhibiting the respectful behaviors discussed earlier in the chapter.

After talking for several minutes, pause, and the speaker will give feedback to the listener on how it felt to receive her respectful communication. Switch roles and repeat.

In the class as a whole, discuss what doing these exercises has taught you about the importance of respect in interpersonal relationships.

Exercise 3. In your social encounters for the next few days, try to focus on the respect and disrespect you receive from others you meet at work, in the stores, on the street, or in professional relationships. What specific behaviors make you feel worthwhile and which ones humiliate or anger you? In the receiving of respect, does it make any difference whether the relationship is a one-shot encounter or an on-going one? Compare your findings about respect and disrespect with your classmates.

Exercise 4. Consider some of the factors which prevent you from being as respectful as you would like. For example, you might use your clients' or colleagues' first names without first checking out what they would like to be called. List the areas where you would like to improve your ways of conveying respect.

Exercise 5. Review the list of ethical guidelines for confidentiality developed by the Colorado Society of Clinical Specialists in Psychiatric Nursing (found earlier in this chapter), and check to what extent your workplace institutes these regulations. What additional guidelines are employed in your unit? To what extent are clients' needs for confidentiality preserved? As a class, share the information from each of your units and learn about the variation in protection of confidentiality in the workplace.

REFERENCES

Calfee, B.E. (1989). Confidentiality and disclosure of medical information. *Nursing management*, 20(12), 20-23.

Colorado Society of Clinical Specialists in Psychiatric Nursing (1990). Ethical guidelines for confidentiality. *Journal of Psychosocial Nursing*, 28(3), 43-44.

Egan, G. (1986). *The skilled helper: A systematic approach to effective helping*. Monterey, Calif.: Brooks/Cole Publishing Company.

Haynes, R.B. (1976). A critical review of the "determinants" of patient compliance with therapeutic regimen. In Sackett, D.L. & Haynes, R.B. (Eds.), *Compliance with therapeutic regimens*. Baltimore: The Johns Hopkins University Press.

Knapp, M.L. (1980). *Essentials of nonverbal communication*. New York: Holt, Rinehart & Winston.

Leininger, M. (1978). *Transcultural nursing: Concepts, theories, and practices*. New York: John Wiley & Sons

Purtilo, R. (1990). *Health professional and patient interaction* (4th ed.) Philadelphia: W.B. Saunders Company.

Riley, J. (1989). Telephone call-backs: Final patient care evaluation. *Nursing Management*, 20(9), 64-66.

Rogers, C.R. (1961). *On becoming a person: A therapist's view of psychotherapy*. Boston: Houghton Mifflin Company.

SUGGESTIONS FOR FURTHER READING

Gazda, G.M., Walters, R.P., & Childers, W.C. (1975). *Human relations development: A manual for health sciences*. Boston: Allyn & Bacon, Inc.

Chapter 9 informs nurse readers how to perceive and communicate respect. The exercises will help nurses to improve their knowledge of respect. The authors include a scale for rating your ability to transmit respect which is helpful for enhancing skill development.

Egan, G. (1977). *You and me: The skills of communicating and relating to others*. Monterey, Calif.: Brooks/Cole Publishing Company.

In chapter 8 Egan describes his views about how respect is conveyed in interpersonal relationships. He provides a checklist useful to the nurse reader in giving and receiving feedback on her ability to show respect.

CHAPTER 6

Genuineness

*"Nothing prevents us from being natural
so much as the desire to appear so."*

Duc de La Rochefoucauld

OBJECTIVES

This chapter will help give you the confidence to assert your right to express yourself in a way that is congruent with your thoughts and feelings. After studying this chapter you will be able to differentiate between genuine and nongenuine behavior and articulate the importance of being genuine with your clients and colleagues. You will enjoy the self-assurance and satisfaction that comes with being genuine.

BENEFITS OF GENUINENESS IN INTERPERSONAL RELATIONSHIPS

Commercial advertising makes millions of dollars claiming that products are "the real thing," "100% all natural," or "the original." If a *person* is genuine what does it mean? Why is it important to be "your natural self" in human relationships?

Realness and congruence are the two synonyms Rogers (1980) used for genuineness, which he claimed is a fundamental basis for the best of communication (p. 15). A basic feature of genuineness, in Roger's view, is presenting your true thoughts and feelings verbally and nonverbally, to another person. It is not only the words you say or how you say them but also your facial expression and body posture that make up genuineness. Being genuine means that you send the other person the real picture of you, not one distorted by being different than how you really think or feel. In the helping relationship with clients, and in mutually supportive relationships with colleagues in the workplace, being genuine does not mean impulsively dumping your reactions on others; it is aggressive to "hit" clients and colleagues with feelings, then "run." In a therapeutic relationship, genuinely presenting your thoughts and feelings to others can be done assertively and constructively.

As nurses, we make an important judgment call in deciding to genuinely share our inner thoughts and feelings with others. The literature advises nurses to be genuine "when it is appropriate to do so." Appropriateness is linked to whether our revelations will benefit our client (or colleague) and/or the relationship. Peck (1978) counsels

"So the expression of opinions, feelings, ideas and even knowledge must be suppressed from time to time in . . . the course of human affairs. What rules, then, can one follow if one is dedicated to the truth? First, never speak a falsehood. Second, bear in mind that the act of withholding the truth is always potentially a lie, and that in each instance in which the truth is withheld a significant moral decision is required. Third, the decision to withhold the truth should never be based on personal needs, such as a need for power, a need to be liked, or a need to protect one's map from challenge. Fourth, and conversely, the decision to withhold the truth must always be based entirely upon the needs of the person or people from whom the truth is being withheld. Fifth, the assessment of another's needs is an act of responsibility which is so complex that it can only be executed wisely when one operates with genuine love for the other. Sixth, the primary factor in the assessment of another's needs is the assessment of that person's capacity to utilize the truth for his or her own spiritual growth. Finally, in assessing the capacity of another to utilize the truth for personal spiritual growth, it should be borne in mind that our tendency is generally to underestimate rather than overestimate this capacity" (pp. 62-63).

It is a risk to be genuine because sometimes it involves expressing negative thoughts and confronting others with our reactions. When we are genuine, whether expressing negative or positive reactions, the message we give to our clients and colleagues is: "You are strong and worthy of my engaging fully with you."

Nurses who are genuine seem to the client to mean exactly what the words they are saying connote, and their accompanying affective nonverbal behavior matches their words (Arnold & Boggs, 1989). When our verbal message doesn't correspond with our facial expression, posture, voice tone, and body language, our clients and colleagues decode the disparity as two distinct and dissimilar messages. It's not hard to imagine that this incongruence of conflicting or mixed messages puts our credibility in question (Arnold & Boggs, 1989, p. 168). It's unlikely that a meaningful relationship ensues when our clients or colleagues suspect our trustworthiness.

As nurses we have expectations about the behaviors that accompany our assumed roles. For example, some of the behaviors expected of the nurse-advocate are providing scientifically current nursing care; serving on committees for standardizing agency procedures; and coordinating all services used by the client in the attempt to restore, maintain, or promote health (Hunter & Engelke, 1983, p. 139). The roles we assume have cultural, gender, and situational performance expectations. These rules are comforting because they provide guidelines for performance. Being *genuine* means remembering that roles are filled by individuals (Nuwayhid, 1984, p. 287) with unique personalities, styles, and ideas. *Realness* means being free from the bonds of the role, and not hiding behind the façade of the role (Egan, 1977, p. 183). Being a person and a nurse at the same time involves spontaneity, and not weighing every word we say or talking in scripts that seem planned or rigid. Congruence includes an openness to sharing without always waiting to be asked, to express directly what's going on inside us without distorting our messages.

Genuineness is a "what you see is what you get" phenomenon; people receiving your genuineness can trust you because they know you are not sending false signals or hiding something from them. It is this building of trust that is the most important reason for being genuine. When we feel we can count on others, that they are reliable, then we start to relax in the relationship. We stop worrying about what they might *really* be thinking and feeling. The energy freed from worrying can be put into the relationship, both deepening and moving it in the direction for which it was established. Being genuine as a nurse is one major step in gaining credibility with clients and colleagues.

Incongruence

When there is a mismatch between a nurse's experience of her thoughts and feelings and her awareness, this incongruence is called denial of awareness or defensiveness (Rogers, 1961, p. 341). For example, you may notice your colleague looks angry. She is stamping her foot, pointing her finger, becoming red in the face, and raising her voice in an accusatory way. However, when you suggest that she is angry she brushes it off and denies her obvious feelings.

When there is a mismatch between a nurse's thoughts and feelings and her communication of this internal experience, it is usually thought of as falseness or deceit (Rogers, 1961, p. 341). For example, you know that you disapprove of the new policy to join your unit with another unit in the hospital. Because you want to make a good impression on your boss you hide your anger and tell her you think the merging of the units is a good idea.

If we pretend our thoughts and feelings are different from what they are, then we will say things that we do not believe in. If we act on thoughts and feelings that we do not have, we give people the wrong impression about us; we lead them astray. In contrast, expressing our genuine thoughts and feelings about issues makes what we stand for crystal clear to our clients and colleagues. The research findings of Rogers (1957) and Shapiro, Krauss & Truax (1969) established that therapist genuineness has positive therapeutic outcomes.

Even if we can control our verbal communication when we are trying to deceive another about our true thoughts and feelings, our nonverbal cues can give us away (Knapp, 1980). Nonverbal leakage behavior can reveal the information we are hiding, or indicate that we are attempting to deceive without indicating specific information about the nature of the deception (Knapp, 1980, p. 140). We are skilled at manipulating our facial expression and our posture to jibe with our verbal message, but the way we move our feet, legs, or hands can betray incongruency with our verbal message—that we are not genuine. Some of the feet and leg movements that might alert others to our incongruence are aggressive foot kicks; flirtatious leg displays; autoerotic or soothing leg squeezing; abortive restless flight movements; tense leg positions; frequent shifts of leg posture; and restless or repetitive leg and foot acts. Revealing hand movements could include: digging our hands into our cheeks; tearing at our fingernails; or protectively holding our knees while smiling and looking pleasant. Knapp reported studies revealing that one of the reasons we may not expend much effort inhibiting or dissimulating feet and hand behavior is that over the years we have learned to disregard internal feedback, and we don't learn to control areas of our bodies in which we receive little external feedback (Knapp, 1980, p. 141). Another way we might reveal our incongruence is by neglecting to include the nonverbal action that customarily would accompany the verbal message. Our omission is a signal to clients and colleagues that something is wrong.

You may be asking yourself how anyone could act any way but genuinely? Occasionally it feels risky to reveal what we think and feel to others. Suppose they do not agree? Suppose they think we are off base or stupid? Sometimes we fear that clients or colleagues might reject us if they do not like what we say. We worry that others might laugh at us, argue with us, put us down, or gossip about us to others. We may be threatened by fears that, if we are honest, a colleague might refuse to work with us or a client may request the services of another nurse.

When feeling vulnerable to rejection, we might modify what we think and feel to make it more acceptable to others. We change in an attempt to give them what we think they wish to hear. In so doing, we begin the entanglement of giving a false impression of ourselves. If others are fooled, they expect the behavior to be repeated and then we are trapped. We can continue to try to act falsely—or confess. If our lack of authenticity is spotted, then others will stop trusting us, question our word, or ask for a second opinion. It is ironic that when we behave insincerely our worst fears of rejection can occur.

When we are genuine there is no guarantee that our clients or colleagues will accept us or agree with us, but they will usually be touched by our willingness to present ourselves as we are, and our courage to risk rejection. Our honesty is reassuring and refreshing. If others choose to withdraw from a relationship with the genuine us, then they leave us with the satisfaction of knowing we have been honest with ourselves. Being genuine is being assertive; it is an action of standing up for our legitimate rights to express our point of view. When we are authentic our concept of ourselves as assertive nurse is strengthened.

Being Genuine with Clients and Colleagues

The following examples illustrate how to be genuine with clients and colleagues.

> For several days you have been nursing a client who has been flirtatious. He has asked for your phone number, seductively locked eyes with you, and made body contact with you as frequently as possible. You are attracted to this young man and would like to take him up on his invitation for a date. However, that would only happen after his discharge, and it is your preference to maintain a professional client-nurse relationship while he is in the hospital.

> **Your thoughts:** You think it is appropriate to meet your client's needs in a professional way and refrain from expressing romantic behavior while in the client-nurse relationship.

> **Your feelings:** You are attracted to this client but worry about embarrassing yourself and him by behaving inappropriately.

The genuine communication to make would be to explain your dilemma to your client and specify how you would like the relationship to be handled while he is in the hospital.

> **Genuine You:** "I would like to accept your invitation to go out with you after you are discharged from the hospital. However, while you are here, I want a relationship where I feel I'm giving you and my other clients my best nursing care. I want to treat all my clients the same because I don't think it's fair to show favoritism to you. Can you understand my position?"

This statement assertively communicates your thoughts and feelings in a way that is in keeping with your personal and professional values, making you trustworthy. If you had refrained from expressing your point of view you would have communicated in a nonassertive and nongenuine way.

> **Nongenuine Unassertive You:** "Well, I might go out with you . . . we'll see."

This message does not make it clear that you want to date your client and it might invite more of the flirtatious behavior you want to avoid.

> **Nongenuine Aggressive You:** "You guys are all the same. You're a chauvinist . . . you treat nurses like play things. Cool it, mister! I've got a job to do."

This approach does not indicate your honest feelings of attraction to your client and it creates bad feelings. You have lost out by not communicating in a professional way.

Consider this situation between colleagues in the workplace:

> A fellow nurse tells you that she has told a client her husband could bring in their cat when he comes to visit his wife. She ex-

---

BENEFITS OF NURSE GENUINENESS FOR CLIENTS AND COLLEAGUES

Nurse genuineness	Benefits for clients and colleagues
• Speaks deep from within without apology	• Feel free to express their true thoughts and emotions
	• Develop a feeling of trust for the nurse
• Expresses what she is thinking, feeling, experiencing in the here and now	• Are provided with information they can use in the relationship here and now
• Shows spontaneity	• Unwind in a relaxed atmosphere
• Conveys openness	• Enjoy a climate of realness

---

plains to you, "I thought it might cheer up Mrs. Kent; she misses her cat so much. You don't mind, do you?"

The truth is you do mind. There are strict hospital rules about not having pets on the unit and you agree with them. You are in charge on this shift and you do not wish any negative repercussions from breaking the rules.

Your thoughts: It is unfair to show favoritism by breaking the rules for one client. There are good reasons for excluding animals from the unit.

Your feelings: You are annoyed that your colleague has made this decision without consulting you since you will bear the brunt of any consequences. You wish to correct your colleague without putting her down.

The genuine way to communicate would be to state your disagreement and disappointment and ask your colleague to reverse her mistake.

Genuine You: "It's unfortunate that you didn't discuss this issue with me first. I feel strongly that we shouldn't show favoritism and I agree with the health unit's rationale for restricting pets from the unit. Will you tell Mrs. Kent that she won't be able to have a visit with her cat while she's in the hospital?"

This assertion makes it clear to your colleague what you think and feel, and does so in a way that respects her feelings.

Nongenuine Unassertive You: "Gee, I don't think we should be allowing a cat on the unit, do you? I guess there's nothing we can do about it now."

By passively allowing the rule to be broken, and not expressing your annoyance and opinions in a clear, direct way, you are denying the expression of your genuine reaction.

NEGATIVE EFFECTS OF NURSE INCONGRUENCE FOR CLIENTS AND COLLEAGUES

Nurse incongruence	Negative effects on clients and colleagues
• Puts up façade or pretense	• Distrust for nurse • Suspicion of nurse
• Withholds how she is thinking or what she is experiencing	• Strained, tense relationship • Valuable information missing from the interchange
• Mismatch between verbal and nonverbal messages	• Decode the message as two distinct and dissimilar ones • Confusion • May only believe the nonverbal message • Question the credibility of the nurse • Find it difficult to maintain meaningful dialogue in the presence of mixed messages
• Is rigid, contrived and acts as if scripted, or how she thinks she should act	• Don't feel they are talking to a real person • Feel that the nurse is trying to impress, rather than reach or connect with, them

---

Nongenuine Aggressive You: "You what? Well, forget it. Go and tell Mrs. Kent that you've made a mistake. And don't ever make that kind of decision without consulting me."

This angry outburst is incongruent with your desire to communicate respectfully with your colleagues.

Being genuine is an assertive act. In expressing our thoughts and feelings we need to take care that they are clear, direct, and respectful of our client's or colleague's position.

Factors Influencing Genuineness

There are three main sources of our genuineness: our self-confidence, our perception of the other person, and environmental influences.

When our self-confidence is blossoming we feel strong enough to risk revealing our true selves. When our self-confidence is withering it is easier to try and impress others with what we think they want to hear, in order to feel accepted and important. Self-confidence is not something we are born with, but a part of our being we need to continually nourish. When we risk being authentic, we feel good about being true to our thoughts and feelings. This good feeling is translated into self-confidence.

When we perceive that others have power and influence over us, we might refrain from being authentically ourselves. If we decide that another person is smarter, more deserving, or more worthy, then we are more likely to show off for these people than relate to them in a way congruent with our thoughts and feelings. Learning to take charge and empowering ourselves to trust our own reactions will help us to perceive others as equals with whom we can dare to reveal our true thoughts and feelings.

Environmental variables also influence our ability to be genuine. In front of a large group in an auditorium, many of us might shy away from revealing our true thoughts and feelings. Limited time may prevent us from being genuine. If we know that expression of our thoughts and feelings could cause a reaction in others that would require more than the available time to work out, then we might wait for a better time to express ourselves genuinely.

To be congruent we need to be aware of our thoughts and feelings (Rogers, 1961). As we get close to ourselves and get to know ourselves better, expanded self-awareness builds and deepens our self-concept. This greater self-awareness is something we need to relate more genuinely to others (Rogers, 1980).

How You Can Evaluate Your Genuineness

You are the most important judge of your genuineness. If you are behaving in ways that are true to your thoughts and feelings, then you will feel more relaxed and self-assured. The comfort that you feel derives in part from the freedom that comes from living in harmony with yourself. Being genuine protects your right to be integrated. In other words, being genuine is being respectful of yourself.

When you are authentic it is likely that others will react positively by communicating with you, seeking out your trustworthy companionship, and, in turn, revealing their true feelings and thoughts. Following are some clues from others to help you evaluate your genuineness.

PRACTICING GENUINENESS

Exercise 1. For the next couple of days observe the genuineness in those you encounter daily. When you feel someone is genuine, stop and ask yourself what it is about their communication that makes you arrive at that conclusion.

Conversely, when you assess someone's communication as insincere, determine what makes him untrustworthy. Was it what he said or the style in which it was delivered? Making these notations will help you discover more about genuineness and will expand your ability to examine your own authenticity.

After you have each done this exercise on your own, get together as a class and compare your findings about genuineness.

Exercise 2. Assess your reactions to being on the receiving end of genuine and nongenuine behavior. What are the differences in how you feel? Which feels better and why? What do your reactions tell you about how you would like to communicate with others?

In the classroom collate your various observations about your reactions to genuine and nongenuine behavior.

Exercise 3. Find a partner with whom to work. One of you will be the speaker and the other the listener. As the speaker, think about an emotionally laden situation that you can discuss. For this part of the exercise the speaker will attempt to be nongenuine: if you feel excited you will downplay it; if you feel sad you will minimize it; if you think you should keep the reins on your temper you will lose control. After 5 minutes of being unauthentic stop your conversation.

As the listener:
1. How did it feel to be receiving nongenuine behavior?
2. What effects did it have on you?
   Give this feedback to your speaker.
   Reverse roles so that each partner can be a nongenuine speaker. In the class as a whole, compare notes on what doing this exercise has taught you about genuineness.

Exercise 4. Continue working with the same partner, one taking the role of speaker, the other of listener. Re-enact the same role play situation as in Exercise 3. This time the speaker will attempt to be genuine in her communication. As the listener, note your reactions to receiving genuine communication from your speaker, and give her your feedback. Reverse roles so that each of you has seen the picture from both sides.

In the process of giving and receiving authentic and false communication, you will have learned a lot about the importance of genuineness in interpersonal communication. In the class as a whole compile what you are learning about genuine communication.

Exercise 5. In your day-to-day activities notice when you are naturally and easily genuine and when you are untrue to yourself. After several days make note of the factors that make it easier for you to be genuine and those which make it more difficult. Assessing your genuineness in this way will make clear where you are congruent and where you need to work harder at being integrated.

Exercise 6. This exercise is the same as Exercise 5 except you observe your behavior at work. Note when you use your courage to be real and avoid hiding behind a professional façade. Observe when it's more difficult for you to be authentic about what you are thinking, feeling, or experiencing. What can you learn about your genuineness in relation to these situations? What information do you get about your genuineness or incongruence from the people in the situation?

After you have done both Exercises 5 and 6, ask yourself if there are any differences in your genuineness when you are on duty and when you are off. What does your answer tell you?

REFERENCES

Arnold, E., & Boggs, K. (1989). *Interpersonal relationships: Professional communication skills for nurses*. Philadelphia: W.B. Saunders Company.

Egan, G. (1977). *You and me: The skill of communicating and relating to others*. Monterey, Calif.: Brooks Cole Publishing Company.

Hunter, M.L., & Engelke, M.K. (1983). Consumerism and preventive health care. In Lindberg, J.B., Hunter, M.H., & Kruszewski, A.Z., *Introduction to person-centered nursing* (pp. 129-143). Philadelphia: J.B. Lippincott Company.

Knapp, M.L. (1980). *Essentials of nonverbal communication*. New York: Holt, Rinehart & Winston.

Nuwayhid, K.A. (1984). Role function: Theory and development. In S.C. Roy, *Introduction to nursing: An adaptation model* (2nd ed.). (pp. 284-305). Englewood Cliffs, N.J.: Prentice-Hall Incorporated.

Peck, M.S. (1978). *The road less travelled: A new psychology of love, traditional values and spiritual growth*. New York: Simon & Schuster Inc.

Rogers, C.R. (1957). The necessary and sufficient conditions of therapeutic personality change. *Journal of Consulting Psychology, 21*(2), pp. 95-103.

Rogers, C.R. (1961). *On becoming a person: A therapist's view of psychotherapy*. Boston: Houghton Mifflin Company.

Rogers, C.R. (1980). *A way of being*. Boston: Houghton Mifflin Company.

Shapiro, J.G., Krauss, H.H., & Truax, C.B. (1969). Therapeutic conditions and disclosure beyond the therapeutic encounter. *Journal of Counseling Psychology, 16*(4), pp. 290-294.

SUGGESTIONS FOR FURTHER READING

Gazda, G.M., Walters, R.P., & Childers, W.C. (1975). *Human relations development: A manual for health sciences*. Boston: Allyn & Bacon, Inc.

Appendix D contains a scale for rating your ability to communicate in a genuine way. Chapter 13 has some useful exercises to help nurses be more aware of different levels of genuineness, and to practice this communication behaviour.

Schulman, E.D. (1978). *Intervention in Human Services* (2nd ed.). St. Louis: Mosby–Year Book.

Chapter 8 describes extensively the skills of empathy, genuineness, and nonpossessive warmth, with definitions, examples, rating scales, exercises, rating sheets, sample score sheets, discussion of nonverbal cues, and self-evaluation. Schulman includes an interesting genuineness rating scale which takes into account the helper's congruence, self-disclosure, and confrontational skills. For interested nurse readers there is a scoring sheet and explanation provided for using this comprehensive rating scale.

CHAPTER 7

Specificity

"If no thought your mind does visit,
make your speech not too explicit."

Hein

OBJECTIVES

This chapter will clarify the meaning of specificity for you. After studying this chapter you will be able to articulate the usefulness and effect of this communication behavior. The exercises will give you experience in using specificity.

WHEN SPECIFICITY IS USEFUL

Being specific means being detailed and clear in the content of our speech. It means being concrete, so that our communication is focused and logical. In contrast, vagueness can be frustrating, and lack of clarity creates distance between people who are trying to communicate (Egan, 1977). As well as clarifying our own speech, the technique of specificity involves assisting clients (or colleagues) to move from broad, elusive areas of discussion to narrower, more pinpointed areas of concern (Northouse & Northouse, 1985, p. 198).

There are some interpersonal situations in which being concrete is especially advantageous. It is important to be specific when we are:
- Explaining our thoughts and feelings
- Reflecting others' thoughts and feelings
- Asking questions
- Giving information or feedback
- Evaluating

This list covers situations that nurses repeatedly encounter with clients and colleagues. Specificity benefits communication in three ways:
- The process of communicating is more satisfying when we are "on the same wavelength" as those with whom we are communicating.

- Each communicator achieves clearer comprehension of their own thoughts and full understanding of the others'.
- The foundation for problem solving is complete and accurate, enhancing the success of further communications in our relationships with clients and colleagues (Arnold & Boggs, 1989, p. 229).

Being Specific When Explaining Your Thoughts and Feelings

There are gradients to any emotion, and it is important to choose the one that says exactly what you want to convey to your listener. For example, in the anger category you might be feeling enraged, frustrated, furious, annoyed, or irritated. Each subtle variation conveys a slightly different mood. Hitting the mark by expressing exactly the right flavor of emotion ensures that your meaning is crystal clear.

If you tell your client that you are enraged with him for being late for his clinic appointment two mornings last week, when you were really only mildly irritated, you may create a gulf between the two of you by overstating your case.

With the emotion of sadness you might feel "blue," depressed, in the doldrums, hopeless, or discouraged. If you tell your co-worker that you are merely out of sorts, when you are really in despair because your child support check has not arrived and your taxes are due, such minimizing of your feelings risks diminishing the intimacy and trust between you.

When we are not specific about describing our thoughts and feelings we invite misunderstanding. Since the purpose of communicating is to enhance the understanding between two people, being indirect or unclear is unproductive.

In addition to hitting the mark about the quality of emotion, it adds clarity to include what specifically makes you feel a certain way. For example, you are happy that your client has initiated practicing his deep breathing and coughing. You convey your pleasure by saying:

"Mr. Weller, I'm pleased that you are doing your deep breathing on your own. I know it's not the most comfortable thing to do right after a cholecystectomy but it will pay off. It's unlikely that you'll get pneumonia and the movement increases your circulation, which helps healing."

Being specific by adding a rationale for your feelings enhances the sincerity of your message. Your explanation has built-in rewards for Mr. Weller. Such a response would make a lot more sense to him than:

"That's great, Mr. Weller. Glad to see you doing your exercises."

In this example it is unclear why you are pleased: because he is a dutiful client? because you will not have to spend time reminding him to do his exercises?

Here is another example from the workplace. You are feeling grateful that your colleague on the night shift has highlighted all abnormal lab results and displayed them clearly for your inspection when you arrive for the day shift. You tell her:

> "I'm thrilled with this chart you prepared, Jo, and grateful for the time it'll save us on the day shift. Your highlighting will streamline our alerting the physicians and indicate at a glance which patients need temperatures done or repeat lab work. Thank you."

This specific articulation about why you feel grateful adds depth and conviction to your feelings. It respectfully conveys your appreciation, more than a glib "Wow" or "Gee, thanks" would have.

Some nurses, clients and families, and colleagues have a preference for logical, rational thinking processes; they are proficient at appreciating, and being specific about, facts. They may not readily consider feelings, or be comfortable dealing with them, (Myers, 1980, p. 163). Since their strength lies in logical, objective thinking, they may lack the vocabulary to be specific when discussing feelings. Those who prefer thinking over feeling tend to decide things impersonally, are more analytical, and will respond more easily to others' thoughts (p. 163). Nurses, clients and families, and colleagues who prefer to decide things on the basis of personal feelings and human values are more attuned to others' feelings and likely have more vocabulary and the comfort to talk about feelings (Myers, 1980; Lawrence, 1982). They tend to be more concerned about the human feelings and values in communication than the factual, objective information.

You will learn more about specificity in relation to expressing your thoughts and feelings in chapter 9, Self-disclosure.

Being Specific When Reflecting Others' Thoughts and Feelings

Listening is not a silent pastime. It is active and vocal. Through your warmth and respect you can show you are attending to what your clients or colleagues are saying. By being specific you can convince them that you have heard and understood the meaning of their dialogue.

When you reflect others' thoughts and feelings you are like a recording, giving them a chance to hear what they are really saying. When helpers respond with clear, concise, detailed statements about others' concerns it helps those with problems clarify them (Gazda, Asbury, Balzer, Childers & Walters, 1984).

For example, one of your clients has given a lengthy description of her son's epilepsy:

> **Mrs. Cant:** "I'm so frightened he'll forget to take his medication that I often call the school nurse to check that he's taken it. And when he's late getting home from school, I worry to death that he's lying on a sidewalk somewhere having a seizure. When he plays soccer I'm right there on the sidelines—not so much cheering as

praying that all that running won't fire off a seizure. My Lord, will it always be like this?"

Here is an example of a specific reflection:

Specific You: "You're wondering if your son will be able to live a normal life, and whether you'll ever be free from worrying about his health and safety."

You can pinpoint the essence of someone's meaning by being specific when they get engrossed relating their thoughts and feelings. This tactic helps them grasp more fully both the sense and the significance of what they are saying.

Contrast the clarity of this response with these nonspecific alternatives:

Nonspecific You: "You must be very tense fretting about your son," or "It sounds like you spend a lot of time worrying."

Neither of these statements captures the exact meaning that Mrs. Cant was trying to convey. Replying accurately and specifically demonstrates that you fully understand your listener. In chapter 8, Empathy, you will learn more about the communication behavior of reflecting others' thoughts and feelings in a concrete way.

Being Specific When Asking Questions

There are times as an interviewer when you might wish to be purposefully unspecific so that the interviewee takes the lead. This open-ended strategy usually occurs at the beginning of an interview ("How may I be of help to you?" or "What is the pain like?"), or at a point in an interview when you want more information ("Could you tell me more about your family? . . . Or exercise habits?").

As clinicians, often we want specific information from our clients. To get exactly what we want, we must specifically ask for it. With a client you may wish to know more about the family health history. If you ask: "Tell me more about your family health," you might get everything from "It's fine!" to "Well, let me see in 1901 my great-grandfather was ill on his sailing venture." A stoic response provides you with no information, and a lengthy response requires sifting through to glean the essential details. Occasionally the client's historical recounting may be jumbled or confused, either because he is unsure of the dates and details or because his emotional reactions to his changed health status are interfering with his clarity. It's helpful to stop undirected digressions, backtrack, and reestablish the point your client is trying to make. This process helps clients become clearer (Murray & Zentner, 1985, p. 97).

It is likely that there are specific aspects of family history that are needed: history of cancer, history of cardiovascular diseases, and so on. Getting to the point and asking for specific information simplifies for the client what you want and increases your chances of getting it. Using the skill of specificity, you can prevent frustration or fruitlessness in the communication encounter. As nurses, if we fail to achieve clarity, our clients may be left in a state of confusion, and may even doubt our ability to contribute to the interaction (Hames & Joseph, 1986, p. 149). Phrases like "I'm not sure I understand that," or "Would you go over that again?" let our clients know we are interested and that we need help in understanding what they want us to know (Sundeen, Stuart, Rankin, & Cohen, 1989, p. 116). Some health and physical assessment guidelines provide systematic questionnaries for clarifying clients' symptoms. The symptom analysis in Bower and Thompson's *Clinical Manual of Health Assessment* (1988) is an excellent reference for pinpointing essential data about changes in clients' health status (Bower & Thompson, 1988, p. 13).

There is more about being specific when seeking information in chapter 10, Asking Questions.

Being Specific When Giving Information or Feedback

As nurses, we are often involved in teaching clients about their treatments, tests, medications, and health behaviors. To provide clients with material that is new to them and avoid the disrespect of boring them, it is important to focus on unknown aspects that they particularly want to know about. A good screening question is "What would you like to know about your treatment (test, medication, diet, and so on)?" Posed in an inviting way, this question makes the client delineate the most important area for him. Jumping right in with a complete and chronological explanation wastes time, might be irrelevant, and may even focus on material that frightens the client.

The same approach can be used with clients or colleagues who want feedback from you. Clarifying the nature of their request at the outset ensures that your feedback will be focused on the area important to them.

For example, imagine a situation in which a newly hired nurse with 6 months post-graduate experience asks you for feedback on her performance as a team leader the past five shifts. At this point you could enthusiastically jump in with praise and advice, but you pause before bombarding her. Instead you respond to her request for feedback with "I'd love to comment on your team leadership abilities. What specific areas would you like me to focus on?" This approach allows her to clarify that her abilities to delegate and to handle unforeseen crises are what she wants you to address. Requesting specificity allows you to focus your feedback so that it is helpful to the other person.

Being Specific When Evaluating

After you have implemented any nursing action, it is important to evaluate its success. Whether you have done some teaching or carried out a treatment, it is important to find out if you have accomplished your goals.

Your evaluation questions can be phrased specifically. Instead of asking a vague question like "How was that?" or "Have you got the hang of it now?" you can phrase your questions to reflect the objectives that necessitated your nursing action.

For example, you could ask your colleague who wants feedback on her team leadership: "Has my feedback on your abilities to delegate and to handle crises been helpful to you?" To the client who wants to know what would be facing him in the week after surgery, you could say: "Did I cover all the points you wanted to know about the recovery phase after your open-heart surgery?" You could ask the first-time father who feels awkward and nervous about bathing his baby: "Has my demonstration on how to bathe your son helped your confidence?" These specifically focused questions help nurses to evaluate whether they have been helpful. You can see that asking these follow-up questions completes the nursing process.

Providing Specific Documentation

Employing specificity to collect information from clients needs to be complemented by systematically recording the data. Clear documentation increases the likelihood that clients will receive the best care. Today, when the courts are holding nurses liable for their own actions, as many as one out of four malpractice suits are decided from nursing documentation in the client's chart. Obviously, good care and avoidance of malpractice are two solid reasons for completing the nursing record in a clear and logical manner (Edelstein, 1990, p. 40). Your nursing records should follow the care plans and indicate that the care you provided responded to specific client needs and was appropriate for specific nursing and medical diagnoses. Where nursing documentation is written with specific problems and outcomes in mind, the nurses' notes provide a concise, chronological, factual, and easy to audit record of clients' progress (Edelstein, 1990, p. 46).

Philpott (1985) outlines 22 reasonable and prudent nursing recording policies, practices, and systems (pp. 126-130). Following are a few of Philpott's key points pertinent to the skill of specificity.

- The complexity of the health problems and the level of risk posed by the client himself, his condition, or by the use of medical, nursing, or other therapies, dictate the detail and frequency of documentation.
- The higher the risk to which a particular client is exposed the more comprehensive, in-depth, and frequent should be the nursing recordings.
- Effective nursing recording is factual, honest, and based on accurate data taken directly from visual, verbal, and/or olfactory cues, and palpation.
- Effective recording shuns bias, avoiding tendencies to prejudge or label patients.
- Effective documentation tends toward quantitative expression, avoiding vague generalizations. For example, with the client who is experiencing

a sleeping problem, nursing recording such as "usual night" or "fair night" offers no useful understanding, wastes charting space and nursing time, and may mask a serious problem. Specific documentation, such as "slept from 0200 hours to 0300 and states she slept soundly and feels refreshed" provides a clear, accurate, and concise picture of the client's situation; it also enhances credibility for the nurse writer.

Professional care is reflected by proficient charting which not only proves what the nurse has done but effectively communicates the client's status and progress, saving time for everyone on the health care team (Reiley & Stengrevics, 1989). American nurses have come up with a number of charting systems that are specific and communicate high-quality client information accurately, completely, and in the most timely and effective way (Reiley & Stengrevics, 1989, p. 54).

PRACTICING SPECIFICITY

One way to really understand the benefits of an interpersonal skill is to experience the negative reactions in a situation when the skill is not being used. The first phase of each of the following exercises provides that opportunity.

Exercise 1. Find a partner with whom to work. One of you will roleplay a nurse and the other will roleplay a client. As the client you want some specific information from the nurse. Decide in advance exactly what information you want and for what reason you want it. During the interview, attempt to be as specific as you can. As the nurse in this roleplay, you will not make any efforts to determine the exact nature of what the client wants to know or why he wants the information; also, you will be unfocused, vague, and unclear. Proceed with a discussion for 4 minutes, and then pause to debrief with these questions as guidelines:

As the client:

1. How did you feel when the nurse neglected to determine what you specifically wanted to know or the reasons you had for wanting the information?

As the nurse:

1. How did you feel when you neglected to determine what your client wanted?

   Switch roles so that each of you has the chance to give and receive vague, unspecific communication.

Exercise 2. Find a partner to do this exercise. In this roleplay you will be nurse colleagues on a unit. One will be the speaker and the other the listener. As speaker, you wish to discuss with the listener a problem you are having on the unit. In relating your situation you will be unspecific, unclear, and vague. As the listener, you will use the skill of specificity to try to determine the nature of the speaker's problem situation. After a 4-minute discussion, debrief using these questions as guidelines:

As the listener:
1. How did it feel to receive unspecific, vague communication from the speaker?

As the speaker:
1. How did it feel to receive specific, focused communication from the listener?
2. Did the speaker's use of specificity lead to any changes in your communication?

   With the entire class, examine what you have learned about the importance of specificity by employing it and by being vague.

Exercise 3. Choose a partner in the class. One of you will roleplay a client who wants some information about his illness and the tests he is undergoing. The other will roleplay the nurse who employs the skill of specificity. Engage in a discussion for 5 minutes and then debrief using these questions as guidelines:

As the client:
1. How did it feel when the nurse made an effort to find out what you needed to know and tried to be clear and focused in her explanation?

As the nurse:
1. What was it like to use the skill of specificity when determining the client's request, giving him information and determining if you had been helpful?

   After debriefing, switch roles so that each of you will have the opportunity to practice and receive specificity.

   With the total class, discuss what using specificity correctly has taught you about that particular skill.

REFERENCES

Arnold, E., & Boggs, K. (1989). *Interpersonal relationships: Professional communication for nurses.* Philadelphia: W.B. Saunders Company.

Bowers, A.C., & Thompson, J.M. (1988). *Clinical manual of health assessment* (3rd ed.). St. Louis: Mosby–Year Book, Inc.

Edelstein, J. (1990). *A study of nursing documentation.* Nursing Management, 21(11), 40-46.

Egan, G. (1977). *You and me: The skills of communicating and relating to others.* Monterey, Calif.: Brooks/Cole Publishing Company.

Gazda, G.M., Asbury, F.R., Balzer, F.J., Childers, W.C., & Walters, R.P. (1984). *Human relations development: A manual for educators* (3rd ed.). Boston: Allyn & Bacon, Inc.

Hames, C.C., & Joseph, D.H. (1986). *Basic concepts of helping: A holistic approach* (2nd ed.). Norwalk, Conn.: Appleton-Century-Crofts.

Lawrence, G. (1982). *People types and tiger stripes: A practical guide for learning styles* (2nd ed.). Gainesville, Fla.: Center for Applications of Psychological Type, Inc.

Murray, R.B., & Zentner, J.P. (1985). *Nursing concepts for health promotion* (3rd ed.). Englewood Cliffs, N.J.: Prentice-Hall, Inc.

Myers, I.B. (1980). *Gifts differing*. Palo Alto, Calif.: Consulting Psychologists Press, Inc.

Northouse, P.G., & Northouse, L.L. (1985). *Health communication: A handbook for health professionals*. Englewood Cliffs, N.J.: Prentice-Hall, Inc.

Reiley, P.J., & Strengrevics, S.S. (1989). Change of shift report: Put it in writing! *Nursing Management, 20*(9), 54-56.

Philpott, M. (1985). *Legal liability and the nursing process*. W.B. Saunders Canada, Ltd.

Sundeen, S.J., Stuart, G.W., Rankin, E.A., & Cohen, S.A. (1989). *Nurse-client interaction: Implementing the nursing process* (4th ed.). St. Louis: Mosby–Year Book, Inc.

SUGGESTIONS FOR FURTHER READING

Readings related to employing specificity in communication

Egan, G. (1977). *You and me: The skills of communicating and relating to others*. Monterey, Calif.: Brooks/Cole Publishing Company.

Nurse readers will learn more about the communication technique of specificity by reading chapter 5. Three elements of concreteness are explained and students can augment their expertise by completing the exercises on specificity.

Gazda, G.M., Asbury, F.R., Balzer, F.J., Childers, W.C., & Walters, R.P. (1984). *Human relations development: A manual for educators* (3rd ed.). Boston: Allyn & Bacon, Inc.

In addition to describing specificity, the authors include a scale for rating concreteness and exercises to help students augment their skill level.

Readings related to effective documentation

Bernzweig, E.P. (1987). *The nurse's liability for malpractice: A programmed course* (4th ed.). McGraw-Hill Book Company.

Blackmer, K.M., (1989). Implementing nursing diagnosis. *Nursing Management, 20*(9).

Cline, A. (1989). Streamlined documentation through exceptional charting. *Nursing Management, 20*(2), 62-64.

Hanson, M.H., Kennedy, F.T., Dougherty, L.L., & Baumann, L.J. (1989). Education in nursing diagnosis: Evaluating clinical outcomes. *The Journal of Continuing Education in Nursing, 21*(2), 79-85.

Miller, P., Pastorino, C. (1990). Daily nursing documentation can be quick and thorough! *Nursing Management*, November, 47-49.

Porter, Y. (1989). Brief: Evaluation of nursing documentation of patient teaching. *The Journal of Continuing Education in Nursing, 21*(3), 134-137.

Schmidt, D., Gathers, B., Stewart, M., Tyler, C., Hawkins, M., & Denton, K. (1990). Charting for accountability. *Nursing Management, 21*(11), 50-52.

CHAPTER 8

Empathy

> "Empathy is the single most revolu-
> tionary emotion I can think of."
>
> Gloria Steinem

OBJECTIVES

By the end of this chapter you will understand what empathy is and be able to explain its importance in interpersonal communication. There are a number of exercises which will give you the opportunity to practice demonstrating empathy with supervised feedback.

Empathy is more complex than the other interpersonal communication behaviors you have mastered so far in this textbook. Empathy requires more rehearsal to ensure that it becomes integrated into your communications repertoire. The benefits of empathy for your clients and colleagues outweigh the investment of time that practicing empathy requires.

What is Empathy?

Empathy is the act of communicating to a fellow human being that we have understood how he is feeling and what makes him feel that way (Dymond, 1949; Hogan, 1969). When we mentally put ourselves in the shoes of another person and then verbally convey to that person that we understand what it must be like to wear those shoes, we are being empathic (Rubin, 1977).

Carl Rogers, an American psychologist, contributed immensely to the meaning and significance of empathy for helping professionals. He died in 1987 and, in honor of his gifts to us, his direct words are quoted to expand your understanding of the meaning of empathy. This passage is from his book *A Way of Being* (1980):

"An empathic way of being with another person has several facets. It means entering the private perceptual world of the other, and becoming thoroughly at home in it. It involves being sensitive, moment by moment, to the changing felt meanings which flow in this other person, to the fear or rage or tenderness or confusion or whatever he or she is experiencing. It means temporarily living in the other's life, moving about in it delicately without making judgements; it means sensing meanings of which he or she is scarcely aware, but not trying to uncover totally unconscious feelings, since this would be too threatening. It includes communicating your sensings of the person's world as you look with fresh and unfrightened eyes at the elements of which he or she is fearful. It means frequently checking with the person as to the accuracy of your sensings, and being guided by the responses you receive. You are a confident companion to the person in his or her inner world. By pointing to the possible meanings in the flow of another person's experiencing, you help the other to focus on this useful type of referent, to experience the meanings more fully, and to move forward in the experiencing" (p. 142).

A synonym for empathy is *communicated understanding*. When we are convinced that another person fully understands us, without judging us for how we are feeling, questioning why we are reacting that way, or advising us to feel differently, it provides us with a wonderful feeling of acceptance. The process of empathy involves the unconditional acceptance of the individual in need of help; judgments and evaluation of feelings are never offered (Pike, 1990, p. 237).

This nonjudgmental reception from a fellow human being is accompanied by feelings of relief and freedom. Once we know we have been understood and accepted, we do not have to struggle to get our point across, nor do we have to justify our reactions to the other person. When we receive empathic responses from our listener it relaxes us by removing fears of being misunderstood or rejected. Acknowledgment of our feelings reassures us that we have a right to be who we are. We may wish to change, and we might change our feelings and reactions in the future, but there is nothing so accepting as having others verbally acknowledge that they understand our feelings at this moment of our life.

Another synonym for empathy is *active listening*. We can listen passively or actively. Listening passively includes attending nonverbally to our client or colleague with the likes of eye contact and head nodding and verbally encouraging phrases "uh huh," "mmhumm," "I see," "yeah," or "I hear you." It is easy to delude ourselves that when we listen passively we truly communicate that we understand our speaker; but because passive listening does not include an actual articulation of the other's feelings, it lacks the conviction and reassurance of active listening. The receiver of passive listening has to assume, hope, or pretend that we have understood him. Active listening removes this guesswork; it specifically provides the speaker with the knowledge that we know how he is feeling— and understand why. The receiver of active listening feels guaranteed that he has been understood.

Natural empathy is a basic human endowment, an intrinsic ability to understand the feelings of another human. Natural empathy contrasts with clinical empathy, a tool or skill which is consciously and deliberately employed to achieve a therapeutic intervention (Pike, 1990, p. 235). The goal of empathy is to aid in the establishment of a helping relationship. It is not empathy by itself that is beneficial, but the intention of the giver and the perception of the receiver.

If empathy is truly a curative factor it must somehow be both communicated to, and received by, the client; it is more than a state of mind or attitude. As a concept empathy is a "value-neutral tool" that can be used for destructive or manipulative purposes. To be used in a therapeutic or curative way, it must be used to accept, confirm, and validate the total experiencing of the other person. It must be used with the intention of helping (Miller, 1989, p. 532).

How to Communicate Empathically

Empathy includes the ability to reflect accurately and specifically in words what our client or colleague is experiencing, drawing on the nonverbal behaviors of warmth and genuineness.

Preverbal Aspects of Empathy

In her review of empathy, Pike (1990) summarized the literature on the mental processes of empathy before the response becomes verbal (p. 237). Empathy is not total transportation into the world of another, with the self being last in the process. "While there is momentary abandonment, the empathizer never loses sight of her own separateness; she is always aware that the feelings of the other are not her own" (Pike 1990). Clinical, therapeutic empathy is not subjective. After experiencing the private world of the client, the nurse achieves some objectivity by tuning into his situation. While she is understanding what the client's situation feels like, the nurse feels tension and discomfort, which prompt her to action. The empathy is transformed into verbal connection with the client for the purpose of being helpful (Pike, 1990, p. 237). This mental shifting requires *flexible ego boundaries* (p. 238). The nurse shifts from her world into that of the client, and then back to a processing part of her mind where she confirms knowledge of the client's feelings and develops a plan of what to say or do that will be in the client's best interests.

Verbal Aspects of Empathy

The verbal part of the skill of empathy is that of reflecting to your client or colleague understanding of his feelings and the reasons for his emotional reaction. It is important that this verbal reflection be accurate, with no exaggeration or minimizing of what the person is telling you. The feeling words you use must match what the speaker intended; the exact nuance and strength of the feeling needs to be expressed. Your reflection of the rationale for the speaker's feelings specifically needs to be what the speaker intended—nothing more and nothing less. The two qualities of verbal empathy that have just been described are *accuracy* and *specificity*.

Being empathic does not mean repeating verbatim what someone just told you. Parroting only irritates the speaker, implying you have not really processed or understood his situation and subsequent reaction. When you respond empathically you should choose your own words and respond in your own style, yet still be accurate and specific. You may be wondering how to accomplish this feat. The following example will illustrate:

> A young patient who has been married for only 6 months has just been told that she has cervical polyps. As she talks, you notice her brow is furrowed, her eyes are glistening and she hesitantly says, "Can you tell me . . . what I mean is . . . I really love my husband . . . and will these polyps . . . I mean, I hope I can still make love with my husband?"

There are several reactions you pick up from this young woman. Her stammering and tremulous speech suggest that she is embarrassed discussing sex. You can most therapeutically deal with her embarrassment by responding in a forthright manner. Her main concern, however, is being able to continue a normal sexual relationship with her husband. You reply empathically with:

> "I can see that you are worried that these polyps you have on your cervix will interfere with your sex life with your husband. Let me explain about cervical polyps, I think I can reassure you."

This response meets the criteria for accuracy and specificity. Your use of the word *worry* accurately reflects the verbal and nonverbal clues you picked up. Reflecting the word *fear* would have been too strong, and using the words *wonder about* or *curious about* (sexual relationship) would have been too neutral for the emotional level she expressed. The feeling words the listener reflects must mirror the nuance the speaker is conveying.

CHOOSING THE "RIGHT" EMPATHIC WORD

Here is a list of adjectives describing feelings of being afraid, tense, or worried (Hills & Coffey, 1982), giving you an idea of the range from which you can select the feeling word or phrase which is "right on."

Afraid/tense/worried:
afraid, agonizing, alarmed, anxious, apprehensive, cautious, concerned, disturbed, dreading, fearful, fidgety, frightened, hesitant, ill-at-ease, in a cold sweat, jittery, jumpy, nervous, on edge, panicky, petrified, quaking, quivering, restless, scared, shaken, tense, terrified, trembling, troubled, uncomfortable, uneasy, wary, worried

The phrase "that those polyps you have on your cervix will interfere with your sex life with your husband" specifically captures the reason for her worries.

By using your own words and phrasing things in your own style, you avoid parroting and clearly demonstrate that you have understood her worries. Having received your understanding before the lesson on polyps will make your client more receptive to the teaching. Hearing understanding from another person is a relief and leads us to believe that what the listener has to say is trustworthy.

Nonverbal Aspects of Empathy

The nonverbal features of empathy are equally as important as the verbal aspects. A singer might correctly enunciate each word of a song yet miss expressing the mood of the piece; thus the song lacks vitality. Just as an audience would feel unconnected hearing an emotionless song, so disengagement can occur when empathy is delivered without warmth and genuineness. It is possible to articulate a technically perfect empathic response that meets the criteria for accuracy and specificity but does not positively affect the other person.

It is only when your empathy is accompanied by warmth and genuineness that the true caring and concern for what your clients and colleagues are experiencing comes across. However, it is important not to overplay your warmth to the point that your intended empathy seems gushy or too sympathetic. Being empathic is not equivalent to feeling sorry for another person. Empathy is free of the judgment of condolence; it is a value-free message showing that you understand the other person's point of view. The warmth you express with empathy should convey genuine caring, not honeyed insincerity. An example might clarify the necessity for an appropriate level of warmth:

> Your colleague has just told you that she is pregnant and therefore upset because she will not be able to continue her full-time nursing career. If you were to smother her with a hug or become overly solicitous, your attentive warmth would come across as sympathy. Sympathy focuses on your own feelings rather than the other's. Being too warm in this situation might suggest that you think her predicament is hopeless. Empathy with the appropriate warmth, such as a concerned facial expression and a gentle touch on the shoulder, tells your colleague that you understand; now she can approach her problem unburdened by your overprotectiveness.

It is essential to feel genuine empathy for another person. If you decidedly do not care about how a client or colleague is feeling, then using an empathic response would be incongruent. Even if the verbal part of your empathy is correct, your nonverbal behavior can give away your lack of caring. Usually our expression of warmth is diminished when we do not genuinely care about the feelings of the other person. This diminished warmth may speak louder than the words of our empathic response, so that the message received is one of not caring. The mixed message of caring words and uncaring nonverbal gestures can only be confusing for clients and colleagues.

In summary, an empathic communication requires a specific and accurate verbal response accompanied by genuine caring and a receivable level of warmth. These attributes of empathy must be packaged in your own natural style of speaking.

When to Communicate Empathically

Rogers (1980) asserted that there are situations in which empathy has the highest priority of the attitudinal elements making for growth-promoting human relationships. When clients or colleagues are hurting, confused, troubled, anxious, alienated, terrified, doubtful of self-worth, or uncertain as to identity, then understanding is called for.

As nurses, every day you encounter clients who are in this kind of pain. You have many opportunities to know your client's most intimate thoughts and feelings. Diers (1990) warned that empathy is intrusive and cautions nurses to ask themselves "How far should I go?" (p. 240). She reminds us that there is a tremendous amount of freedom related to empathy. "Empathy is a concept by intellection, like 'justice' or 'love', as opposed to a concept by observation like 'chair' or 'bottle'. Such concepts are seductive because there is so much room to play around" (p. 241). It is your clinical and ethical judgment that guides you when to verbalize empathy. One workshop leader had some advice which might help you: "Whenever we enter another's mind, we must remember to be respectful and take off our shoes."

High (1989) reminds nurses that we have as much responsibility for our clients' need to express their feelings on intimate matters as we do for their privacy. We might ask ourselves: "How much should I encourage my clients to tell me? Am I at risk of crossing the line between facilitating communication (with my empathy) and aggressively pursuing their private reactions?" Being empathic can be helpful or invading, and as nurses we must strive to use our empathic skills with the intent of being helpful.

Diers argues: "Empathy is a dangerous notion if it is thought to be mindless, experiental, existential connectedness. Surely every patient encounter requires an openness to the other's experience, for only when one is open to another can one perceive needs. But surely, not every encounter will benefit from empathy; some will require theory, or applied experience, or even translation or consultation" (p. 241).

The Benefits of Empathy for Clients and Colleagues

Clients and colleagues share their thoughts and feelings with you for the purpose of being understood; otherwise why would they bother to reveal themselves? As a listener, it is not good enough to have an understanding about how your clients or colleagues feel without verbally sharing that empathic understanding explicitly and accurately. Communicating your understanding has many payoffs for your clients and colleagues, and for your relationships with them.

Empathy increases the feeling of being connected with another human. This positive feeling of belonging helps reduce negative feelings of loneliness and isolation. Although it has often been said that we are ultimately alone in our journey through life, empathy is a bridge that connects us, giving confidence and hope. The knowledge that you understand your clients and colleagues helps them continue on their way, secure that their feelings have been acknowledged as normal human reactions. The companionship you extend through empathy, however brief the engagement, creates a human bond that adds to your client's or colleague's personal strength. Rogers put it simply: empathy dissolves alienation (1980, p. 151).

Empathy can contribute to feelings of increased self-esteem for those to whom you extend it. The fact that you take the time to listen, hear, process, and reflect what your client or colleague said makes them feel important. Caring enough to show that you understand makes others feel significant and worthwhile.

"It is impossible to accurately sense the perceptual world of another person unless you value that person and his or her world, unless you, in some sense, care. Hence, the message comes through to the recipient that 'this other person trusts me, thinks I'm worthwhile. Perhaps I *am* worth something. Perhaps *I* could value *myself*. Perhaps I could care for myself' " (Rogers, 1980, pp. 152-153).

Your empathy demonstrates that you accept how your clients and colleagues feel and contributes to their trust that you genuinely accept them as they are. Your withholding of judgment or advice deepens this trust. Empathy is a skill you can use to deepen your relationships with clients and colleagues. When you unconditionally accept others as they present themselves they can relax and feel free to be themselves. Your acceptance helps your clients and colleagues to accept themselves.

A consequence of empathic understanding is that the recipient feels valued, cared for, and accepted as the person that he or she is (Rogers, 1980, p. 152). " . . . true empathy is always free of any evaluative or diagnostic quality. The recipient perceives this with some surprise: 'If I am not being judged, perhaps I am not so evil or abnormal as I have thought. Perhaps I don't have to judge myself so harshly.' Thus, the possibility of self-acceptance is gradually increased" (p. 154). Finely tuned understanding by another individual gives the recipient a sense of personhood, of identity (p. 155), and Rogers showed us that empathy gives that needed confirmation.

Your empathy can help your clients and colleagues move on to new feelings and change their behavior. The acceptance your empathy offers frees your clients and colleagues from having to defend or rationalize their feelings; as a result, they are able to experience alternative reactions, freed of any clinging to defensive feelings. When you do not give empathy then your clients and colleagues feel they have to justify their feelings.

Receiving empathy helps them to be open and move on to different ways of experiencing. It is perfectly natural for people to change their reactions as new information is processed or if old data are reexamined in a new light. The acceptance you provide through empathy helps your clients and colleagues to remain flexible enough to move to a new awareness. Just as being stuck in one place retards self-growth, so having the option to move on or change fosters self-growth.

"In our personal and professional lives we are often in relationships with individuals who must make difficult decisions about their lives. More often than not, that person does not need more information, certainly does not need a judgmental presence, probably does not want the answer or the decision taken from them. What they require from us is real presence that will support them, empower them, and give them the courage to decide" (Marsden, 1990, p. 541).

In some instances your empathic reflection will help your clients or colleagues to comprehend more fully how they are reacting. Hearing your reflection of their feelings may increase their self-awareness. Not only is this enlightenment satisfying but it can widen their perspective of their whole situation. Consider this example:

You have just empathically reflected to Douglas, one of your clients in the diabetic clinic, that he sounds jealous of his roommate's good health, freedom to eat and drink what he wants and to party till all hours.

> **Douglas:** "Yes, you're right! That's exactly how I'm feeling. I hadn't realized how it gripes me that he isn't restricted like I am. I guess I really am jealous that he doesn't have the medical expenses that I have, not to mention the time-consuming treatments I have to put up with. No wonder I'm so short with him when I see him having a good time. In fact sometimes I'm quite miserable to him . . . I'd better not let this situation get out of hand."

Your empathic labeling of his feeling of jealousy increased Douglas' understanding of his behavior and himself. The literature on empathy reports that psychotherapists high in empathy, genuineness, and warmth elicited greater self-exploration in their clients (Shapiro, Krauss & Truax, 1969).

The insight and expanded self-awareness sometimes triggered by your empathic responses can help your clients and colleagues decide how to handle a situation. Knowing how one feels about a situation and how those feelings are affecting one's way of coping with a situation are important factors in deciding on a course of action. Good problem solvers take their own feelings into account when confronted with any situation, problem, or issue (D'Zurilla & Goldfried, 1971). Having knowledge of our feelings helps us determine whether the situation should be changed in order to feel better, or whether it is more appropriate to change our feelings and outlook on the situation so as to feel better adjusted.

In the situation above, now that Douglas is aware of his jealousy of his roommate's health and freedom, he can use this self-awareness to help him handle his situation. Douglas could consider all kinds of possibilities. In terms of changing his situation he could get a roommate with a chronic illness so that he would not feel jealous or he could brainstorm ways to minimize the restrictions in his diabetic regimen so that he could live his life more naturally. In terms of changing his feelings, he could stop comparing himself with others and augment his gratefulness for the lifestyle he can lead; or he could stoke his jealousy until his roommate can no longer tolerate his hostility and decides either to leave Douglas or fight back.

Knowledge of their feelings and awareness of the impact these emotions have on their situation, provided by your empathic response, gives clients and colleagues more information with which to generate effective solutions.

Your empathy can lead to clients listening to themselves more empathically. The non-valuative and acceptant quality of the empathic climate enables clients to take a prizing, caring attitude toward themselves (Rogers, 1980). Being understood makes it possible for clients to listen with greater empathy toward their own reaction to what they are experiencing. This greater understanding and prizing of themselves opens new facets of experience which bring into their awareness a more accurate picture of themselves and a clearer self-concept (p. 159).

Research has demonstrated that empathy accounts for improvement in psychotherapy clients. (Cartwright-Dymond & Lerner, 1963; Truax, *et al*, 1966; Shapiro, Krauss & Truax, 1969). Rogers (1980) cited research from the late 1960s and the early 1970s that in the study of therapist/client relationships, clients who eventually showed more therapeutic change (in comparison with those who showed less) received more of the therapist's qualities of empathic understanding, acceptance, and genuineness (pp. 276-277). Therapist empathy was the most significant of factors distinguished between more and less effective therapists (Lafferty, Beutler, & Crago, 1989). Lafferty's research findings support the significance of the therapist's empathy in effective psychotherapy. Patients of more effective therapists felt more understood than patients of less effective therapists (p. 79).

It can be argued that empathic responses from nurses can enhance healing and well-being in all clients. Illness and hospitalization cause fear, dependency, and upheaval in clients' daily lifestyle and relationships; whether the health problem is surgical, medical, obstetrical, or psychiatric. An empathic nurse can tune into her client's feelings in a helpful way (Rubin, Judd & Conine, 1977).

Fine and Therrien (1977) argued that empathy in health professionals could improve the success of the complete clinical problem-solving process and client compliance.

Benefits of Being Empathic for the Nurse

The above points clarify how your employment of empathy can benefit your clients and colleagues. There are also benefits to you—the nurse who empathizes. The most obvious payoff is the warm feeling of compassion you get when you help someone feel understood and accepted. Knowing that you have taken the opportunity to make a client or colleague feel better provides immense satisfaction and can augment your feelings of competence.

As a nurse you want to collect enough information from your clients to accurately assess their concerns and develop the best nursing care plan for treating their health problems. When clients feel accepted by you their trust will allow them to open up and provide the information necessary for you to accurately assess their situation. Having sufficient data to make a correct nursing diagnosis is the first and most important step in the systematic problem-solving approach to nursing care. Whether clients' problems are physical, emotional, or both, empathy can be employed to acquire sufficient and comprehensive data.

Empathy can be shown at all stages of the problem-solving process. When developing a plan of care it is essential to determine how your client feels about the proposed treatment schedule and to empathically reflect your understanding. Acknowledging clients' reactions to treatment regimes, and where possible adjusting plans accordingly, is likely to increase compliance behaviour.

As a nurse you will want to know if your nursing care has been effective. There are many objective measures of success, but one important yardstick is how your client feels about the treatment outcome. Clients may be sufficiently satisfied and wish to terminate treatment, or they may want to try an alternative plan to achieve their desired outcome. Clients' input has implications for how to proceed in the client-nurse relationship. Showing empathy lets your clients know that you understand and acknowledge their evaluation of progress.

In your working relationships, being empathic with colleagues augments cohesiveness. Showing that you understand your colleagues not only makes working together more enjoyable, but helps you prevent and work out difficulties in your relationships.

Overcoming Blocks to Empathy

Clearly, empathy has many positive benefits for our clients and colleagues and also has a payoff for us. If we are not conveying empathy at appropriate opportunities in our relationships with clients and colleagues, then it is likely we are relating in ways that are nonhelpful or damaging. What *are* we doing if we are not communicating empathically when it is warranted, and how can we switch to communication that is more caring?

There are several activities that might result in our failing to express empathy. One trap is to judge our clients or colleagues. If we question the appropriateness of their thoughts and feelings then we effectively shut off the unbiased and accepting part of our communication. Being truly empathic means being able to put aside our opinions and tune into how the other person is feeling.

It would be absurd to suggest that we should cancel all judgmental thoughts. It is human to have preferences and opinions. We are taught throughout life to be selective in our tastes for food, art, clothing, and people. This discriminating is second nature to most of us. We use it every moment of our lives in deciding what to wear in the morning, selecting a strategy to solve a work problem, or choosing what to eat for supper. It is highly likely that most of us cannot turn off this judgmental thinking in our interpersonal relationships.

Most times our judgments serve a useful purpose in our lives. However, when we verbalize our judgments about another's thoughts and feelings we only make them feel criticized and labelled. Clients and colleagues feel like their case is closed when they have been judged; as though acceptance is impossible. Being judged engenders feelings of rejection and defensiveness. Clients and colleagues tend either to withdraw from us to protect themselves from further pronouncements, or to aggressively challenge us in an attempt to defend their thoughts and feelings. Whichever response occurs, the verbalized judgment has served to arrest any therapeutic communication.

The following example illustrates the benefits of empathic communication and the detrimental effects of being judgmental.

Your client is going for a colposcopy examination the next day and says to you:

"I'm scared to death of this copos . . . how do you say it? . . . exam tomorrow . . . the whole idea spooks me . . ."

You could respond with:

Nonempathic You: "Oh! It's nothing to worry about. You'll be just fine. Lots of our patients have one. By the way, it's pronounced colposcopy."

This response negates your client's fear and belittles her anxieties about this unknown procedure. It is unlikely that this response would make your client feel that you took her feelings seriously. Instead of feeling acknowledged she likely feels misunderstood and put down by your judgmental reply.

You might have responded with:

Empathic You: "The thought of having a colposcopy exam is really frightening for you. What can I do to relieve some of your fears about it?"

This empathic opening acknowledges her fears about the test, and the accompanying offer demonstrates your desire to help alleviate her fears. It is likely that she will be relieved by this nonjudgemental acceptance of her feelings. Your empathy makes it safe for her to trust you further by asking questions or revealing more of her feelings. Whereas a judgemental response closes lines of communication, an empathic reply opens them up.

An example involving a colleague may illustrate further.

You have just started evening shift on your ward after several days off and the nurse team leader on the day shift remarks:

"Boy! Count yourself lucky to have been off for the past 3 days. It's been like a zoo here! We've had two deaths and five admissions and we've been short-staffed the whole time. I'm wiped out!"

You could respond with:

Nonempathic You: "Well, the time passes quickly when you're busy, and after all, you've been trained to handle hectic situations . . . that's what they pay us for."

This reply undermines your colleague's feelings. Your judgment that she should be coping dismisses her feelings as inconsequential and even inappropriate. A noncaring response like this would only serve to make your colleague hostile and defensive, and certainly lead to a strained working relationship.

A more understanding response would be:

Empathic You: "No wonder you're tired. It sounds like you've had to handle 3 times the usual workload with the admissions and deaths . . . and all without enough help. When's your well-deserved time off coming?"

This empathic reply makes your colleague feel she has been heard. There is no doubt that you understand what she has been coping with while you were away. All she desired was for you to register how it has been for her. This response fits that bill.

When we judge others we effectively ignore their point of view. Instead we shift the focus to what we feel or think and emphasize our perspective. As helping professionals we feel sad when we hurt clients or colleagues by ignoring or upstaging them. The desire to communicate in a caring way is motivation to use empathy. Being nonjudgmentally empathic requires the desire to show acceptance and the will to focus and concentrate on the concerns of others.

Remember this idea so that as a helping professional you can take care of yourself: it takes courage to be empathic (Pike, 1990). "Entering into a patient's world as if it were his own exposes the nurse to the possibility of pain, despair, anger, fear and hopelessness. Courage is especially called for in situations where the nurse is powerless to cure the patient's distress, pain, or suffering" (p. 238).

The greater the nurse's maturity and experience, the greater is her usable vault of knowledge, attitudes, and learning for enhancing her empathy. But the nurse needs one important key to open the vault: access to feelings (Pike, 1990, p. 238).

Empathy is assertive because it takes into account the other's thoughts and feelings and protects your rights to communicate in a caring way. It is responsible to be empathic because it ensures that your client feels acknowledged enough to engage in all aspects of the nursing process.

SIX STEPS TO COMMUNICATING MORE EMPATHICALLY

How can we nurture our ability to reliably convey empathy on a consistent basis? The following guidelines are based on a systematic problem-solving approach. If you desire to be empathic, then these six steps will be helpful.

1. Clear your head of distracting agendas. In your busy life you will have many thoughts going through your head, such as personal worries, pressure from expanding work, or perhaps feelings of discomfort related to talking with a client or colleague. To the extent that you can put these aside, do so. If you are able to focus on the person you are with you will streamline communication. Paying attention to your speaker increases the chances that you will deal with their situation more thoroughly and more effectively. Listening empathically means not having to return time and time again to get complete information, and that means one less thing on your long list of things to do. Teach yourself to concentrate (Raudsepp, 1990).

2. Remind yourself to focus on your speaker. Remember that your priority is to listen and hear your client or colleague so that you can verbally convey your understanding. Remind yourself that your purpose is to tune in to what the speaker is saying. Some people find that a physical gesture, such as removing their glasses or adopting a definite listening stance reminds them to focus. "Don't interrupt," reminds Raudsepp (1990).

3. Attend to your client's or colleague's verbal and nonverbal message. Hear the words your speaker is using to describe how he is feeling, and the reason for his reaction. Also look for what your speaker is saying nonverbally. Take in the whole message that your client or colleague is sending you.

4. Ask yourself "What does this person want me to hear?" Attempt to pick out the most important message being delivered. What is the predominant theme for your client or colleague? Is his anguish the strongest feeling? Is joy the prevailing emotion? Your answer should be what your speaker wants you to hear, and that very seed is the embryo for your empathic response.

5. Convey an empathic response. Verbally reflect your speaker's feelings and the reason for them, ensuring that your response meets the criteria for accuracy and specificity. Pay attention to your nonverbal communication. Convey the amount of warmth you deem appropriate and ensure that the expression is congruent with your intentions to be understanding and accepting.

6. Check to see if your empathic response was effective. The purpose of being empathic is to make others feel relieved (that we understand them) and cared for (by our genuine interest in their situation). Check it out with your speaker. Does he nod his head? Does he smile or tell you in other ways that he is delighted you have understood him? Does your speaker visibly relax by letting go of tension or by engaging you in further conversation? These clues will inform you that you have been successful.

If your attempt to be empathic has missed the mark, your speaker will let you know in several ways. More assertive clients or colleagues will tell you outright: "No, that's not quite how I'm feeling . . . It's more like this . . . ." Others may just slowly withdraw from opening up any more with you. It is acceptable most times to explicitly ask your speaker if your empathy is on target. Questions like "Is that how you are feeling?" or "Have I understood how it is for you?" are effective.

When to Convey Empathy

It is helpful to be empathic any time someone shares their thoughts and feelings with you. An empathic reply can be used on its own or with another message or communication strategy. For example, empathy can be used with:

Statements

"You feel frustrated because the clinic is not open in the evenings when it would be more convenient for you to come and have your blood pressure checked. Because there have been several requests for extended hours, I will be raising this issue with our head nurse."

In addition to knowing your plan to follow up his complaint, it is re-assuring for this client to have his personal feelings about the situation acknowledged.

Questions

"Yes, I can see that you are pretty excited about being discharged from the hospital earlier than you had expected. Have you had time to arrange for your babysitter to start earlier and give you a hand with your two-year-old and your new baby?"

Your empathic beginning *potentiates* the effect of your concern for your client's discharge plans.

Alternate Points of View

"You feel pretty adamant that your pack-a-day smoking habit won't harm your health, since your grandfather smoked and lived to be 95. I have a different way of looking at smoking since I've recently known several clients who have died of lung cancer. The statistics do indicate a high positive correlation between smoking and lung cancer."

Most clients and colleagues hear our side of an argument if we give equal recognition to their point of view.

Explanations

"Being moved to a double bedroom has really upset you and you feel that your privacy has been invaded. Switching rooms truly was our last alternative. We need a single room to carry out isolation techniques for an infectious client in order to protect everyone on the unit."

By first acknowledging your client's feelings it helps him accept more fully the rationale for your decision.

Invitations for More Information

With a client:

"You're worried about the sharp pains in your kidney area. Have you had any other unusual signs and symptoms lately?"

With a colleague:

"From your point of view our new charting system is cumbersome and pretty frustrating. Do you have any suggestions for streamlining the recording of our nurses' notes?"

Most people engage more fully in our request for additional information when they hear that we understand what they have already told us.

Missing opportunities to convey empathy can create a gulf in which the speaker feels ignored by the listener. When we do not hear others a new struggle is created for them. They are disappointed and shocked at not being understood and in turn either withdraw with wounded feelings or fight to convince us of their feelings. When empathy is not proffered our clients and colleagues feel cheated, frustrated, and decidedly not heard. Including empathy with other communication strategies lets our clients and colleagues know beyond a doubt that they have been heard and understood.

In any therapeutic relationship it is important that our partner feels cared for. The client-nurse relationship is one in which we have established ourselves as helpers. That label means that we acknowledge and make public our desire to support others. Empathy is one concrete way to show our caring.

Practicing Empathy

Exercise 1. This exercise provides you with several hypothetical situations in which clients or colleagues express thoughts and feelings to you. On your own, write down an empathic response to each of the examples. Remember to meet the criteria of being accurate and specific.

After you have written your initial empathic response, critique it and suggest some alternative ways of phrasing your first try to make it more empathic. In your improved response try to convey complete understanding and phrase it in your natural way of speaking.

Example 1:

A nurse colleague said: "I'm not going to be able to get through that job interview with Mrs. Jones for the position of assistant head nurse. I just know I'll be so uptight that I'll blow it like I did the last time."

First attempt at empathy: "You're feeling pretty nervous about that interview."
Critique: This reply lacks specificity. Including a reference to the fact that it is a job interview would have acknowledged the importance of the event for your colleague. Referring to the reason for her worry about the interview would have made a more complete and accurate empathy response.
Suggested alternative: "You're feeling pretty nervous about your job interview for the assistant head position and worried that you might botch it like you feel you have before."

Example 2:

A client says: "My first child was retarded. I'd like to have another child . . . but . . . what if that child turns out to be retarded as well?"

First attempt at empathy: "Yeah, it is a big chance to take, isn't it—getting pregnant, I mean."
Critique: This is more of an opinion than an empathic response and it might feed into her worry. Being more accurate by including a reference to her feelings would make this reply more empathic. Verbalizing her reasons would meet the criteria for specificity.
Suggested alternative: "You have mixed feelings about having another child. On the one hand you'd like another baby, but you're frightened that you may have another mentally impaired child."

Example 3:

A client tells you: "I didn't have to take any pain medication last night for my injured back . . . And I slept right through the night. It was the first good sleep I've had in four nights."

First attempt at empathy: "That's great! I'm glad you're sleeping better!"
Critique: This statement is more a judgment than a reflection of the client's feelings. The implied feelings are relief (at not having to take the medication) and joy (at sleeping well). These feelings, and the reasons for them, need to be included to make the response empathic.
Suggested alternative: "Boy! What a relief for you to have been comfortable enough to do without your analgesic, and you look overjoyed that you slept so well."

Now it is your turn! For each of the following situations attempt a written empathic response. Then critique your attempt and suggest how it could be improved.

Example 4:

A client on unit 2 says to you: "I don't know what to do. My wife is a patient on unit 3 . . . she's just had another small stroke and I don't know how to help her."

Your first attempt at empathy:
Your critique:
Suggestions for improvement:

Example 5:

A client says to you: "My husband died a year ago. It's been the longest and saddest year of my life."

Your first attempt at empathy:
Your critique:
Your suggestions for improvement:

Example 6:

A client says to you: "I had a real scare today. My chest x-ray has a spot on it and my doctor has called in a specialist to see what it is. I'm so worried because she told me that cancer can't be ruled out until I've had further tests."

Your first attempt at empathy:
Your critique:
Your suggestions for improvement:

Example 7:

A newly hired nurse colleague says to you: "Things are just beginning to fall in place for me since I moved here. I now have a nice place to live in . . . and a reasonable rent. I'm starting to make some friends and beginning to feel comfortable here working on the unit."

Your first attempt at empathy:
Your critique:
Your suggestions for improvement:

Example 8:

An 18-year-old client says to you: "I had really hoped to go to university in the fall but now that I'm stuck in this traction I can see that I'm not going anywhere! The only thing I'll be studying is the ceiling. What a rotten waste of time. Why did this accident have to happen to me?"

Your first attempt at empathy:
Your critique:
Your suggested alternative:

Example 9:

A colleague says: "I'm really fed up with having to run all the way down the hall to answer the telephone on evenings when there's no unit clerk on. Last night it rang 5 times when I was trying to give out my medications at the other end of the unit. Each time I had to lock up my med cart and hurry back to the nurses' station. It's a waste of time and I can't put up with this inconvenience any more."

Your first attempt at empathy:
Your critique:
Your suggested alternative:

Example 10:

A client is looking forlorn and says: "Oh! I'm just so blue today. I miss my little boy so much . . . he's only 4 . . . I just talked to him on the phone. He wants to know when I'm coming home . . . I wish I could tell him but all these tests they're doing on me will take so long. I sure will be glad when they are finished and I can return home and be with him again."

Your first attempt at empathy:
Your critique:
Your suggested alternative:

After you have completed the above examples on your own, get together with the rest of your class and compare different responses. It will be interesting to see how many different ways an empathic response can be phrased and still meet the criteria of accuracy, specificity, naturalness, warmth, and genuineness.

Exercise 2. This exercise gives you the chance to experience the differences between passive and active listening. Find a partner with whom to work. One of you will be the speaker and the other the listener. The speaker will talk on any subject about which she has strong feelings.

In the first part of the exercise the listener will listen passively, and in the second part she will listen actively. For the first part of this exercise the listener will display attentive nonverbal listening and will offer encouragers such as "uh huh," "yes," "I see," and the like. Carry out part one of this exercise for 4 minutes and then proceed to part two.

In the second part the speaker will proceed as she did in part one. But this time the listener will listen actively by responding with empathic statements at every appropriate opportunity. Proceed with this second part of the exercise for 4 minutes.

After completing both parts one and two answer the following questions.

As speaker: What differences did you notice between receiving passive and then active listening?

As listener: What differences did you notice between listening passively and listening actively?

Switch roles so that each partner will have the chance to both give and receive passive and active listening.

Together as a class, pool all the ideas you have gleaned about empathy from doing this exercise.

Exercise 3. In the next few days observe how others listen to you. Note how you feel when you receive passive listening in contrast to active listening during your conversations with people in your day-to-day activities. What have you learned about empathy from your observations?

Exercise 4. Over the next week attempt to make an empathic reflection each time someone expresses their thoughts and feelings to you. Try these empathic responses with your grocer, your landlady, the person beside you on the bus, your children and neighbors—everyone you encounter. This exercise is hard work but it will provide you with extensive practice in being empathic.

A highly empathic person is socially perceptive of a wide range of personal cues and appears to have an awareness of the impression he makes on others (Hornblow, Kidson & Jones, 1977). What do you notice about your effect on others when you are empathic? How do others behave when you are empathic with them?

After you have completed this exercise, ask yourself what it has

Name of Listener: _____ Date: _____

Name of Observer: _____

EMPATHY RATING SCALE

Response #	Accuracy: matched intensity?	Specificity: rationale included?	Naturalness: own words?	Warmth: verbal? nonverbal?	Genuineness interest & caring conveyed?
1.					
2.					
3.					
4.					
5.					
6.					
7.					

Figure 8-1

EMPATHY RATING SCALE

Criteria for empathy rating scale

1. Accuracy: Does the intensity of the listener's words match the
                      speaker's intended message?

2. Specificity: Does the listener include the rationale for the
                      speaker's feelings?

3. Naturalness: Does the listener avoid parroting? Does the listener
                      reflect the speaker's message in her own naturally
                      worded style?

4. Warmth: Does the listener convey verbal and nonverbal
                      warmth with her empathic response?

5. Genuineness: Does the listener convey that she is really interested
                      in, and cares about, what the speaker is saying?

---

taught you about empathy. Compare your findings with those of your colleagues in your class.

Exercise 5. Take some of the most commonly felt emotions (such as sadness, fear, anxiety, joy, anger, and so on) and for each emotion make a list of the range of words that have similar meanings. Divide the class into small groups and ask each group to take one of the concepts. Have a contest to discover which group will come up with the most synonyms for its feeling concept. Afterwards, compile the lists from all the groups and make copies for all the students. These references will be handy in the future when you are searching for just the right word.

Exercise 6. This exercise gives you a chance to receive supervised feedback on your ability to be empathic. Work in groups of four. One will take the role of speaker, one the role of listener, and the other two will be the observers. The speaker will choose a topic about which she has strong feelings. The listener's task is to demonstrate empathic listening to what the speaker has to say during a conversation lasting 4 minutes. The observers will use the Empathy Rating Scale (see Figure 8-1) to evaluate the speaker's ability to be empathic. Tape recorders or video monitors, if available, provide a valuable asset for self-observation.

Roles should be rotated so that each person in the group has the chance to be speaker, listener, and observer.

The information on the Empathy Rating Scale you will receive as listener will outline your strengths and areas where you need to improve in your ability to communicate empathically. For example, the Empathy Rating Scale may draw your attention to the fact that you neglect to include the rationale for the speaker's feelings, even though you meet the criteria for accuracy, warmth, naturalness, and genuineness. This exercise can be repeated at intervals after practicing empathy so that over time you can see the pattern of improvement.

REFERENCES

Cartwright-Dymond, R., & Lerner, B. (1963). Empathy, need to change and improvement with psychotherapy. *Journal of Consulting Psychology, 27* (2), pp. 138-144.

Diers, D. (1990). Response to: On the nature and place of empathy in clinical nursing practice. *Journal of Professional Nursing,* 6 (4), 240-241.

Dymond, R.F. (1949). A scale for the measurement of empathic ability. *Journal of Consulting Psychology,* 13, pp. 127-133.

D'Zurilla, T.J., & Goldfried, M.R. (1971). Problem solving and behaviour modification. *Journal of Abnormal Psychology,* 78 (1), pp. 107-126.

Fine, V.K., & Therrien, M.E. (1977). Empathy in the doctor-patient relationship: A skill training for medical students. *Journal of Medical Education,* 52 (9), pp. 752-757.

High, D.M. (1989). Truthtelling, confidentiality, and the dying patient: New dilemmas for the nurse. *Nursing Forum,* 24 (1), 5-10.

Hills, M. & Coffey, M. (1982). *On delivering care: An interpersonal skills training manual for nurses.* University of Victoria, B. C., Canada: Unpublished manual.

Hogan, R. (1969). Development of an empathy scale. *Journal of Consulting and Clinical Psychology,* 33 (3), pp. 307-316.

Hornblow, A.R., Kidson, M.A., & Jones, K.V. (1977). Measuring medical students' empathy. *Medical Education,* 11, pp. 7-12.

Lafferty, P., Beutler, L.E., & Crago, M. (1989). Differences between more and less effective psychotherapists: A study of select therapist variables. *Journal of Consulting and Clinical Psychology,* 57 (1), 76-80.

Marsden, C. (1990). Real presence. *Heart & Lung,* 19 (5), 540-541.

Miller, I.J. (1989) The therapeutic empathic communication (TEC) process. *American Journal of Psychotherapy, XLIII* (4), 531-543.

Pike, A.W. (1990). On the nature and place of empathy in clinical nursing practice. *Journal of Professional Nursing,* 6 (4), 235-140.

Raudsepp, E. (1990). Seven ways to cure communication breakdowns. *Nursing 90,* 20 (4), 132-142.

Rogers, C.R. (1980). *A way of being.* Boston, Mass.: Houghton Mifflin Company.

Rubin, F.L., Judd, M.M., & Conine, T.A. (1977). Empathy: Can it be learned and retained? *Physical Therapy,* 57 (6), pp. 644-647.

Shapiro, J.G., Krauss, H.H., & Truax, C.B. (1969). Therapeutic conditions and disclosure beyond the therapeutic encounter. *Journal of Counseling Psychology,* 16 (4), pp. 290-294.

Truax, C.B. et al, (1966). Therapist empathy, genuineness, and warmth and patient therapeutic outcome. *Journal of Consulting Psychology,* 30 (5), pp. 395-401.

SUGGESTIONS FOR FURTHER READING

Carkhuff, R.R., Pierce, R.M., & Cannon, J.R. (1980). *The art of helping* (4th ed.). Amherst, Mass.: Human Resource Development Press, Inc.

Chapter 3, "Responding," contains the material on empathy. The text is clear reading for students of interpersonal communication. The accompanying drawings help emphasize the points. There is a useful chart outlining the various levels of intensity for different categories of feelings.

Egan, G. (1982). *The skilled helper: Model, skills, and methods for effective helping* (2nd ed.). Monterey, Calif.: Brooks/Cole Publishing Company.

In chapter 4, Egan demonstrates how accurate empathy helps clients explore and clarify their problems. Later, in chapter 6, he helps readers develop their empathy skills to the level of advanced empathy where the helper verbalizes the feelings only implied by the helpee. The many examples are designed to help nurse readers to augment their skill level.

Gazda, G.M., Walters, R.P., & Childers, W.C. (1975). *Human relations development: A manual for health sciences*. Boston: Allyn & Bacon, Inc.

Empathy warrants two chapters in this textbook. In both, the exercises are carefully designed to help readers augment their skills of perceiving and effectively communicating empathy. The authors provide an empathy rating scale which nurse readers could use to assess their ability to be empathic with others.

Stotland, E., et al. (1978). *Empathy, fantasy and helping*. Beverley Hills, Calif.: Sage Publications.

For the nurse who has become interested in empathy, this book will enlarge her knowledge of the subject. This text is a summary of experimental studies of empathy; it is not a "how to" book. It is clearly written and expands the reader's awareness of issues in measuring empathy.

CHAPTER 9

Self-Disclosure

> *"Loving is scary, because when you permit yourself to be known, you expose yourself not only to a lover's balm, but also to a hater's bombs! When he knows you, he knows just where to plant them for maximum effect."*
>
> S.M. Jourard

OBJECTIVES

Self-disclosure is another interpersonal communication behavior that you can use to show your clients and colleagues you understand them. By the end of this chapter you will understand what is meant by self-disclosure, and appreciate how this skill can be used to advantage in your relationships with clients and colleagues. You will have a chance to enhance your self-disclosing in the exercises at the end of this chapter.

SELF-DISCLOSURE IN PERSONAL AND PROFESSIONAL RELATIONSHIPS

Disclose means to "un" close or to open up. To self-disclose, then, means to open up our "self" to others. When we self-disclose we reveal our thoughts and feelings and make known to others some of our personal experiences. Throughout your life you have used self-disclosure to let others know about you in order to develop a closer relationship.

Self-disclosures can take any number of forms: complaining, boasting, gossiping, expressing political or religious views, and sharing endearments, secrets, or dreams. In social relationships self-disclosures are traded back and forth until the partners establish a mutually agreed upon plateau. Intimate relationships are characterized by more private revelations than those shared between superficial acquaintances. The give and take of self-disclosing can occur with or without formal spoken rules. A specific request for deeper closeness, or an observed withdrawal of the usual pattern of sharing, influences the relationship to readjust the established level of intimacy.

Guidelines for Self-Disclosing in the Helping Relationship

The client-nurse relationship demands some special considerations for the employment of self-disclosure. As a helping relationship, it is established for the benefit of the client; in other words it is a client-centered relationship. It follows that anything you reveal about yourself—your thoughts, feelings, and experiences—should be revealed for the benefit of your client.

You need to consider the why, what, when, and how of self-disclosing with your clients.

Why Should Nurses Employ Self-Disclosure With Clients?

Whereas in a social relationship you might self-disclose to allow others to understand you better, the opposite is true in the professional client-nurse relationship. Self-disclosure is a skill that you can use to show clients how much you understand them because of your similar thoughts, feelings, or experiences. The intent of a self-disclosure is to be empathic: to show that you really understand your client because you have walked a similar path. An effective self-disclosure can transmit all the benefits of empathic responses outlined in the previous chapter.

Because self-disclosure is a sharing of your personal self with a client, it can deepen the bond between you. While still within the parameters of a professional helping relationship, your self-disclosure lets your client know you are a normal human being.

What Should Nurses Reveal to Clients in Self-Dislosures?

As nurses we have to use our judgement about what specifically we will reveal to clients. Two questions to answer before self-disclosing are: "Is what I am planning to reveal likely to demonstrate to my client that I understand him?" and "Do I feel comfortable (safe from repercussions and embarrassment; legally and morally secure) about revealing this information to my client?" Both questions should receive a solid affirmative response before you self-disclose to your client.

When you self-disclose it is important to set up a client-wins/nurse-wins situation. If your client wins, your self-disclosure makes him feel understood. If you win, you feel good that you have been skillful in making your client feel better. If your client loses, it is because your self-disclosure is irrelevant so that he is distracted from his major issue and left feeling misunderstood. If you lose, it is because your self-disclosure leaves you feeling uncomfortably exposed or embarrassed.

When Should Nurses Use Self-Disclosure with Clients?

The purpose of a therapeutic self-disclosure is to let your client know that he has been understood. It augments an empathic reply and deepens the trust between you and your client. When you wish to augment your level of understanding and strengthen the client's trust, and you feel comfortable revealing the content of your self-disclosure, then self-disclosure would be right for both you and your client.

How to Self-Disclose in the Helping Relationship

To successfully implement a helpful self-disclosure you need to follow all the guidelines for conveying empathy outlined in the previous chapter. Here is a concise list of those steps:
1. Clear your head of distracting agendas
2. Remind yourself to focus on your speaker
3. Attend to your client's (or colleague's) verbal and nonverbal message
4. Ask yourself: "What does this person want me to hear?"
5. Convey empathy, beginning with an empathic response followed by a self-disclosure

It is usually better to self-disclose after you have conveyed an empathic response. Using an empathic response first keeps the focus on your client or colleague before shifting it to you. Your self-disclosure enhances and augments your empathic reflection. Beginning with an empathic response and following up with a self-disclosure deepens your speaker's conviction that he has been understood. As with empathy, the final step is:
6. Check to see if your empathic response and self-disclosure were effective

In short, the steps for implementing self-disclosure are:
1. Listen
2. Reply empathically
3. Self-disclose
4. Check it out

Examples of Helpful and Nonhelpful Self-Disclosures

For the following situation an acceptable empathic reply has been provided. Following this example several ineffective self-disclosures are provided, with a rationale to explain their limitations. And lastly, an acceptable complete response is proffered.

Situation One: With a Client

A client, Mrs. Kern, has just relayed the following information to you: "I was so scared this weekend when I had Jack at home on a pass from the hospital. He started coughing and got all red in the face . . . and then he bent over with this violent chest pain. I thought he was going to die. Luckily his nitroglycerine was right on the window sill. As soon as I gave it to him he calmed down right away. His pain left within minutes, thank goodness!"

1. Listen. This lady wants to hear messages related to the fright she suffered because of her husband's pain and the relief she experienced when he recovered.

2. Reply empathically. Before employing your self-disclosure you would convey an empathic response such as:

> "Gosh! I guess you were scared your husband might have a fatal heart attack when he doubled up like that with his chest pain. It was probably twice as frightening because you were at home without the security of all the hospital emergency equipment. What a relief for you when the nitro' worked . . . ."

This satisfactory empathic introduction would be followed up with a self-disclosure.

3. Self-disclose. The following examples will help you differentiate between satisfactory and unsatisfactory ways of implementing self-disclosure.

Unsatisfactory: Response One

> ". . . I remember hearing about my grandfather having chest pain, and I recall them saying that my grandmother used to have some hair-raising moments. They lived in the country and even the telephone system was unreliable. . . ."

This attempt at self-disclosure is inadequate because it is not your personal experience and does not demonstrate to Mrs. Kern that you really understand what she had suffered over the weekend. This attempt is more a disclosure of your grandmother's experience, and would likely confuse and distract Mrs. Kern.

A self-disclosure should convince Mrs. Kern that you have been where she is, felt the way she is feeling, and experienced what she is experiencing. Only a revelation of a personal experience will persuade the speaker that your understanding is authentic.

Unsatisfactory: Response Two

> ". . . Scares like that are really traumatic. I, too, had a frightening situation on the weekend. The fire alarm went off and I was the only nurse on the floor. I almost panicked, but like you, I kept calm and luckily it turned out to be a false alarm."

This response competes with Mrs. Kern's. One important feature of a self-disclosure is that the content must be pertinent to the speaker's situation. If your self-disclosure is beside the point or, worse still, unrelated, then the message for Mrs. Kern will get is that you do not really comprehend her situation. This response has little to do with Mrs. Kern's horribly anxious moments with her husband. Shifting gears to talk about your unrelated experience will likely convey the message to Mrs. Kern that you are trying to upstage her. She might be jarred into refocusing on your plight and become the helper instead of the helpee.

Unsatisfactory: Response Three

". . . Yes, I sure know how terrible it can be watching someone suffer excruciating chest pain right before your eyes. Last week there was a woman on the unit who suffered an episode of extreme chest pain, and like you I was anxious and worried. This lady had three children at home and you really wondered how they would cope if she died. She was a single parent, so they said . . . guess her husband left her years ago . . . a drinker, even abused her I've heard. You know, it makes you wonder. . . ."

Response three is far too vague and tangential. The irrelevant material is distracting and detracts from any caring intended by the response. The whole purpose of a self-disclosure is to reassure your client or colleague that you understand their plight because you have had a similar experience yourself. The self-disclosure should be brief and focused on the important issues pertinent to the speaker's situation. For Mrs. Kern, it would be important to relate your understanding of her fear and relief as succinctly as possible. The more focused your self-disclosure, the more clearly your understanding will be transmitted.

Satisfactory Response

". . . My dad had severe angina, too, and I had some pretty anxious times when he would turn ashen and look so tortured when his chest pain got excruciating. When all I could do was just stand by and hope that the nitro' would work, I used to feel so desperate and helpless. Did you feel that way this weekend?"

This response meets the criteria for an effective self-disclosure because it empathically demonstrates that you have had a similar personal experience with a loved one. Beyond a doubt your revelation is relevant to Mrs. Kern's. This self-disclosure is brief and focused so Mrs. Kern would perceive immediately that you are absolutely tuned in to how she felt being alone with her ill husband.

4. Check it out. This fourth response meets an additional criterion for self-disclosure: it is tentative. The question "Did you feel that way this weekend?" invites Mrs. Kern to talk more about her feelings. It refocuses on her and allows her to confirm or expand how she felt. A question like this helps you check to see whether your self-disclosure has hit the mark. By inviting Mrs. Kern to comment, you appropriately return the focus to her reactions about her situation.

A complete and fully acceptable self-disclosure to Mrs. Kern could be worded this way:

> "Gosh! I guess you were scared your husband might have a fatal heart attack when he doubled up like that with his chest pain. It was probably twice as frightening because you were at home without the security of all the hospital emergency equipment. What a relief for you when the nitro' worked. My dad had severe angina, too, and I had some pretty anxious times when he would turn ashen and look so tortured when his pain got excruciating. When all I could do was just stand by and hope that the nitro' would work, I used to feel so desperate and helpless. Did you feel that way this weekend?"

This response integrates the steps of listening, responding empathically, self-disclosing, and checking it out. It is absolutely clear that you have understood Mrs. Kern and are interested in discussing her situation with her.

Situation Two: With a Colleague

> A fellow nursing student, Joan, says to you: "I'm just thrilled! I've had the most wonderful day on the neuro unit where I'm doing my practicum. I'd been paying close attention to this young client's pupillary response and blood pressure. I kept checking his vital signs, and I was sure I could detect a rising trend in his blood pressure and some sluggishness in his pupillary reflex. I decided to point out my observations to the neurosurgeon who came by on his rounds. He checked out my concerns and promptly arranged for my client to go to surgery. In the O.R. they removed a life-threatening hematoma. I felt so pleased that my careful attention helped save his life. Days like this make all the hard work and studying worth it."

1. Listen. The message your classmate wants you to hear is that she is proud of her astuteness and grateful that her diligence helped save her client's life.

2. Reply empathically. Before self-disclosing you would convey an empathic response such as:

> "Wow! No wonder you're ecstatic! Thanks to your vigilance your client's life was saved. You look thrilled that your astuteness paid off so dramatically. It was life or death, and you're grateful that you picked up on the subtle changes in his vital signs. . . ."

This satisfactory empathic introduction would be followed up with a self-disclosure.

3. Self-disclose. The following examples will help you differentiate between some satisfactory and unsatisfactory ways of implementing self-disclosure.

Unsatisfactory: Response One

". . . My sister had the same experience when she was a student nurse. It was 5 years ago now, but it meant so much to her that she still talks about how excited she felt. She happened by a client's room and saw him choking. She did the Heimlich and of course rescued the man. . . ."

This attempt at self-disclosure is inadequate because it is not your personal experience and does not demonstrate to Joan that *you* really understand her moment of achievement. Your story about your sister would not convince Joan that you have been where she is, felt what she is feeling, or experienced what she is experiencing. A personal disclosure of your own is the best way to persuade Joan that you understand her. Joan may interpret response one as a competitive remark, a story to upstage her own.

Unsatisfactory: Response Two

". . . I know just how you feel. I had a great day, too. I got my whole assignment finished, and all the orders caught up by noon. So, then I was able to take the clients out for a walk. They enjoyed the break and the fresh air, so I too feel like I accomplished something today."

Your situation is not one of life or death and does not compare to Joan's. The irrelevance of response two would create a gulf between you and Joan, rather than bring you closer together through understanding. Your feeling of accomplishment is not equivalent to Joan's because she was directly responsible for saving a life.

Your self-disclosure must be relevant to the speaker's situation to show that you completely grasp the significance of her reaction. If your self-disclosure is off the mark, as this response is, it tells Joan that you do not really comprehend what she has told you.

Unsatisfactory: Response Three

"I know how thrilling it can be to save someone's life. Last summer I saw a boat out on the water in front of our cottage . . . you know the spot right near the small island . . . well, it was there a long time. I could see this person waving both arms overhead back and forth. I remembered that Jan had told us that arm waving like that was the international distress signal. It turned out to be two young girls who were joy riding in their parent's motor boat and had run out of gas. They had no paddles and no life jackets. And one of them was quite sick. She was a diabetic and she'd had some beer and too much sun, and she desperately needed her insulin. We brought them back to shore and got them to safety, so I know what it's like to have saved someone's life."

Instead of feeling understood with this response, Joan would likely feel bored and irritated. If your speaker has to wade through unimportant details and sift through irrelevant recollections, it can be exasperating. It is considerate to word your self-disclosure as briefly and clearly as you can. Succinctness will cause your speaker to understand your message sooner, not later or never, as in the example above.

Satisfactory Response

". . . I've had that proud feeling of knowing that if it hadn't been for me my client might not have lived. When I was on floor 4J, I discovered a client having a myocardial infarct. I called the code and started CPR . . . and he lived! Isn't it reassuring to know that you can remember what you've studied and apply it correctly in the real world?"

This response meets the criteria for an effective self-disclosure because the similarity of your experience makes it relevant. It is brief and focused so that your colleague Joan immediately receives your message that you have understood her.

4. Check it out. The tentative question at the end is an effective technique for checking out with Joan if your self-disclosure corresponds with her experience. Your question returns the attention to Joan, where it should be. Joan has the chance to elaborate further on how she is feeling. This response does not upstage her excitement but adds to it. By sharing your relevant experience you have made her feel understood.

A complete and accurate self-disclosure that includes the four steps could be phrased like this one:

"Wow! No wonder you're ecstatic! Thanks to your vigilance your client's life was saved. You look thrilled that your astuteness paid off so dramatically. It was life or death and you're pleased that you picked up on the subtle changes in his vital signs. I've had that proud feeling of knowing that if it weren't for me my client might not have lived. When I was on floor 4J I discovered a client having a myocardial infarct. I called the code and started CPR . . . and he lived! Isn't it reassuring to know that you can remember what you've studied and apply it correctly in the real world?"

This response combines the steps of listening, responding empathically, self-disclosing, and checking. Your client or colleague feels heard, understood, and respected when you actively listen with empathy and self-disclosure, and then close off by turning the conversation back to your speaker.

It is responsible to self-disclose because you bring your own relevant experiences to the interaction. When you self-disclose you are assertively safeguarding the other's right to be understood and preserving your right to communicate in a caring way.

PRACTICING SELF-DISCLOSURE

Exercise 1. In the natural course of your life during the next few days note the self-disclosures that people reveal to you. Are these self-disclosures relevant, brief, and personal? Are they conveyed to make you feel understood? Note your reactions to these self-disclosures from colleagues, sales people, teachers, or friends. Consider what characteristics of their self-disclosures led you to feel cared for and what features jarred you and made you question the genuine interest of the self-discloser.

After you have done this exercise individually get together as a class and compare your findings about the communication behavior of self-disclosure.

Exercise 2. This time observe your own self-disclosures with others. Note your intentions when you self-disclose to people you contact. Is it for their benefit or yours? Remark on the characteristics of your self-disclosures. Are they your own personal experiences? Are your self-disclosures brief and focused? Do you end them with a tentative question?

From your observations, assess your ability to effectively self-disclose. Where are you doing well and what improvements could you strive for in your employment of self-disclosure?

Exercise 3. For this exercise work in groups of three. One of you will be the speaker, another the listener, and the third the observer. As speaker, choose a topic with which your listener is familiar. This way it is more likely that she will have had some similar experiences so that she can realistically make a self-disclosure.

As speaker your task is to talk for 5 minutes about this topic, conveying your thoughts, feelings, and reactions. The listener's task is to attempt to implement a self-disclosure at every appropriate opportunity. The observer will make note of the listener's self-disclosures and give feedback about how her self-disclosures meet the following criteria.

Criteria for a Complete Self-Disclosure
Empathic Response:

Was an empathic response included before the self-disclosure?

Self-Disclosure:

Was the self-disclosure personal? Was it brief, focused, and relevant?

Checking:

Did the listener complete her self-disclosure with a tentative question as a way of validating with the speaker?

After 5 minutes stop and debrief with these questions:

As Listener:

1. How did you feel employing the skill of self-disclosure?
2. What aspects were awkward and which went smoothly for you?

As Speaker:

1. How did the listener's self-disclosures make you feel?
2. From your point of view is there anything the listener might have done differently to make you feel more understood?

As Observer:

1. What aspects of the listener's self-disclosures were done well?
2. What suggestions can you make to help her improve?

Rotate roles so that each of you has a chance to be speaker, listener, and observer.

This exercise provides you a chance to think about self-disclosures from many different angles. What has your contemplation taught you about the important communication behavior of self-disclosure? Compare your thoughts with those of your colleagues.

Exercise 4. Like any new skill we learn, whether typing, tennis, or dancing, the most progress is made when we practice. To improve your ability to self-disclose, attempt to include a self-disclosure wherever appropriate in your day-to-day encounters with others.

Take the opportunity to evaluate yourself. Critique your self-disclosures using the criteria outlined in Exercise 3. Also make note of the response you receive from your speaker. Did your self-disclosure result in your clients or colleagues opening up more about their experiences? Did your speaker look pleased and convinced that you understood?

Remember to congratulate yourself on your successes. Be clear about how you want to improve and visualize yourself successfully meeting your goal.

SUGGESTIONS FOR FURTHER READING

Adler, R.B. (1977). *Confidence in communication: A guide to assertive and social skills.* New York: Holt, Rinehart & Winston.

Adler discusses the importance of self-disclosure in our social relationships. He includes a diary-type chart for readers to assess whether they express the full range of their emotions in the most satisfactory way. Adler emphasizes the assertiveness of self-disclosing.

Egan, G. (1977). *You and me: The skills of communicating and relating to others.* Monterey, Calif.: Brooks/Cole Publishing Company.

Chapter 3 will help nurses become more knowledgeable about self-disclosure in social relationships. Egan suggests some factors that prevent us from disclosing more fully. There are some excellent exercises to help nurses become more aware of themselves, which is the first step in self-disclosing.

Evans, D.R., Hearn, M.T., Uhlemann, M.R., & Ivey, A.E. (1979). *Essential interviewing: A programmed approach to effective communication.* Monterey, Calif.: Brooks/Cole Publishing Company.

This whole textbook is set up in a programmed learning approach to coach helpers to learn effective interpersonal communication skills. Chapter 9 on self-disclosing walks students through the most effective responses.

Stewart, J. (1977). *Bridges, not walls: A book about interpersonal communication* (2nd ed.). Reading, Mass.: Addison-Wesley Publishing Company.

In section VI on self-disclosure, Stewart includes two papers by Sidney M. Jourard and John Powell. These essays are beautifully written and open up readers' awareness of the significance of self-disclosure. These readings provide nurses with some philosophical aspects to the issue of self-disclosing in interpersonal relationships.

CHAPTER 10

Asking
Questions

*"A fool may ask more questions in an hour than
a wise man can answer in seven years."*

English Proverb

OBJECTIVES

By the end of this chapter you will be able to describe the important
points to keep in mind when asking questions of clients and colleagues.
The information in this chapter will help you improve your effectiveness
in questioning by suggesting which techniques to hold on to, which to discard, and what new approaches to add to your repertoire. The exercises at
the end of the chapter make it possible for you to assess your ability to
ask questions skillfully.

THE IMPORTANCE OF ASKING QUESTIONS EFFECTIVELY IN
NURSING

As a professional nurse, you will spend about half of your working time
asking questions of clients and colleagues. Anything you spend this much
time doing you should do extremely well.

Adeptness at asking questions is a fundamental requirement of a
competent and considerate nurse. The more effective you can be in asking
questions, the more time you will save yourself and others, the more pertinent and useful information you will collect, and the more effective your
interviewing experience. Effective questioning will ensure that you collect the data you need to provide quality nursing service.

From the time your client enters your care until the completion of
your helping relationship you will be asking him questions. You will ask
him about the nature of his concern so that you can agree on a nursing

127

diagnosis. Finding out what he hopes to achieve with the help of your nursing services requires effective questioning. You will discover his preferences for a treatment plan and frequently check with him about its effectiveness. Determining his readiness for termination of your relationship, and his readiness to take care of his own health concerns after discharge, demands that your questioning skills be clear and focused.

You might be thinking that the client-nurse relationship is mostly composed of questioning! Well, to a great extent it is. Therefore, it is crucial that you attain proficiency in this fundamental nursing communication behavior.

In your role as a nurse your main reasons for asking questions are to secure data that are essential to provide quality care to your clients and to ensure the smooth running of your nursing unit. For both these purposes there are six questions you need to answer to ensure you secure the facts you need.

The Why, What, How, Who, When, and Where of Asking Questions

If it is important for you to secure the information you want, then it is worthwhile spending the time planning the strategy which is most likely to secure this essential data.

The Why of Asking Questions

Before you open your mouth to make inquiries you should be sure about *why* you need the information from your client. If your question is rooted in personal curiosity or uncertainty (you decide to ask everything you can think of with the hope that what you need will be included), then you are unlikely to get what you want—or know you have it when you get it—and in the process you may offend your client. Before you speak, silently answer this question: "How will the information I am seeking direct me in helping my client?" If you can justify the question, then ask it!

If there is any doubt that your client may not understand your reasons for asking, then explain them to him in advance. For example:

In your investigations of your client's fall off a ladder you want to learn about his safety habits in general to determine if he is in danger of future home accidents. Before barraging your client with what might seem to be unrelated or even nosy questions, it would clarify to say something like:

> "I'd like to ask you some questions about your safety precautions with the ladder and about your home safety measures in general. Because about 80% of accidents occur in the home, my questions might trigger some ideas that could make your home a safer place to work and live. Are you agreeable to exploring this area with me?"

Here is another example: Within the past year, your 79-year-old client has been brought to the emergency department three times after fainting. The cause of the fainting has not been unearthed, and your observations about her thinness and lack of vitality make you wonder whether inadequate nutrition might be at the root of her fainting. The following statement would clarify the purpose of your questions:

> "We still don't know what is causing your fainting, Mrs. Jones, and we want to investigate every likely source. One possible cause could be a lack of the nutrients essential to keep you going. I'd like to ask you some questions about your diet to find out whether you are getting all you need from the foods you eat. Is that okay with you?"

Both these examples illustrate how you can prepare your client for your line of questioning. When clients understand your purpose they are more likely to be open and reveal information, in contrast to being guarded because they are uneasy about your intentions.

The **What** and **How** of Asking Questions

What you will ask and *how* you will ask it are the next considerations in your strategy. When you have determined *why* you require the information, then you must plan *what* to ask to ensure you are clear in your intentions and *how* to phrase your question in a way that invites your client to respond.

What you say must be phrased clearly, and a logical progression to your questions is helpful. They should be phrased in a way that shows your respect for your client's privacy and personal information. Any judgments you have about the responses should not be spoken.

For example, imagine that you require some information about your client's overall activity level and day-to-day schedule in order to help him fit in his colostomy hygienic care. Having explained your purpose and secured his permission your next step is to proceed with your inquiry. You choose to proceed in a systematic order with:

> "Let's begin with your mornings. Could you outline what you do, hour by hour, on a typical weekday morning, from the time you get up until lunch time?" This question outlines for your client exactly what you want to know. He can focus on the mornings and it is apparent that you will proceed to other times in his weekly schedule.

Consider another example. You are completing a health history on a client newly admitted to your surgical unit. Because he will be having an anaesthetic you need information about his past health status, past illnesses, and familial health history. Your unit employs a concise preoperative assessment tool to efficiently glean this extensive material from clients. Having secured your client's permission, after explaining the purpose of your line of questioning, you proceed with:

> "As you know, this is a lot of material to cover. To streamline things I'm going to use this guideline our unit has developed. It's a good checklist to ensure that we cover everything. Please ask me if there's anything I say which isn't clear to you. Beginning with your childhood, did you ever have diphtheria? . . . or whooping cough? . . . or rheumatic fever?"

Explaining your format helps your client accept what might otherwise seem like a barrage of unrelated questions.

Any material which a client provides is of a personal nature, and some areas are more sensitive than others. For some clients, talking about sexual activity or birth control practices may be difficult. For others, talking about personal hygiene or alcohol consumption may be embarrassing. Some clients do not feel comfortable revealing their self-care practices, and others hesitate to reveal family issues or job-related information. As a nurse you cannot know in advance which topics might be difficult for any particular client, and so you must keep in mind that any information a client reveals about himself, his significant others, or his health care practices might be sensitive for him.

There are some steps you can take as a nurse to put your client at ease and make him feel more comfortable in revealing this information. One thing you can do is reassure him about the confidentiality of your relationship. This step should be taken right at the beginning of an interview or at the earliest point in the client's admission to your service. If you wait until later it can be awkward, and by that point you may have lost opportunities for uncovering important information.

Confidentiality has a wide range of meanings and you must be honest and clear with your client so that he understands exactly what the parameters are. Does it mean that you will not repeat what he said to anybody? Does it mean that you will verbally pass the information to a trustworthy colleague but not write it in his chart? Does it mean that you will convey your client's information to team colleagues at his client-care conference? Or does it mean that the confidential information will be written in your client's chart for other team members to read and be aware of? Exactly what your client may reveal will likely be determined by what you, his nurse, intend to do with the information he contemplates telling you.

It is essential that you and your client have an identical understanding of the meaning of confidentiality. Sundeen, Stuart, Rankin, and Cohen (1989) remind us that a client may feel betrayed if he was under the impression that the client-nurse relationship was confidential, and then discovered that you have revealed what he considers personal information to another health team member or written it in his chart (p. 187).

Another thing you can do to increase your client's comfort is to treat all areas you discuss with equal respect and a professional approach.

Making the effort to ensure that your client has privacy, and the time to respond unhurriedly, will facilitate his replying openly and fully. Being equally relaxed and straightforward, whether discussing sexual matters, family health history, bowel habits, or exercise patterns, will contribute to putting your client at ease. If you flush, wriggle in your chair, lose eye contact, or lower your voice, your client will quickly get the message that this topic is a sensitive one for you and any embarrassment for your client will be escalated. To improve your ability to be at ease when asking questions in a variety of areas you will find rehearsal with friends or colleagues helpful.

The Who of Asking Questions

Who to ask is another important consideration. When your client is able to speak for himself he is the best person to approach. There may be occasions when you need information about your client that he might not be able to provide. There are times when the observations of significant others shed light on your client, and this perspective is valuable to have. For example, if your client has been on a mood elevating medication, you may wish to have his wife's observations of any changes in addition to your client's sense of the effectiveness of the drug. Or one of your clients with multiple sclerosis may have had a weekend pass at home and you may wish to get family members' perspectives of his abilities to manage at home, in addition to your client's report. Whenever you consult your client's family members or friends about the client himself, it is most courteous and respectful if you do so with the knowledge, and where possible in the presence, of your client. In some agencies it is the policy to secure written consent from clients before questioning significant others and previous or concurrent health care providers. To respect client confidentiality and protect the legality of your actions, it is important that you make yourself aware of such policies.

There are times when clients cannot answer questions. For example, unconscious, aphasic, or psychotic clients, are not able to provide information which might be important in their recovery. As the nurse you will have to do some detective work in such cases to discover the essential people from whom to get this information.

The When and Where of Asking Questions

When and *where* to carry out your questioning is your next consideration. The physical setup of many hospitals and clinics makes it difficult to secure a completely private place to interview your client. However, you should make every effort to arrange for a time and place where you will not be interrupted by phone calls, noise, other clients, agency activity, or visitors. Arranging such a time and place may require your utmost patience since both you and your client have days filled with scheduled and unscheduled activities. It does not usually pay to rush an interview or talk about sensitive issues in an open ward area. Clients have every right to privacy and a sense of unhurried attention from you—the nurse.

Keeping in mind these six aspects of question asking will improve your effectiveness by making you a systematic and sensitive interviewer.

Common Tactical Errors in Asking Questions and What to Do About Them

The broad strategies outlined in the preceding section will be valuable in guiding your inquiries in a general way. When it comes to the nitty gritty of speaking you will find the following suggestions about avoiding or overcoming poor techniques a helpful reference.

The Long-Winded Buildup

In efforts to explain the purpose of our line of questioning to our clients and colleagues we sometimes go overboard. When we provide a rambling, detailed introduction we run the risk of confusing or boring the other person. When providing an explanation of the rationale for our questions the KISS principle is best: Keep It Short and Simple!

Wrong way:
> **Long-winded You:** "Mr. Haddon, I'd like to ask you some questions about your allergies so that we can eventually work out a lifestyle plan that will allow you to avoid or minimize the stressful reactions you suffer from the various things that irritate you. As you know, repeated allergic reactions can be stressful for the body when it has to constantly fight to return bodily functions to normal. When you are in an allergic reactive state your body is in the alarm phase and is working overtime trying to return things to normal. When you feel miserable because of the allergies, you also feel tense and anxious, and maybe even at times frightened that your allergic reactions will get out of control. It's only when we have all the information that we can help you plan the best ways to avoid your irritants. Shall we begin?"

A long-winded buildup like the one above can put off the client who understands the purpose and wants to get down to business of the task. Openers that are redundant, wordy, and too detailed are diversions that detract from the task.

Right way:
> **Focused You:** "Mr. Haddon, I'd like to ask you some questions about your allergies so we can eventually work out a lifestyle plan that will allow you to avoid or minimize your stressful reactions to the various things that irritate you. Your chart indicates you have both food and environmental allergies. To begin, could you itemize your known food allergies?"

This concise opening spells out your purpose and how and why you will be asking Mr. Haddon your particular questions. The clarity and brevity of this statement neither bores, frightens, puts down, nor confuses the client.

The Thunder Stealer

Our questions sometimes take the form of asking clients their opinions about the cause of their health problems, their preferences for effective treatment, or what degree of cure or alleviation of the problem they think should be sought. It is respectful to give our clients the opportunity to offer their ideas, especially when we have requested their perspective. In our enthusiasm we sometimes jump in with our views and opinions before giving our clients a chance to speak. This zealousness on our part can be intimidating for clients and prevent them from expressing their real views. Jumping in and upstaging clients can anger some of them. Many clients feel hurt that we would barge ahead, expounding our beliefs, without having the courtesy to hear their point of view about their health care situation.

Wrong way:
  Upstaging You: "Well, Miss Ricco, together we have agreed upon six possible steps you could take to minimize your facial blemishes. I am interested in knowing what you think of each of these options. I know which I would recommend. Definitely get rid of any oil-based skin care products you have and start using oil-free products. Don't you agree that this change would prevent your pores from clogging up? And you'd likely agree you should buy the special soap Dr. Best recommended, wouldn't you? I think you should go for our second option too. . . ."

Miss Ricco soon would have the message that you are not in any way interested in her views. Usurping every chance for your client to speak is frustrating and demeaning. Stealing our clients' thunder gives them the message that we think what we have to say is more important and that they should depend on us for direction. This picture is out of line with today's well-informed health consumer and a health care system which is striving to get people to take charge of their health care responsibilities.

Right way:
  Considerate You: "Well, Miss Ricco, together we have agreed upon six possible steps you could take to minimize your facial blemishes. I am interested in knowing what you think of each of the options we've talked about."

The nurse who is genuinely interested in discovering what Miss Ricco really thinks about the treatment options would stop here and let her proceed. Clients have preferences that motivate them to choose certain health behaviors; and barriers like cost and time, which mitigate against other treatment choices. Clients have a responsibility for their health care, and as nurses we can encourage their participation by giving them a chance to speak and listening to them when they answer our questions.

The Multiple Choice Mixup

As interviewers we sometimes get carried away and assault our clients with a barrage of questions. After receiving a string of questions our clients become confused and do not know what information we are looking for or where to begin answering.

Wrong way:

> **Bombarding You:** "Mrs. Parker, there are some things we need to know to help you through your labor, delivery, and postpartum stay with us. Have you discussed what kind of delivery you prefer? Have you and your husband met with your physician and gone over all the options? What I mean is, have you decided on whether you will receive analgesics and/or any type of anaesthetic during labor? Do you know the various types: general, spinal, perineal block? And next we need to know your plans for breast feeding. Have you decided on that yet?"

Whew! Mrs. Parker's head would be spinning as she tried to keep pace with this bombardment. Just as she would have formulated a response to one question, you were off to the next, probably making her feel distracted, confused, and irritated.

Right way:

> **Clear You:** "Mrs. Parker, there are some things we need to know to help you through your labor, delivery, and postpartum stay with us. I'd like to review your plans for pain management during labor and for feeding your baby. Are you comfortable enough to go over these two areas now?" You pause to check out her readiness. "First, are you planning to use any type of pain controlling agent during your labor and delivery?"

Mrs. Parker has been given one question to answer in this example. She knows there are more questions forthcoming, but she knows exactly what you are seeking when a single clearly worded question is posed.

Incomprehensible Cryptic Codes

As nurses, we get accustomed to medical terminology and develop our own shorthand to abbreviate long, unwieldy medical terms. Using this jargon among professionals is fine, but using it with clients only adds to their confusion. Clients have a right to receive questions which are worded clearly in language they can understand.

Wrong way:
    Cryptic You: "I've come with your digoxin, Mr. Winters. Before I give it I need to check out your apical and radial pulses and estimate your oedema. Have you had any angina, palpitations, or SOBOE this morning? We want to prevent chemotoxicity."

Mr. Winters would almost need a medical dictionary to decipher your questions! Using medical jargon might make him feel stupid or uncomfortable. And just as bad, you might receive incorrect information from clients who give answers to questions they do not understand because they are embarrassed or confused.

Right way:
    Clear You: "Mr. Winters, I've come with your heart medication—digoxin. Before I give it I need to check your heart rate over your heart with my stethoscope and at your wrist. Have you had any chest pain this morning?" After pausing for an answer, you ask: "Have you noticed any fluttering or fast beating of your heart this morning?" After receiving his answer you ask: "Have you had any shortness of breath at any time this morning?"

Asking questions in plain English increases the probability that your client will understand what you are asking and, in turn, give an appropriate response.

The Offensive Misuse of "Why"

As nurses we do a lot of detective work trying to determine why a client got sick, why he is upset, why he does not follow his treatment regimen, and so on. These "whys" are all legitimate questions, but when it comes to asking it is usually best to refrain from using "why" too frequently with clients because it tends to make them feel threatened. To avoid such an aggressive tactic it is better to rephrase the question so it is softer and more receivable.

Wrong way:
    Threatening You: A client is slamming his pillow against his bed frame. "Why are you doing that, Mr. Kent?"

A teenager is using his crutches incorrectly. "Why aren't you weight bearing more?"

A diabetic woman is having three toes on her left foot amputated: "Why don't you take better care of your feet?"

An elderly widower is sad: "Why are you letting life slip by you instead of getting back into things?"

Each of these "why" questions is aggressive, blunt, and almost attacking. Each one might force the client to be defensive, curt, or in some way protective. Withdrawal or hostility in the client diminishes the chances for an open and honest response.

Right way:
   Gentle You: To the client who is slamming his pillow against his bed frame: "What is making you upset, Mr. Kent?"

To the teenager who is using his crutches incorrectly: "What is it that prevents you from weight bearing more?"

To the diabetic woman who is having three toes on her left foot amputated: "What factors make it difficult for you to take better care of your feet?"

To the elderly widower who is sad: "What are some of the things that keep you sad and prevent you from getting involved in things you used to enjoy?"

Each of these questions goes after the same information as the questions above, but they are less aggressively phrased. Because these questions do not put the client on the spot they invite the client to respond.

Open and Closed Questions

Closed questions are focused and posed to elicit a specific and brief response from a client. Open questions invite the respondent to elaborate in whatever direction he chooses. A skilled nurse interviewer knows when to use each type of question.

Wrong way:
   Closed You: A client has just returned from the x-ray department where he underwent a barium enema, a procedure he was dreading. You ask: "Did your barium enema procedure go okay?"

This question only requires a "yes" or "no" and does not invite your client to elaborate further about his experience.

In an initial health history you ask your client: "Do you eat a well-balanced diet?"

The "yes" or "no" response to this type of question would tell you little about his nutritional intake.

Your 63-year-old client is going to be transferred to an extended care facility. You ask: "Are you looking forward to going to Haven's Point?"

This approach gives your client little choice about how to answer.

Right way:
> **Interested You:** A client has just returned from the x-ray department where he underwent a barium enema, a procedure he was dreading. You ask: "How did your barium enema procedure go for you?"

> In an initial health history you ask your client: "What does an average day's food intake for you look like?"

> Your 63-year-old client is going to a long-term care facility. You ask: "How do you feel about leaving here and going to live at Haven's Point?"

These three examples are open-ended questions that would require your client's elaboration. The information obtained by these questions would give you fuller comprehension of your client's perspective.

In nursing practice, we err more frequently on the side of posing closed questions where open-ended ones would provide more useful information. However, we are sometimes too general when we should be more focused in our question asking. Therefore it is worthwhile to examine your question-asking practices to see if there are times when you might make your questions more focused.

The Mystery Interview

When we ask questions of our clients they respond with the belief that as skilled clinicians we are sorting, sifting, and analyzing their data in order to contribute to their nursing care plan. It makes the client feel connected and respected when we give him feedback on our problem-solving process.

Wrong way:
> **Abrupt You:** You have been doing an initial health assessment with a client admitted for extreme and rapid weight loss. The time allotted for the interview is over and you say to your client: "I've got to go now. I'll see you later and we can continue our interview then."

Clients feel left out when we end an interview without giving them any indication of our assessment.

Right way:

> **Clear You:** If it is necessary to end an interview before you can complete your assessment you can say something like: "We've talked about your weight loss problem a fair amount today. In order to know all the factors which might be contributing to your weight loss I need to get some more information from you at our next interview. Until we meet again this afternoon, could you be thinking about anything you can recall, anything unusual that happened to you at the time you first started losing weight?"

Even though this closing remark does not provide your client with a definite summary, it keeps him up-to-date with your clinical assessment of his problem. Informing our clients of what is happening, including our plans and what they can expect next, provides helpful transitions so that they can map progress, feel included, and minimize worrying about erroneous assumptions.

If you employ the suggestions in this chapter your question asking will be assertive and responsible. You will respect your right to secure client information you need to complete the nursing process, yet maintain the dignity of your client.

PRACTICING ASKING QUESTIONS

Exercise 1. For this exercise you get to watch TV or listen to the radio! Over the next week or so observe the skills of TV and radio interviewers. Make note of what interviewers do well and where you think they could improve.
- Are their introductions long-winded or focused?
- Do they give interviewees a chance to express their opinions before jumping in with their views?
- Are their questions succinct and clear or are they a barrage of seemingly unrelated topics?
- Do they phrase their questions in clear English or do they use technical jargon which might confuse the interviewee?
- Are "why" questions used aggressively or is the interviewer nonthreatening?
- Are open-ended questions used appropriately?

At the end of the week compare what you have learned about effective ways to ask questions with your colleagues.

Exercise 2. For this exercise work in threes. One person will be the interviewer, one the interviewee, and one the observer. The interviewee will choose to be interviewed about anything she likes; for example, her interest in chess, windsurfing or birdwatching, the latest paper she is writing for one of her courses, or a new product she is planning to buy. The interviewee must let her interviewer know what her topic is before the interview begins.

For 8 minutes the interviewer will ask questions about the topic her interviewee has chosen. During the exchange the observer will make note of how effectively the interviewer asks questions. At the end of 8 minutes she will have feedback on the strengths of the interviewer and where the interviewer could improve.

The questions in Exercise 1 can be used as guidelines for giving feedback. Tape recording this exercise will give you a chance to review your work more thoroughly.

The group of three should change roles so that each gets the chance to try all roles.

What has this exercise taught you about the skill of asking questions?

Exercise 3. Client-nurse situations are not the only occasions where we ask questions. We can learn a lot about our question-asking skill level from how we interact with friends, family, and colleagues at work. Over the next week or so, make notes on the effectiveness of your question asking. What do you like about your approach to asking questions of your friends and family and peers? What are some changes you could make to improve your competence?

Observe how others ask questions of you and notice what is effective and what is unclear or uncomfortable.

Exercise 4. As you go into your clinical units take some extra time to assess your skill level in asking questions of your clients. Prepare for your interviews by paying attention to the *why, what, how, who, when,* and *where* of asking questions. As soon as possible after an interview with a client stop and reflect on how effective you were. Review the common mistakes and make note of where you excelled and where you need to improve.

If possible, tape record this interview with one of your clients and critique your question-asking ability afterward. Having the verbatim account of your question asking is the most ideal learning situation. You must have your client's total agreement to record an interview, including his permission about who can listen to the tape. Some clients prefer to review a tape-recorded interview before releasing it to nurses. Some agencies require nurses to obtain written consent before tape recording an interview with a client. It is important to erase the tape after you have critiqued your interviewing skills and to follow through by informing your client that you have done so.

Exercise 5. As a nurse working on an orthopedic unit you are nursing a newly admitted, elderly female client, Mrs. Haley, diagnosed with Alzheimer's disease and a broken left hip. This evening her son and daughter-in-law and her frail elderly husband, with whom she lived before her recent admission, have come to the unit to visit your client. It is your responsibility to investigate how your client fell and broke her hip.

Working on your own, choose and write down what your first three questions would be. Be able to defend
- **Why** you chose to ask those questions
- **What** exactly you would ask
- **How** you would ask it
- **Who** you would ask
- **When** you would pose your questions
- **Where** you would ask your three questions.

When you have finished writing down your three questions on your own compare the similarities and differences in your approaches as a whole class. This exercise focuses on your question-asking and problem-solving skills. What has this exercise taught you about the relationship between question-asking and problem-solving?

REFERENCES:

Sundeen, S.J., Stuart, G.W., Rankin, E.A., & Cohen, S.A. (1989). *Nurse-client interaction: Implementing the nursing process.* St. Louis: Mosby–Year Book.

SUGGESTIONS FOR FURTHER READING

ARTICLES

Copp, L.A. (1990). The spectrum of suffering. *American Journal of Nursing,* 90(8), 35-39.
  This humbling article reminds nurses about one question to ask our clients who have pain: what have they found helpful to ease their pain? Often this simple question is not asked and valuable information about client coping, as well as an opportunity to acknowledge client responsibility for successful problem solving is overlooked.
Harvey, K. (1990). The power of positive questioning. *Nursing Management,* 21(5), 94-96.
  This intriguing article proposes that nurses risk asking questions in ways that promote affirmative responses and agreement in certain situations.
High, D.M. (1989). Truth telling, confidentiality, and the dying patient: New dilemmas for the nurse. *Nursing Forum,* 24(1), 5-10.
  This excellent article challenges nurses to reevaluate their conceptualization of confidentiality in relation to the privilege of nursing terminally ill clients. Balancing clients' need to talk intimately is their right to privacy and respect. High poses this question for nurses: "What do you let your patients tell you?" The relevance of this query has implications for the art of question asking in nursing.
Riley, J. (1989). Telephone call-backs: Final patient care evaluation. *Nursing Management,* 20(9), 64-66.
  This article proposes a way for nurses to monitor clients' post-discharge welfare in this day of short-stay admissions to acute care facilities. One important step in implementing this program is to teach nurses what information to secure from recently discharged clients and how to ask questions in an unbiased way.

BOOKS

Benjamin, A. (1974). *The helping interview* (2nd ed.). Boston, Mass.: Houghton Mifflin Company.
  Benjamin covers the uses and abuses of questions, types of questions, and timing of questions. His frequent examples illustrate effective and ineffective questioning.
Bradley, J.C., & Edinberg, M.A. (1982). *Communication in the nursing context.* New York: Appleton-Century-Crofts.
  In chapter 5, the authors illustrate effective information gathering techniques and demonstrate how to use these skills effectively in the interview situation. How to overcome common pitfalls in interviewing is useful reading for students of interpersonal communication.
Evans, D.R., Hearn, M.T., Uhlemann, M.R., & Ivey, A.E. (1979). *Essential interviewing: A pro-*

grammed approach to effective communication. Monterey, Calif.: Brooks/Cole Publishing Company.

Chapter 3 guides readers through correct and incorrect methods of inquiry. The points to remember about effective inquiry at the end of the chapter are a handy reference.

Fayram, E.S. (1986). Implementation. In J.W. Griffith-Kenney, & P.J. Christensen (Eds.), Nursing process: Application of theories, frameworks, and models, (pp. 212-218). St. Louis: Mosby–Year Book.

This chapter outlines the pertinent questions for nurses to consider when assessing the validity and viability of a client's nursing care plan.

Ivey, A.E. (1983). *Intentional interviewing and counseling*. Monterey, Calif. Brooks/Cole Publishing Company.

Chapter 3, Questions: Opening Communication, discusses in which situations the various types of questions work best. The examples and exercises help the reader to practice effective question asking.

Sierra-Franco, M.H. (1978). *Therapeutic communication in nursing*. New York: McGraw-Hill Book Company.

The examples of dialogue illustrate how to be nondirective and highly directive in an interview. The advantages of both approaches are explained.

Stewart, C.J., & Cash, W.B. (1982). *Interviewing: Principles and practices* (3rd ed.). Dubuque, Iowa: Wm. C. Brown Company, Publishers.

The chapter on questions and their uses is for the advanced student. Extensive detail is provided to help interviewers master different types of questions, phrasing, and sequencing of questions.

CHAPTER 11

Expressing Opinions

"People are usually more firmly convinced that their opinions are precious than that they are true."

George Santayana

OBJECTIVES

This chapter exposes you to some opinions about expressing opinions! You will have the opportunity to explore your views on expressing opinions and in so doing be prepared for those occasions when your opinions are solicited by clients or colleagues. You can practice expressing opinions in a respectful way by doing the exercises at the end of this chapter.

THE DIFFERENCE BETWEEN GIVING ADVICE AND EXPRESSING OPINIONS

Expressing opinions as a nurse refers to the act of disclosing what you think or feel about health care situations affecting your clients or colleagues. Expressing opinions is assertively interactional; that is, your opinions are offered as additional information for your client's (or colleague's) problem-solving and decision-making process. In contrast, giving advice is a unilateral process of solving problems or making decisions for others (Hames & Joseph, 1986). Offering advice prevents clients from becoming independent and gives colleagues the idea that you might think they are incapable of self-direction (Hames & Joseph, 1986, p. 132).

Expressing opinions can be part of providing clients with a fuller picture to make choices about their health and treatment plans. Clients have a moral right to information and "if they exercise that right by asking questions or seeking information, there is a duty to provide that information" (Freel, 1990, p. 572). Expressing opinions is not telling clients (or colleagues) what to do, but giving them the benefit of your point of view.

It includes clients in their health decision making and avoids both the dependency of clients relying on the nurse and the anger and blame when the nurse's advice is rejected at some point.

WHEN TO EXPRESS YOUR OPINIONS AS A NURSE

There are three situations when clients and colleagues seek your nursing counsel. These occasions are when they are at a decision point about:

Whether to Provide or Withhold Information:

For example, clients may wonder whether they should expose information about their condition to a physician or another family member. Colleagues may be in a quandary about whether to reveal information to a client and/or his family, and to colleagues or supervisors. A fellow student may be undecided about whether to confide in her nursing instructor about a personal problem.

Whether to Comply with a Treatment Plan or Resist It:

Some clients may have conflicting doubts and hopes about their health problem and might be unsettled about whether to follow a treatment plan or attempt to survive without it. For example, fellow nurses may have mixed feelings about adhering to a new unit policy or nursing procedure. A student colleague may be in a dilemma about whether to comply with a residence curfew.

Which Strategies to Implement in Order to Get the Desired Outcomes:

For instance, clients who know what expected health status they are aiming for may not be able to decide which treatment plan to follow. Colleagues at work may know exactly what outcomes they want but need some help in deciding what actions they can take that will most likely ensure that they reach their goal. A classmate may be lost about what approach to take to ensure that she gets a high grade on her next assignment.

As a nurse, your views may be sought by clients or colleagues at any one of these decision points. Your opinions provide them with information which can be incorporated into their decision making.

Although they are referring to the psychotherapeutic helping relationship, Jensen, Josephson & Frey (1989) have some pointers about sharing information with clients that would apply to the client-nurse helping relationship. Nurses could share their opinions about any of the above three situations when there is uncertainty about outcome, both negative and positive effects of the options, or when one course is not necessarily superior to the other (Jensen, Josephson & Frey, 1989, p. 379). Providing your opinions as a nurse can create a situation for discussing any one of the above decision points, and provide an opportunity to truly collaborate about your client's health care. Both of these mutual acts will strengthen your relationship.

Your Feelings about Expressing Opinions

Before proceeding any further, take a pencil and jot down your responses to these questions.

1. How do you feel when someone expresses his opinion to you without your seeking it?

2. How do you feel when someone refrains from giving you his opinion when you have sought his counsel?

After you have expressed your feelings about these questions, then compare your reactions with those of colleagues in your class.

Many of us feel differently about opinions we have sought versus viewpoints we did not seek. In our culture, where we place a high value on liberty and the freedom to act as we choose within the limits of the law, it is likely that many of us feel some resentment when another person takes it upon himself to influence us without our consent. Some of us are more willing to consider opinions that we have agreed to receive. This knowledge of human nature suggests a principle for expressing opinions: whenever possible secure the receiver's consent before lending your persuasion. Your opinions that fall on resistant ears are not likely to be considered by an unwilling receiver.

Many of you will have indicated that you expect to be given opinions from someone whose counsel you have sought and that you feel cheated when denied. When we ask lawyers, physicians, and teachers for their professional opinions, we expect them to provide us with some guidance. And so it is with our clients and colleagues who seek our points of view in our professional capacity as nurses.

Here are two more questions about expressing opinions.

3. How do you feel when a client (friend, family member, or work colleague) who has asked for your opinion does not act on the views you expressed?

4. How do you feel when a client (friend, family member, or work colleague) incorporates your opinions into his actions?

You may respond that you have no strong feelings about whether another acts on your opinions. Some may experience pride or relief that another acts on their counsel, and hurt or disappointment when they do not. The strength of your feelings may be related to how much you derive a sense of power or control over another person's actions. To what extent does your self-esteem as a nurse depend on a client or colleague doing things your way versus knowing you offered him your wisest counsel so that he had adequate information on which to base his decision?

The degree to which we allow others the freedom to make their own decisions is revealed in the extent to which we care more for their autonomy and well-being than whether our opinions are revered. As nurses, we must keep in mind what expectations regarding seeking opinions our clients come with and, more importantly, what agendas we carry around about offering others our viewpoint.

HOW TO EXPRESS YOUR OPINIONS IN AN ASSERTIVE WAY

As a nurse you will be called upon in your professional life to express health care opinions by your clients and colleagues, and in your personal life by friends, family, and even perfect strangers! Because you are an educated, professional nurse, there will be innumerable times when you will be tempted to express opinions to clients and friends or family about their health care. You will feel more confident about handling these situations if you have worked out some principles to stand by for expressing opinions. Here are some guidelines:

Get the Consent of Your Receiver Before Expressing Your Opinions

To avoid generating feelings of hostility or resentment in your clients or colleagues, ask if they are interested in hearing your viewpoint. Here are several phrases you can use to complete this courteous step that can flow naturally into your conversation:

"A former client told me a good way to get around a situation like yours. Would you like to hear that suggestion?"

"I've just read an article that had some excellent ideas on how to solve your problem. Do you want to hear what it had to say?"

"Last year I had the same difficulties you are now having. By trial and error I learned some great ways to get rid of the problem. Would you be interested in hearing how I worked things out?"

"I've seen many people with a similar problem to yours. I have some recommendations for you that have come from those experiences. Would you like to hear them?"

"I've thought about this issue for a long time and I have some opinions I'd like to express to the team if you'd like to hear them."

Clients or colleagues from whom you are requesting permission to proceed will let you know whether they want to hear your ideas. Those who are verbal and direct will reply with a definite "yes" or "no." Those who are less direct will send you nonverbal signals that will tell you whether to proceed or refrain from sharing your conclusions. If they look away, change the subject, or argue that their situation is unique, they are warning you to back off and keep your opinions to yourself. If they give interested gestures, it is your clue to continue.

Make Allowances for the Uniqueness of Your Client or Colleague

We give opinions based on the knowledge that our ideas have worked in similar situations with like people and circumstances. However, it is impossible for us to know all the circumstances and personal factors that would facilitate our ideas working with a particular person in his specific situation. Consequently, we should avoid being dogmatic when expressing our opinions. We should be somewhat tentative about offering our persuasions to show our consideration of the other's special circumstances.

Avoiding strong phrases like: "I really think you should," "You really ought to," or "It should be clear to you that this is the direction to take . . . ," will make your views more receivable so that they can be incorporated in your client's or colleague's problem-solving.

When offering your opinions you can include one of the following phrases which will give others a fair chance to accept or reject your ideas:

". . . Do you think this idea will help in your situation?"
". . . What do you think about these recommendations?"
". . . How do you think this suggestion will fit your lifestyle?"
". . . How does my slant on your situation strike you?"
". . . Can you adapt any of these ideas to your situation?"

Include the Rationale for Your Viewpoint

Your clients and colleagues expect you to have opinions about health care and work- or school-related issues. Giving your rationale is a responsible way to defend your position. It ensures that sufficient data is available for clients and colleagues to make the final decision.

Here are some phrases that you might use to include your rationale with your opinions to clients:

"In my view, options 2 and 4 would be the most likely to get the results you are looking for. Which options do you favor?"

"If you have the money, I think going to the clinic in Healthtown is the best resource for what you're after. If finances are strained you might wish to consider one of the self-help groups here in town. What do you think?"

"If I were feeling as desperate as you seem to be, I think I would go for the quick-start option rather than the slower one. After some respite in your symptoms you could shift over to the regular stream. How does that plan sound to you?"

"I hesitate to suggest plan A because all your social supports and family are out of town. Plan B would ensure that you get some regular supervision while you are learning the technique. What are your preferences?"

"In my clinical experience, using the prepared formula has proven to be more successful than the one clients have to mix from scratch. That's my opinion. Does that help you make a decision?"

"I really don't know which way would be better for you. In my experience there have been clients that have been happy with both treatment choices. The final choice gets down to personal preference since both options are solid in every respect. So my advice is 'choose the one you like!' "

In all these examples the nurse has offered a reason to defend her preferences and turned the final decision back to her client. If we want clients to take charge of their own health care, we can offer them our professional opinions yet make it clear that the final responsibility is theirs.

With your colleagues on the health care team you might include your rationale in the following ways:

"Because Mrs. Jones is beginning to improve I think it would be a mistake for us to transfer her just now. Maybe Mrs. Hanes could be moved first so that Mrs. Jones would have an extra week of physical therapy? What do you think?"

"Our Kardex system is outdated. I think we should adopt the system written about in the latest issue of the *American Journal of Nursing*. It describes how to keep all the pertinent information updated and right at your finger tips. I'll bring the article in so that you can see how useful it might be for us."

"I think we should ask the instructor to go over the section on neuroanatomy one more time before the exam. It's worth 40% and she only spent one lecture period on it. What do you think?"

"I think we should go back to the old system of having the night nurse doing the preps for the clients going to surgery at 0730. Leaving it until days is too rushed, don't you think?"

"We are run off our feet over meal times and inundated with volunteers when the unit is crowded during visiting hours. I think it would be better to arrange to have the volunteers come at meal times to help us with feeding, don't you?"

"I think we should have a first-year student representative on the faculty curriculum committee in addition to the second-year rep. We need a student there to get our perspective across to the faculty, don't you think?"

"Since you ask, Dr. Kenson, I have been Mr. Jones' nurse for the last week and a half, and I feel strongly that he could be discharged sooner than you are recommending. His condition is stabilized and the home care nurses could see him daily for his injection and dressing change. He is very anxious to get back to his own surroundings and begin to take up his life again, especially to start a bit of writing on his home computer. What do you think?"

"Thanks for the chance to give my input to the safety committee. In the 3 months I've been here there has not been a fire drill, and I notice that the two exit lights on our unit aren't lit. I think we could all benefit from regular fire drills and scheduled inspection of the equipment. Would you agree?"

These examples demonstrate how to give your opinions assertively and still consider your colleagues' viewpoint. Giving your opinions does not mean coercing your colleagues to adopt your ideas. Providing a rationale for your point of view and inviting others' opinions makes the decision-making a collaborative process.

It is possible that the decision-making climate set by nurse managers influences the style of decision-making used by staff nurses with their clients. In a study of nurse problem solving, Schmieding (1990) discovered that the majority of head nurse actions did not involve the staff nurses in any way. Nurses who are committed to a mutual problem-solving approach with clients would likely want the same kind of respect and collegiality as in a participative management climate. Nurses can influence how decisions are made by keeping alert and assertively making and taking opportunities to express their opinions as another source of information for workplace decision-making process. Bushy & Smith (1990) encourage nurses to become politically proactive and lobby for changes we would like in the health care system. Developing political savvy is an extension of being assertive and expressing our opinions in relationships with clients and colleagues in the workplace.

Expressing your opinions is assertive and responsible. It protects your right to have your point of view included in the decision making and respects others' rights to know what you are thinking. By including your views you are ensuring that another piece of information is available to the decision makers.

PRACTICING EXPRESSING OPINIONS

Exercise 1. For this exercise work in threes. One of you will roleplay a client with a problem about which she is seeking the nurse's opinion. Another will roleplay the nurse in this interaction. The third will be the observer and give feedback.

For 4 minutes the "client" will make clear her request for the nurse's opinions and the nurse will attempt to express her views assertively. Debrief with the following questions:

As the observer:
1. Did the nurse gain the client's permission to express her opinions?
2. Did the nurse take into account the client's unique circumstances when she expressed her opinions?
3. Did the nurse provide a rationale to defend her opinions?
4. Overall, how assertive was the nurse in expressing her opinions to her client?

As the client:
1. How did you react to the nurse's offering of her opinions?
2. What did you like about the nurse's approach to sharing her views?
3. What suggestions for improvement would you make?

As the nurse:

1. What is your assessment of your ability to assertively express your opinions from your participation in this exercise?
2. What did you like about how you expressed your opinions?
3. What suggestions for improvement would you make?

Switch roles so that each of you has a chance to be client, nurse, and observer.

Exercise 2. Repeat exercise 1 but this time one of you will roleplay a colleague (nurse, physical therapist, physician, clergy) instead of a client who wants the nurse's opinions on an issue. Proceed as outlined in Exercise 1.

After completing both exercises discuss your feelings about expressing your opinions to colleagues and clients. What similarities and differences are there for you? What accounts for any differences you notice?

Exercise 3. Over the next few days note the way others express their opinions to you. Check out if they ask your permission, consider your particular situation, how tentative they are, and whether they provide a rationale. Your reactions to receiving advice from a variety of people will tell you a lot about how to effectively express your opinions.

As a class compare and contrast your observations and conclusions about expressing opinions.

Exercise 4. Over the next few days observe how you express your opinions to others in your day-to-day encounters. Assess the assertiveness of your approach. Congratulate yourself on your effectiveness and make note of where you need to improve.

REFERENCES

Bushy, A., & Smith, T.O. (1990). Lobbying: The hows and wherefores. *Nursing Management, 21*(4), 39-45.

Freel, M.I (1990). Truth telling. In J.C. McCloskey & H.K. Grace (Eds.), *Current issues in nursing* (pp. 567-575). St. Louis: Mosby–Year Book.

Hames, C.C., & Joseph, D.H. (1986). *Basic concepts of helping: A holistic approach* (2nd ed.). Norwalk, Conn.: Appleton-Century-Crofts.

Jensen, P.S., Josephson, A.M., & Frey, J. (1989). Informed consent as a framework for treatment: Ethical and therapeutic considerations. *American Journal of Psychotherapy, XLIII*(3), 378-386.

Schmieding, N.J. (1990). Do head nurses include staff nurses in problem-solving? *Nursing Management, 21*(3), 58-60.

SUGGESTION FOR FURTHER READING

American Nurses Association (1990). Maximize involvement in workplace decision making. In American Nurses Association, *Survival skills in the workplace: What every nurse should know* (pp. 27-34). Kansas City, Miss.: The Association.

This chapter expands nurses' awareness of the larger organizational structure in the workplace and provides practical suggestions for strengthening their professional influence.

CHAPTER 12

Confrontation

*"Nothing so needs reforming
as other people's habits."*

Mark Twain

OBJECTIVES

By the end of this chapter you will have a clear understanding of confrontation, including how confrontation can benefit you and your clients and colleagues. Your increased understanding of its benefits will make you feel more confident about using confrontation with clients and colleagues. The exercises at the end of the chapter will provide you an opportunity to improve your ability to confront others.

DIFFERENT KINDS OF CONFRONTATION

Confrontation is an interpersonal process used by nurses to facilitate the modification and extension of others' self-image (Ackerhalt, 1987, p. 269). One type of confrontation is a nurse's deliberate invitation for clients and colleagues to examine incongruities or distortions between feelings, beliefs, attitudes, and behavior (Acherhalt, 1987; Egan, 1977; Stuart & Sundeen, 1991). This type of confrontation, designed to make others aware of incongruencies, can be offered by nurses when, for example, clients or colleagues are saying one thing and doing another, or obviously feeling one way and exhibiting the opposite emotions. Pointing out these discrepancies can be an invitation to expand their self-awareness. This dimension of confrontation is a gift of feedback and is covered in Chapter 15.

Here is an example of a confrontation to expand self-awareness:

John tells you he only smokes a few cigarettes a day. He has yellow stains on the fingers of his left hand, he smells of smoke, and wheezes upon inspiration. His wife says he smokes two packs a day.

Nurse: "John, I am concerned about conflicting information your smoking. The stains on your fingers, the smell of smoke on your clothes, and the sound of your breathing indicate that you smoke more than a few cigarettes a day."

Confrontation that involves an explicit request for a behavior change along with feedback is the focus of this chapter.

WHEN CONFRONTATION IS APPROPRIATE

There are two parts to confrontation: the first is making the other aware of the unproductiveness or destructiveness of his behavior, and the second is making a suggestion about how he could behave in a more productive or constructive way. There are two situations that warrant confronting clients or colleagues: when their behavior is unproductive or destructive to them, and when their behavior invades our rights or the rights of others. In confronting others we are attempting to get them to change in a way that protects their self-interests or is more considerate of others.

Some nurses shudder at the thought of confronting another person. It conjures up images of a heated argument. For most nurses, verbal attacking conflicts with their image of themselves as level-headed professionals.

To avoid looking aggressive, many times we refrain from saying anything about others' unproductive or destructive behavior. Later, we watch our client or colleague get into trouble because of his misdirected actions and then we feel guilty and regret that we did not take the opportunity to speak up. In other situations we fume because we do not quite know how to confront someone who has violated our rights or the rights of others and we stew in frustrated helplessness.

Neither of these two extremes—aggressiveness or unassertiveness— is acceptable to a nurse who wants to feel confident and act competently. There *is* a way to confront others that makes you feel like you are effectively doing something about troublesome behavior. It is possible to confront people in such a way that they are unlikely to be offended. Moreover, they may appreciate your perspective and opinions.

THE C.A.R.E. CONFRONTATION

When confronting your clients or colleagues it is important to do so in a caring way that shows concern for *both* your feelings and theirs. Outlined below is a caring way to confront others. (The format for this comprehensive confrontation is adapted from Bower & Bower, 1976.)

1. **Clarify** the behavior that is problematic. Be specific about the aspect of your client's or colleague's behavior that is self-destructive or destructive to others. The behavior to be changed should be the focus so that it is clear you are attaching no hurtful labels to your client or colleague.
2. **Articulate** why their behavior is a problem. Your articulation may in-

clude how their behavior is likely to hinder them or irritate others or how it makes you feel.

3. **Request** a change in your client's or colleague's behavior. Your suggestions should be offered tentatively and respectfully.

4. **Encourage** your client or colleague to change by emphasizing the positive consequences of changing or the negative implications if no change occurs.

EXAMPLES OF C.A.R.E. CONFRONTATIONS

The two situations outlined below demonstrate how you can confront someone in an assertive way without being aggressive.

Situation One

Your apartment mate is untidy. He leaves his clothes strewn around the bedroom you share, and the bathroom looks like a pharmacy. Frequently his notes and textbooks are laid out all over the apartment. Although he does a major tidy-up about every 2 weeks, he slides back into his messy ways and you have to put up with his disarray for the rest of the time. Not only is this mess esthetically displeasing to you, it makes you hesitate to invite friends over. You confront your roommate with:

Clarify
"John, you have your clothes spread out over the bedroom and all your notes and articles for your paper are strewn around the living room and on the kitchen table.

Articulate
I'm feeling annoyed that you are messing up the shared space in our apartment.

Request
I'd like you to keep your personal belongings in your area of our den.

Encourage
That way it'll be more spacious for both of us in the apartment and I'll feel free to invite friends over without worrying whether the place is a mess."

Presented with this respectful and assertive confrontation John will most likely comply and change his behavior. If such a confrontation does not result in the desired behavior change you have the option of indicating a negative consequence such as: "If you don't become neater, I will: hire a maid and charge you; or find another roommate; or move out."

Situation Two

Your colleague Janet is upset. She has been trying to lose weight for the past 6 months. You notice that she has a pattern of starting off successfully on Mondays, and by the end of the week she has gorged herself on her favorite fattening foods. Afterwards she fasts for several days and then overeats again. You think that these feasts and famines are not helpful for Janet and that it would be better if she distributed her calories more evenly.

After you have asked her permission to express your views, you confront Janet about her unproductive behavior in this way:

Clarify

"Janet, I notice you do well on your diet at the beginning of the week and then you have ups and downs of eating more than you want to or eating so little that you are starving.

Articulate

I think one reason you are unsuccessful in losing weight is because you don't have an adequate intake of calories on a consistent basis.

Request

Perhaps if you figured out a daily calorie intake that would make you feel satisfied and give you the energy you need, you may not binge as often.

Encourage

If you weren't so hungry you might stop overeating and be more likely to lose weight. If you can cut out the overeating you won't feel guilty and have to starve yourself. What do you think?"

The respectful and clear way this confrontation is delivered is likely to invite Janet to consider your idea and possibly implement it. An accusatory confrontation would only be ignored.

Confronting Clients or Colleagues

We can often see how another person's behavior is not safe or in keeping with their goals. Each of us has blind spots about how some of what we say or do is predisposing us to emotional or physical harm, or is incongruent with our professed values or attitudes. As a nurse colleague, or a nurse in a helping relationship with a client, we can offer an objective perspective on how others can change and act in a way that will serve their best interests. The following examples use C.A.R.E. confrontations to offer clients and colleagues ways to enhance their goals and avoid emotional or physical dangers.

Situations in Which Your Client's Behavior Is Self-Destructive or Unproductive

1. Mr. Jones, finance officer for a large corporation, is your 35-year-old client who suffered a massive myocardial infarction 3 weeks ago. Yesterday he was moved from ICU to the cardiac step-down unit. Today he ordered a telephone for his room so that he can conduct business from his bedside. You overhear him asking his secretary to come to the unit to take dictation from him.

Your nursing knowledge warns you that Mr. Jones is escalating his work schedule too quickly and that his workaholic habits may detract from his heart's healing or even put him at risk for another heart attack. You want him to slow down his re-entry into the business world and gradually build up his stamina. You strongly believe that a gradual increase in his workload will augment his chances for a successful recovery. You make this confrontation to Mr. Jones:

> "[C] Mr. Jones, I overheard you making arrangements for a room phone and for your secretary to come and take dictation. I can imagine that you must be eager to get back into the swing of things at work after being away for almost a month. [A] However, jumping in too quickly and taking on too much responsibility at this point in your recovery will likely make you tense and the stress on your heart may increase. [E] Your chances for a successful and complete recovery will be better if [R] you ease back into work more slowly. I suggest that you cancel the phone for your room and limit your work with your secretary to 15 minutes a day for this week and then gradually increase. [E] If you build up your stamina slowly you'll reduce the risk of another heart attack. What do you think?"

2. John, an 18-year-old client on a surgical ward, has just had a repair of a torn achilles tendon. After his lesson on crutch walking with the physical therapist you notice that John is weight bearing too heavily on his affected leg. In doing so he is increasing the chance of his sutures weakening and putting strain on his tendon, thus preventing healing. You confront John with:

> [C] When you put any weight on your injured leg [A] you are risking adding further injury to your tendon. If you weaken your tendon you may not recover full use of your leg. [R] I'd like you to practice using your crutches so that you only place weight on your good leg. [E] That way you'll ensure maximum healing of your injury. Will you try that please, John?"

Situations in Which Your Colleague's Behavior Is Self-Destructive or Unproductive

1. On the medical unit in your hospital you and Judy have been working together on the evening shift for the past 3 evenings. Judy has been complaining of a strained back which she has attributed to turning, positioning, and transfering the heavy clients on the unit. You have noticed that Judy takes little or no precautions to protect her back. After you have secured her permission to express your views, you decide to confront her about her negligence in the following way:

> "[A] Judy, it sounds like your back is bothering you quite a bit. [C] I've noticed that you don't use good body mechanics when you are

turning our heavy patients, and you tend to take the clients' full weight on your own without help from one of us or the Hoyer lift. [E] I think you could save your back from a lot of discomfort and injury if you [R] took the precautions of getting help and using protective devices. What do you think?"

Note the different order of this C.A.R.E. confrontation. The reordering makes it sound more natural in this case, yet it still contains the essential elements.

2. Your classmate, Toni, has not been achieving the grades to which she has been accustomed on her nursing exams. Toni is complaining about the severity of the exams and the tough marking of her instructors. You are aware that Toni has not been studying as much as she could since she began dating two fellows at the same time and going out practically every night. She asks you what she is going to do. You decide to confront her about her recent unproductive behavior:

> "[E] Toni, I know you are capable of achieving better marks even if the teachers are hard markers. [C] It's just since you've been going out so frequently on weeknights that [A] your grades have been less than what you used to receive. [R] Maybe if you invested the same time into your studies that you did at the beginning of the term [E] your marks would improve and reflect your capabilities. What do you think?"

In each of these four situations the client or colleague has been confronted about something he is doing or not doing that causes physical or emotional problems in his life. The confrontation points out the specific behavior that is problematic and proposes a clear alternative, which is checked out with the client or colleague.

Let us examine some situations in which you use the skill of confrontation to deal with behavior disrespectful of your rights or the rights of others.

Situations in Which Your Client's Behavior Is Bothersome to You or Others

1. Mr. Rickett is a 53-year-old cardiac patient who has been aggressive in the 3 days he has been on the unit. He has complained about the food, the room, and the other clients, and today he has been angry and abusive with you in the corridor. He complains that you are the slowest nurse he has ever encountered and that you don't know what you are doing. He has picked on your appearance, questioned your credentials, and repeatedly insulted your nursing care. His aggressiveness is embarrassing, time consuming, and unpleasant for you. You want his hostility against you to cease and you would like to discover the source of his aggression so that together you can recreate a better relationship. You confront him when you are in the privacy of his room:

"[R] Mr. Rickett, we need to talk about how we can get along better. [C] I have been receiving so much criticism from you today that I can only assume that you are very upset. [E] I would like to change things so that you are happy with your care and not being so critical of me [A] because it upsets me and makes me want to keep my distance from you. [E] I hope you are willing to work together with me on turning things around for the better?"

2. Miss Daly is a client who is 4 days postoperative on a surgical floor. She has been up to the showers for the past 2 days. Yesterday another client noticed that someone had left towels strewn all over the bathroom, spilled dusting powder, and left makeup pads and used tissues on the counter. Today you discover Miss Daly in the shower room creating a mess. She is about to leave without cleaning it up when you confront her:

"[C] When you leave your things all around the bathroom [A] it makes it inconvenient and unpleasant for other clients who also need to use the shower and bathroom facilities. [R] Please clear away your toiletries and put your garbage and towels in the bins. If you need any help to do this, please let me know or ask the cleaning staff. [E] Tidying up after you will make it nicer for everyone else, don't you agree?"

Situations in Which Your Colleague's Behavior Is Unpleasant for You or Others

1. You have been working the night shift for the past five nights. In the three previous mornings your nurse relief has been about 15 to 25 minutes late. You are not free to leave the unit until she arrives because there is only one nurse on duty. Her tardiness puts your own personal schedule off by making you late getting home to see your family before they head off to school and work. You decide to confront her:

"[C] Rena, I want to speak to you about your coming in 15 to 25 minutes late in the mornings. [A] It puts my whole routine out of whack because I've been getting home too late in the mornings to see my family. [R] I would like you to arrange to be here at 0730 from now on so that [E] I can give you the report without being too rushed and still get home on time. Can you do that?"

2. Margaret is a new graduate working on a psychiatric unit with you. You notice that each time Margaret has an interview with a client she goes into the session with a coffee only for herself and a cigarette, and puts her feet up on the desk. You know this casual behavior makes clients feel insulted and disrespected and gives them the impression that Margaret is less than interested in their case. Since the clients have not had the nerve to challenge Margaret you decide to say something to her about her behavior.

"[C] Margaret, I couldn't help notice that when you interview some of the clients you have a very casual style, with a coffee cup and cigarette in your hand and your feet up on the desk. [A] I think your manner may give the impression to some clients that you aren't taking them seriously. Since I know you are interested in your work and like to do a good job, I thought you'd be interested in the impression your casualness gives (Await approval from Margaret before continuing). [R] Perhaps if you offered your clients a cup of coffee, too, and didn't put your feet up [E] you would show your clients your real interest in them. What do you think?"

The C.A.R.E. confrontation provides a way of confronting others when either their best interests or yours are threatened. C.A.R.E. confrontations allow you to take action in a calm, controlled, assertive way. They prevent you from being immobilized in a situation where you want to be confrontative and permit you to confront without being aggressive.

PRACTICING CONFRONTATION

Exercise 1. For each of the situations below attempt a C.A.R.E. confrontation. After you have prepared a response get together as a class and discuss your different approaches. Compare your suggestions with those at the end of this exercise.

1. Mr. Steiger, your 38-year-old client, suffers chronic bronchitis. You have noticed him smoking in the patients' lounge and as you enter his room you can smell cigarette smoke coming from the bathroom. Your nursing knowledge tells you that his smoking is self-destructive. How would you confront him?
2. Your client, 60-year-old Mrs. Cantor, has severe pitting edema of the ankles. She has been taught to raise her legs on a chair when sitting, and to wear elastic stockings from toe to midthigh. You have observed that Mrs. Cantor is not wearing her stockings and each time you have seen her in the chair her feet have been on the floor. How would you confront her about her self-destructive behavior?
3. You and Jane started working on the diabetic clinic 6 months ago, after your graduation from nursing. Jane confides to you that she feels she does not have the respect of her team members and that she feels that her opinions are not listened to or acted on. You have noticed that Jane takes a passive stance on the unit: she is overly cautious about her suggestions and speaks quietly. When she presents an idea she often puts it down first. You are pretty certain that some of her unassertive behavior accounts for her ideas not being picked up by the team. How would you confront her about her unproductive behavior?
4. Dr. Morton, the intern on the medical floor, has been unprofessional in his relations with you. He has teased you and made lewd jokes about you. He refuses to consult you about clients for whom you are directly

responsible but goes to other nurses for this information. You want his embarrassing joking to stop and you want him to consult you about your clients. How would you confront him?

Suggested C.A.R.E. confrontations

1. "[C] Mr. Steiger, I have observed you smoking on several occasions in the past couple of days. [A] Smoking causes you to produce more phlegm and that makes you cough more and become short of breath. [R] I would like you to stop smoking [E] so that your lungs will have a chance to clear and your breathing will become easier. If you don't stop smoking, then you are at risk for a serious lung infection."
2. "[C] Mrs. Cantor, I notice that you aren't wearing your elastic stockings and your feet are on the floor instead of being raised on the stool. [A] Wearing your elastic stockings helps prevent blood clots from forming. [R] I strongly recommend that you wear your stockings and raise your legs on a stool [E] so that you prevent any more serious complications of your heart disease."
3. "Jane, I think you have some sound ideas about client management. [C] I notice that when you present your ideas you seem to hesitate and speak softly and uncertainly about your views. When you start off by saying 'this idea may not work . . . ' [A] it's almost as if you set the team up to discount your suggestions before they have heard them. [R] I think the value of your suggestions would be highlighted if you just gave your ideas in a more positive way. [E] Then you and the team would both benefit."
4. "[C] Dr. Morton, making me the brunt of your sexist jokes is [A] distracting and demeaning and I ask you to stop it. [R] I'd like you to consult me about my clients when I am the primary nurse involved. [E] If you can relate to me that way I'm sure we'll develop a good working relationship. And I can assure you that you'll get the essential information about your clients from me in a clear and concise report."

If you require more examples refer to Exercise 3 in Chapter 3, Mutual Problem-Solving in Nursing, for situations in which clients have broken a mutually arrived at agreement.

Exercise 2. For this exercise work in threes. Each one of you should rotate through the roles of confronter, confrontee, and feedback giver. The confrontee will ignore the confronter as she attempts to tell you how she spent her weekend. The confrontee does not attend and does not show respect for the confronter. After several minutes the confronter will use a C.A.R.E. confrontation to get the confrontee to listen more attentively.

As the confrontee:

1. In what ways was the confrontation successful?
2. What suggestions would you make to the confronter to help her be more assertive in making a confrontation?

As the confronter:

1. Which aspects of completing a C.A.R.E. confrontation were easier for you to master?
2. Where did you run into difficulties?
3. What suggestions do you have for improving your ability to confront?

As the feedback giver:

1. Did the confronter *clarify* the behavior that was unpleasant?
2. Did she *articulate* why it was bothersome?
3. Was her *request* for change clear and realistic?
4. How did she *encourage* her confrontee to make the changes she requested?
5. Overall, how assertive was the confrontation?

Switch roles so that each of you has the opportunity to be confronter, confrontee, and feedback giver.

Exercise 3. In the next few days observe how others make confrontations to you. What do they do that makes you feel respected? Are they clear in their message to you? What do they say that leaves you feeling put down or angry? You can learn a lot about how to improve your own confrontations by observing the effect of others' confrontations on you.

After you have collected your own data, compare your findings with those of your classmates. What have your observations taught you about the most effective ways to confront others?

Exercise 4. Attempt to practice confrontation in real life, whether at school, on the units, or in social situations. How effective are you at making C.A.R.E. confrontations? Have you discovered that by using this format you avoid both aggressiveness and unassertiveness? Do these guidelines for confronting provide you with more confidence?

REFERENCES

Ackerhalt, J. (1987). Nurse-client relationship In J. Haber, P.P. Hoskins, A.M. Leach, & B.F. Sideleau, *Comprehensive psychiatric nursing* (3rd ed.) (pp. 255-280). McGraw-Hill Book Company.

Bower, S.A., & Bower, G.H. (1976). *Asserting yourself: A practical guide for positive change.* Reading, Mass.: Addison-Wesley Publishing Company.

Egan, G. (1977). *You and me: The skills of communications and relating to others.* Monterey, Calif.: Brooks/Cole Publishing Company.

Stuart, G.W., & Sundeen, S.J. (1991). *Principles and practice of psychiatric nursing* (4th ed.). St. Louis: Mosby–Year Book.

SUGGESTIONS FOR FURTHER READING

Bower, S.A., & Bower, G.H. (1976). *Asserting yourself: A practical guide for positive change.* Reading, Mass.: Addison-Wesley Publishing Company.
  These authors have created a readable and practical book on how to be assertive. Three of the chapters have a heavy emphasis on confrontation. The authors introduce the D.E.S.C. script

for confrontation from which the C.A.R.E. confrontation was adapted. The concise and humorous writing style and cartoons add to the pleasure of reading.

Egan, G. (1982). *The skilled helper: Model, skills, and methods for effective helping* (2nd ed.). Monterey, Calif.: Brooks/Cole Publishing Company.

In chapter 7 Egan describes several methods of confrontation that can be employed in the client-counsellor relationship. Many examples are given to explain the pros and cons of confrontation.

Evans, D.R., Hearn, M.T., Uhlemann, M.R., & Ivey, A.E. (1979). *Essential interviewing: A programmed approach to effective communication.* Monterey, Calif.: Brooks/Cole Publishing Company.

Chapter 8 concisely outlines the essential points to remember when confronting others. Nurse readers can improve their skills by doing the many exercises in the programmed learning chapter.

Martin, D.G. (1983). *Counseling and therapy skills.* Monterey, Calif.: Brooks/Cole Publishing Company.

For the nurse reader who wishes to advance her skill in confrontation, chapter 4, Confronting Experience, will prove useful. Many of the problems that can arise during a confrontation are described and suggestions for avoiding and handling them are provided.

....

: **CHAPTER 13** :

....

Refusing
Unreasonable Requests

"It is kindness to refuse immediately what you intend to deny."

Publilius Syrus

OBJECTIVES

This chapter will reconfirm your belief in the importance of your right to refuse unreasonable requests from clients and colleagues. You will augment your comfort level and confidence in taking the assertive action of refusing requests which impinge on your rights as a nurse. The exercises provide you with the opportunity to receive feedback on how effectively you refuse unreasonable requests.

WHAT ARE UNREASONABLE REQUESTS?

As nurses we receive requests from others for information, emotional support, and assistance. Week in and week out we are asked to carry out activities that will help our clients and colleagues. Each request we receive is deemed reasonable in the eyes of the person making the request. In most instances, requests from our clients and colleagues seem legitimate when we think about the request in an objective way. However, when a request is made of *you,* you must consider how it affects you personally, because you are the one being asked to fulfill the request. *It is up to you to determine if a request is reasonable or not.*

A request may be unreasonable if it impinges on your right to nurse in a way that is in keeping with your ethics, values, or beliefs. Unreasonable requests are ones that escalate your negative feelings and impinge on your right to feel good about the work you are doing. Frequently you are asked to perform tasks that are disrespectful of your safety or physical capabilities. It is unreasonable to respond to requests which put you in the position of possibly hurting yourself or physically and emotionally stretching yourself to the point that you feel stressed, overloaded, or irritable.

As nurses we have the right to work in a way that allows us to give our best nursing care to clients, promotes the most congenial relationships with our colleagues, and gives us feelings of satisfaction, safety, and comfort doing our job. Chenevert puts our rights as nurses in perspective: "Nurses are responsible people. We have dwelled so long and so hard on our responsibilities we are often surprised at the prospect of having rights ourselves (1990, p. 108)." She outlines our ten basic rights as nurses:

1. You have the right to be treated with respect.
2. You have the right to a reasonable work load.
3. You have the right to an equitable wage.
4. You have the right to determine your own priorities.
5. You have the right to ask for what you want.
6. You have the right to refuse without making excuses or feeling guilty.
7. You have the right to make mistakes and be responsible for them.
8. You have the right to give and receive information as a professional.
9. You have the right to act in the best interest of the patient.
10. You have the right to be human (Chenevert, 1990, p. 109).

Requests for our information or ideas, attention or affection, physical power or skills all take time, energy, and commitment to fulfill. We need to check our resources before agreeing to any request. When we take on a request that overtaxes us, we lose out because we become overloaded and others lose out because we are ineffective when we are feeling burdened. Before saying "yes" to a request we need to check to see if it is reasonable for us to accept. If we decide it is unreasonable, then we must refuse. It is far better to refuse than to capitulate and risk a serious error. Failure to refuse can end up making you a sorry excuse for a nurse (Chenevert, 1990, p. 118).

Mackay reveals that successful business people tap into their own state of mind before saying "yes" to important requests for their time, money, or expertise. "In the final analysis, what your inner voice tells you is the best advice you can get" (Mackay, 1990, p. 249). For making decisions in the world of business, Mackay underlines the importance of being honest enough to understand and predict our reactions if the unexpected happens. "If you know you can't handle the bad stuff, if you're not ready to make a total commitment, then you're not ready to say yes, whatever it is" (Mackay, 1990, p. 251). This is advice that we shouldn't refuse.

Saying "No" Assertively

The skill in saying "no" is to refuse the request in an assertive, as opposed to an aggressive or unassertive, style. By being assertive we protect ourselves by declining a task we cannot comfortably handle and we respect the other's rights by refusing in a polite, matter-of-fact manner. Our desire to help clients and colleagues and our wish to be seen as helpful nurses often interfere with our ability to say "no" clearly and simply.

We sometimes fumble with wishy-washy excuses in attempts to avoid taking on the request. This unassertive behavior makes us feel guilty and helpless and we offend the asker with our weak and irrelevant attempts to justify our refusal. A simple "no" would suffice and save both people embarrassment.

Sometimes our unnecessary or irrational guilt feelings about saying "no" make us refuse the request in a hostile, defensive manner. This aggressiveness makes us feel ashamed that we have behaved unprofessionally, and our requester feels put down or hurt by our explosiveness. Clearly, refusing a request in an unassertive or an aggressive way does not protect our interests or those of our clients or colleagues. The assertive refusal to an unreasonable request is the only way to show respect for ourselves and others.

Saying "no" to unreasonable requests is a way of saying "yes" to yourself. Just as clients are unique individuals and you struggle to consider their individuality when providing nursing care, when you protect your rights by refusing unreasonable requests you are respecting your uniqueness. You are saying "yes" to your values, "yes" to your style of doing things, "yes" to your ways of perceiving situations, and "yes" to your ways of judging and deciding. It is freeing to remove your energy from unreasonable requests and invest it into your visions and goals.

Some Examples of Refusing Requests Assertively

Here are some examples of effective, assertive ways of saying "no," in contrast to some ineffective, aggressive, and unassertive ways.

Example 1

It is Tuesday. Your nurse colleague, Elsa, asks you to work this weekend for her. Your in-laws are coming to visit and you have made plans to give them a tour of some of the excellent countryside restaurants this weekend. Your family has been looking forward to this visit and it is unreasonable for you to work on this particular weekend. In the past Elsa has changed her rotation and worked a weekend for you.

An assertive refusal:
 Elsa: "Could you please work this weekend for me? Rob phoned long distance and he's invited me to go to New York to spend the long weekend with him. I'm so excited! Can you do it?"

 Assertive You: "No, Elsa. I'm not able to switch this weekend. My in-laws are visiting from out of town and we've made reservations to do things. I hope you can find someone to switch. I can see you're really looking forward to going to New York to visit Rob."

This refusal is direct and clear. You are definite, yet you soften the refusal with the inclusion of the explanation for your refusal and your empathic hope that she can secure a replacement.

But Elsa is determined and persists in her attempt to persuade you to switch.

Elsa: "I know you've got company coming, but they are just in-laws and you get to see them often. I haven't seen Rob for 3 months. I know it's last-minute, but Rob just found out he could be free and he called me as soon as he could. Oh, please, won't you work for me?"

Assertive You: "No, Elsa. I am not available to switch with you this weekend."

You continue to be clear and definite. Elsa is pleading and trying to make you feel guilty so that you will give in to her. Your response successfully protects your rights to have a weekend with your family and attends to her rights to be treated respectfully.

Elsa does not stop. She wants you to switch so she plies you with more guilt.

Elsa: "Remember I switched weekends with you in the spring when you wanted to go to your cousin's wedding? You agreed then that you owed me one. Well, now I'm collecting! I need you to pay me back this weekend."

Assertive You: "Elsa, I am unable to work this weekend for you."

This response continues to be clear and unwavering so that Elsa is given a definite answer. Its matter-of-factness is congruent with your desire to avoid becoming hostile or weakened. Although you hope Elsa will find a replacement, it is unreasonable for you to be that person this weekend.

Elsa is starting to get your assertive message.

Elsa: "Okay, okay. I see you've got plans you can't break. It's just that I'm desperate. I'll ask one of the other nurses if she can switch with me."

By being assertive you have prevented yourself from doing two things you did not want to do: work the weekend and come across as defensive or indecisive to your colleague Elsa.

An unassertive refusal:

Elsa: "Could you please work this weekend for me? Rob phoned long distance and he's invited me to go to New York to spend the long weekend with him. I'm so excited! Can you do it?"

Unassertive You: "Gee, Elsa. I don't think so . . . I'm sorry."

This response does not sound convincing. Elsa would get the message that you are not *really* sure you can switch with her. It sounds like you are still debating with yourself, and Elsa will likely try to convince you to switch.

Elsa: "I haven't seen Rob for 3 months. I know it's last minute, but Rob just found out he could be free and he called me as soon as he could. Oh, please, won't you work for me?"

Unassertive You: "Gee, Elsa, I don't think I can. I'm sorry. I've got my in-laws coming and we've made plans. I don't think so, Elsa."

You still have not given a definite "no" and Elsa will likely keep asking you as long as she figures there is hope.

Elsa: "Remember I switched weekends with you in the spring when you wanted to go to your cousin's wedding? You agreed then that you owed me one. Well, now I'm collecting! I need you to pay me back this weekend."

Unassertive You: "Yes, that's true. I guess I owe you one. Yes, I'll switch with you for this weekend."

By being unassertive and indefinite you have agreed to a request that is unreasonable for you to take on. Giving in will most likely leave you feeling angry and your in-laws will be disappointed you have let them down. When we are unassertive we forfeit our rights.

An aggressive refusal:
Elsa: "Could you please work this weekend for me? Rob phoned long distance and he's invited me to go to New York to spend the long weekend with him. I'm so excited! Can you do it?"

Aggressive You: "Don't you know I've got my in-laws coming to visit this weekend? There's no way I can switch with you."

This abrasive, offensive reply shows no understanding of Elsa's predicament. Whereas a simple refusal would have sufficed, this response makes you appear unfriendly and inconsiderate.

Elsa is not put off and continues to try to convince you to change.

Elsa: "I haven't seen Rob for 3 months. I know it's last minute, but Rob just found out he could be free and he called me as soon as he could. Oh, please, won't you work for me?"

Aggressive You: "I can't help it if you haven't seen Rob for 3 months. That's your problem. I've got my own problems with my in-laws coming."

Elsa: "I know you've got company coming, but they are just your in-laws and you get to see them often."

Aggressive You: "They are just as important to me as your absentee boyfriend is to you. Maybe if you got together more often you wouldn't be so desperate now."

Your insensitivity to Elsa's predicament and your judgmental, accusatory remarks will considerably damage your relationship with your co-worker. Aggressive responses are often disproportionate and fired by our irrational anger and guilt.

Elsa persists!

Elsa: "Remember I switched weekends with you in the spring when you wanted to go to your cousin's wedding? You agreed then that you owed me one. Well, now I'm collecting! I need you to pay me back this weekend."

Aggressive You: "I gave you plenty of notice—not 3 days like you're offering me. If you think I can drop my plans, you're crazy!"

Elsa: "Well, I'll be damned if I ever do you a favor again. Some friend-in-need you are."

You may have won the battle by refusing an unreasonable request, but you have lost the war of conducting yourself in a considerate and professional manner. If the bad feelings created by being aggressive can ever be resolved, it will take an inordinate amount of energy and time.

Example 2

It is the evening shift on the surgical floor where you are working. So far there has been one death, an admission, and there are three clients to prepare for surgery the next day. Mr. Gowers, a 70-year-old client, had eye surgery 2 days ago and has orders to remain immobile. He is unable to see what is going on around him through his heavy eye bandages. When you are making your medication rounds he asks you to write a letter for him to his nephew.

An assertive refusal:

Mr. Gowers: "Could you help me write a letter to my nephew tonight? I just remembered it's his twentieth wedding anniversary and I want to let him know I'm thinking of him. He is like a son to me. I'd do it myself but I can't see, and his anniversary is this week."

Assertive You: "Mr. Gowers, I will not be able to help you to write your letter tonight as the unit is too hectic with the number of people to prepare for surgery. I can see it is important for you to get your best wishes off to this special nephew of yours in time for his anniversary. I'd be happy to ask another client to help you since the staff, even our volunteer, is tied up tonight."

This definite response makes it clear to Mr. Gowers that you are unable to do what he wants. Your expression of understanding about his urgency and your suggestion of an alternative solution would make him aware of your concern. You have protected your rights not to take on a task when you are already overloaded, and you have shown your client you are interested in his situation.

An unassertive refusal:
Mr. Gowers: "Could you help me write a letter to my nephew tonight? I just remembered it's his twentieth wedding anniversary and I want to let him know I'm thinking of him. He is like a son to me. I'd do it myself but I can't see, and his anniversary is this week."

Unassertive You: "Uh . . . well, um, I'm not sure I can, Mr. Gowers. We're pretty busy here tonight, but I'll try. Maybe on my coffee break I'll get a chance. I'll see."

You know that you are so busy that you will be lucky to get a decent coffee break. And you know that if you have time for coffee you need to go off the unit and clear your head so that you will come back refreshed. You know you should not take on this extra task and you are already feeling more tense because it is one more thing on your long list of things to do. You have not protected your rights for a reasonable workload, and you have conveyed a lot of ambivalence to Mr. Gowers, perhaps leaving him feeling that he is imposing on you.

An aggressive refusal:
Mr. Gowers: "Could you help me write a letter to my nephew tonight? I just remembered it's his twentieth wedding anniversary and I want to let him know I'm thinking of him. He is like a son to me. I'd do it myself but I can't see, and his anniversary is this week."

Aggressive You: "If you think I've got time to sit down and take dictation, Mr. Gowers, you're mistaken. I'll be lucky to get out of here by midnight, and that's just with doing the basics."

This hostile rejoinder protects you from doing an unreasonable assignment, but it leaves Mr. Gowers feeling devastated. He is likely feeling guilty for asking you and embarrassed at your angry refusal. Neither of you wins in an aggressive refusal.

Example 3

A physician arrives late to the afternoon prenatal clinic. Today is especially busy because more expectant mothers have kept their appointments than usual. One of your nurses is ill, leaving you short-staffed to make sure the clinic runs smoothly. In addition, you are responsible for all the prenatal teaching. The physician tells you he has missed his lunch and asks you to get him something to eat.

An assertive refusal:

Dr. Watts: "Will you go across to the deli and pick me up a salami on rye? I missed lunch because I was so busy this morning."

Assertive You: "No, Dr. Watts, I can't go across to get you lunch. Like you, today I am swamped with the workload."

This assertive response clearly conveys your refusal. It is polite and matter-of-fact. You have upheld your rights to do your job and treated your colleague respectfully.

An unassertive refusal:

Dr. Watts: "Will you go across to the deli and pick me up a salami on rye? I missed lunch because I was so busy this morning."

Unassertive You: "Um . . . uh, well, Dr. Watts, we're kind of busy here today, but, well, I suppose if I do it fast it won't take too much time. Do you want it toasted or plain? Pickles? Mustard? . . ."

Your unassertiveness is probably leaving you feeling pretty angry and disappointed in yourself. It is clear to everyone that you do not wish to get your colleague's lunch. Being unassertive this way you lose time and face.

An aggressive refusal:

Dr. Watts: "Will you go across to the deli and pick me up a salami on rye? I missed lunch because I was so busy this morning."

Aggressive You: "Nurses aren't handmaidens anymore, Dr. Watts. You'd better get with the times. We're all busy, yet we managed to get our own lunches. I'm not being paid to go and fetch food for you."

Wow! You protected your rights with this response but in the process you were rude to a colleague by the way you over-reacted and attacked him. Such accusatory aggressiveness only serves to escalate bad feelings. A simple refusal would have been in order.

Example 4

You are in the process of giving morning nursing care in the cardiovascular step-down unit. Mr. Taber, one of your clients, is a 53-year-old man who suffered a myocardial infarction 3½ weeks ago. He has experienced an uneventful and safe recovery. Two days ago his cardiologist ordered that Mr. Taber could increase his activity level to washing himself and sitting in a chair for 15 minutes each morning and afternoon.

Mr. Taber has not increased his activity level and indicates he is afraid to move too much for fear of having another heart attack. During his morning bath he asks you to wash his arms and legs for him. He is able to do this activity for himself; in fact, it would stimulate his circulation and gently increase the workload on his heart to help strengthen it. It is unreasonable for you to bathe him because it would detract from his healing.

An assertive refusal:
    Mr. Taber: "I think you'd better help me with my morning wash. I don't want to over exert myself and risk a fatal heart attack. Could you do my arms and legs before you go?"

    Assertive You: "No, Mr. Taber. I will not be helping you wash your arms and legs any more. Just go slowly at it and the gentle movement will actually help improve your circulation and strengthen your heart. I will be in the room while you are washing. Just call me if you want me."

This reply sets the record straight from the beginning. Its clarity is enhanced by the explanation of the logic for doing his own self-care. You protect your right to nurse in a way that is in his best interests and you provide him with the reassurance that you are close by if he needs you.

An unassertive refusal:
    Mr. Taber: "I think you'd better help me with my morning wash. I don't want to over exert myself and risk a fatal heart attack. Could you do my arms and legs before you go?"

    Unassertive You: "Well, Mr. Taber, you know you are supposed to be doing most of your wash yourself now. But, uh, since you're nervous I'll help you with your legs, okay?"

By giving in to this request you will be ignoring what is important for him to do in his efforts to recover. You can fool yourself into believing that you are helping him out; however, your stance indicates your need to be seen as helpful and your inability to say "no" clearly. Neither of you wins.

An aggressive refusal:
    Mr. Taber: "I think you'd better help me with my morning wash. I don't want to over exert myself and risk a fatal heart attack. Could you do my arms and legs before you go?"

    Aggressive You: "Stop babying yourself, Mr. Taber. You've got to accept the fact that your heart is okay and go on living. I'm not going to feed your unfounded fears by washing you. You're on your own today."

This refusal is a put-down. It belittles his fears and puts pressure on him to accept his condition before he is ready to. Such aggressiveness adds to a client's bad feelings. Your insensitivity leaves your client feeling hurt and you knowing you have been ruthless and uncaring.

Saying "No" Effectively

Quite likely these examples have made you aware of some "dos" and "don'ts" when refusing unreasonable requests. Here are some suggestions to add to your observations.

DO:
- State your refusal very near the beginning of your reply so that your requester hears a clear, direct answer right away
- Indicate concisely the reason for saying "no" *if* it strengthens your refusal
- Communicate your understanding of the requester's desire for help so that he feels you understand his predicament even if you cannot solve it
- Suggest an alternative source of help if it seems appropriate
- Think about your response, then speak in a forthright, calm, polite manner
- Maintain a matter-of-fact, consistent way of refusing in the face of an aggressive requester

DO NOT:
- Begin your refusal with a list of lengthy excuses which an aggressive requester will argue so logically that you will be forced to concede
- Stammer, pause, hem and haw, hesitate, or burst out your refusal, revealing that you are unsure
- Lose eye contact for lengthy periods, shift uncomfortably, or convey other nonverbal discomfort revealing your hesitancy
- Raise your voice or give other bodily clues of being enraged. It is your right to refuse and you do not need to become hostile to protect this privilege

PRACTICING REFUSING UNREASONABLE REQUESTS

Exercise 1. For each of the following situations write out an assertive refusal. Compare your responses with those of your colleagues and pool your suggestions to come up with the most assertive refusal.
- A client asks you for your home number so that he can call you "if he needs any follow-up advice." In the interests of your privacy, it is your policy not to give out your telephone number to any clients.
- A colleague with whom you are working the night shift asks you to keep an eye on the clients and an ear out for the telephone and night supervisor while she has a nap. You think this request is unreasonable because you are both being paid to do the job and if there is any trouble two staff members will be needed.

- A client wants you to facilitate bringing his 3-year-old son into the hospital to visit him. The rules of this unit are that no children under 12 years of age are allowed because of the high risk of infection. He says he is a single parent and really misses his son.
- A client is being observed for withdrawal from street drugs. She asks you if she can go down to the cafeteria with her visitor to have a cup of coffee. Your preference is for her to remain on the unit where you can have frequent contact with her.
- Your nursing supervisor requests that you wear your nurses' cap. There is no hospital policy enforcing this request and many nurses do not wear caps. You can cite two studies which document that nurses' caps are one of the greatest sources of infection. Furthermore, you feel strongly that it is discriminatory to be the only professionals in the hospital who wear caps.
- A client who comes once a week to receive an injection from you asks you if he could come 15 minutes later in the future. Moving back his appointment would inconvenience you, because it would mean you would be late leaving work and not make your bus connections.
- A colleague who lives in the same area of the city asks you if he can get a ride to and from work with you. That quiet time in the car by yourself is your only peaceful moment in the day. You would find it stressful to have to make conversation with another person during the commuting time.
- The health care team has decided it will try to persuade a resistant client to receive a blood transfusion in order to save her life. As a nurse on the team, it is expected that you will participate in this coercion. Such a decision is against your beliefs about clients' rights to make independent decisions about their health.
- A client in traction on your orthopedic unit is bored with the food at the hospital. He asks you to bring him in a "supreme whopper" on your way into work. The client has no dietary restrictions. You are reluctant to agree to this request because you do not want to show favoritism to any particular client.

You can also use this exercise to verbally practice making refusals. One person in the vignette can roleplay the client, another the nurse, and a third can give feedback to the nurse on her ability to refuse assertively.

Exercise 2. For this exercise work in threes. One will make a request, another will refuse the request, and the third will give feedback. The requester can ask for anything and she should persist in her attempts to get what she wants. Aggressiveness in the requester is encouraged for the purposes of this exercise. The refuser will attempt to give an assertive refusal and will try to maintain that stance in the face of the requester's aggressiveness. The observer will give feedback to the refuser about her ability to refuse in an assertive way. The observer will point out where the refuser could have been more assertive or less aggressive. In debriefing, these questions can be used as a guide.

As the refuser:
1. Were you able to achieve and/or maintain an assertive refusal?
2. Where did you have difficulty being assertive?
3. What could you do to overcome these blocks and be more assertive in your refusals?

As the requester:
1. In what ways did the refuser convince you that she meant "no"?
2. Where and how could she improve her assertiveness in making refusals?

Make sure you each get a turn in each role and debrief after each role change.

Exercise 3. Over the next week make notes of how you make refusals to others. What do you think is effective and what could you do to improve?

Exercise 4. In the next week observe how others handle requests you make of them. Especially note how others refuse your requests. What is assertive about how they make their refusals? How do others make you feel when they refuse your requests? What is it others do to make you feel respected and understood? What is it they do to make you feel humiliated or embarrassed?

From observing others, what have you learned about effective and ineffective ways to refuse unreasonable requests?

REFERENCES

Chenevert, M. (1985). *Pro-nurse handbook: Designed for the nurse who wants to thrive professionally.* St. Louis: Mosby–Year Book.

Mackay, H. (1990). *Beware the naked man who offers you his shirt.* New York: Ivy Books.

SUGGESTIONS FOR FURTHER READING

Bower, S.A., & Bower, G.H. (1976). *Asserting yourself: A practical guide for positive change.* Mass.: Addison-Wesley Publishing Company.
   In chapter 6, "Sample scripts for standard situations", Bower and Bower provide word for word scripts for saying "no" to unreasonable demands. They have developed a useful format for saying "no" that can be a handy guide any time you wish to refuse unreasonable requests.

Chenevert, M. (1978). *Special techniques in assertiveness training for women in the health professions.* Saint Louis: Mosby–Year Book.
   In chapter 7, "How to tell a turkey to stuff it", Chenevert describes many realistic nursing situations in which she emphasizes how to avoid "letting every turkey trot all over you until you lose control and try to make hash out of all of them at once" (p. 70). Her humorous writing style helps her excellent points hit home.

Herman, S.J. (1978). *Becoming assertive: A guide for nurses.* New York: D. Van Nostrand Company.
   Herman has several examples of saying "no" to doctors, instructors, and clients in chapter 5, "Applying assertive behaviour: How to be the assertive you."

Jakubowski, P., & Lange, A.J. (1978). *The assertive option: Your rights and responsibilities.* Champaign, Ill.: Research Press Company.
   The authors provide an excellent figure and text explaining the dysfunctional thoughts that prevent people from saying "no."

Phelps, S., & Austin, N. (1975). *The assertive woman*. Fredericksburg, Va.: Book Crafters and Impact Printers. The authors tackle the issue of refusing requests from several angles in chapter 7, "Saying No". The examples are those of everyday living and are designed to help readers say "no" without feeling guilty. There is a handy checklist to determine whether you should be saying "no" more frequently. Nurses could adapt this idea to develop a similar list for the workplace.

CHAPTER 14

Requesting Support

"People must help one another; it is nature's law."

Jean de La Fontaine

OBJECTIVES

As a student nurse, and later as a graduate nurse, there will be many occasions when you will need support to do your work. This chapter provides you with guidelines for making your requests for support in a way that they are most likely to be successful. You will learn how to be specific about your needs for support and how to plan an assertive strategy. The exercises will give you the opportunity to practice assertive ways to request support.

THE RELATIONSHIP BETWEEN SOCIAL SUPPORT AND HEALTH

The literature suggests there is a positive relationship between the presence of social support and good health. Dimond and Jones (1983) summarized numerous medical studies providing evidence that support prevents susceptibility to illness, diminishes the symptoms of illness, promotes earlier recovery from sickness, and enhances well-being. It has been hypothesized that social support acts as a buffer to maintain or regain health (Cobb, 1976; Gottlieb 1983; Pilisuk & Froland, 1978). Social support has been linked to positive mental health. Mueller's literature review cited evidence linking inadequate social support with psychiatric illness (1980). In a sample of 170 Chinese Americans Lin, Ensel, Simeone, and Kuo (1979) demonstrated that social support accounted for more variance in psychiatric symptoms than stressful life events, occupational prestige, and marital status combined.

Much of the earlier social support literature has been related to clients or potential clients. Recently more is being written about workplace

174

support to help employees contend with occupational tensions and stresses. Some of this literature concerns support for nurses and represents a beginning acknowledgment of the necessity and benefits of support in the workplace for nurses.

The nursing literature of the 1970s and up to the mid-1980s abounded with descriptions of the stressful nature of nursing practice in a variety of clinical settings (Smith, 1986). Accompanying these portrayals was a flood of articles claiming that workplace support groups are an effective way to combat stress. The following list delineates the purported benefits of workplace support groups for nurses and other health care professionals:

- Controls or decreases staff turnover (Gray-Toft & Anderson, 1983; Baider & Porath, 1981; Webster, Kelly, Johst, Weber, & Wickes, 1982; Weiner & Caldwell, 1983; McDermott, 1983);
- Reduces stress/teaches stress reducing strategies/prevents burnout (Gray-Toft & Anderson, 1983; Scully, 1981; Webster, Kelly et al., 1982; Deming, 1984);
- Increases job satisfaction/increases morale (Gray-Toft & Anderson, 1983; Weiner & Caldwell, 1983; Hay & Oken, 1972; Deming, 1984; McDermott, 1983);
- Teaches methods of conflict management (Scully, 1981; Hay & Oken, 1972);
- Assists nurses to work as a team/improves intercollegial communication/encourages working as a unit (Scully, 1981; Taerk, 1983; Baider & Porath, 1981; Webster et al., 1982; Weiner & Caldwell, 1983; Goetzel, Shelov, & Croen, 1983);
- Provides an opportunity to consult about clients/promotes nursing knowledge (Scully, 1981; Taerk, 1983; Webster, 1983; Diminno & Thompson, 1980; Hay & Oken, 1972);
- Provides supervision (Scully, 1981);
- Improves the quality of care provided (Jacobs, 1982; Taerk, 1983; Webster et al., 1982);
- Improves ward atmosphere (Taerk, 1983; Baider & Porath, 1981; Deming, 1984);
- Helps nurses relate to clients more positively (Baider & Porath, 1981; McDermott, 1983);
- Increases confidence in their roles/increases participation in meetings (Baider & Porath, 1981; Webster et al., 1982; Deming, 1984);
- Instills positive influence on nurses' lives away from hospital (Weiner & Caldwell, 1983);
- Helps nurses cope with sensory overload (Skinner, 1980); and
- Allows emotional release of feelings (Skinner, 1980; Diminno & Thompson, 1980; Hay & Oken, 1972).

Although these reports on the benefits of workplace support groups for nurses were descriptive and retrospective, they attested to the enthusiasm for workplace support groups. During the current nursing shortage in America, workplace support has taken on new importance. Employers immersed in recruitment have examined the key attractions for nurses. One of the recurrent demands potential nurse employees vocalize is for a supportive work environment (Corcoran, Meyer, & Magliaro, 1990; Spitzer-Lehmann, 1990; White, 1990; Callahan, 1990; Sanford, 1990; Geissler, 1990; Kinsey, 1990; Franks & Hayden, 1990). What is found is that nurses tend to select units and stay working in them where they deem the work environment supportive and the professional development of the staff is valued (Doering, 1990, p. 223).

DETERMINING THE SUPPORT YOU NEED AT WORK OR SCHOOL

In the broadest sense of the word, *support* is anything that helps you to work more effectively and feel better about how you are functioning. This general notion of support is vague and will not help you articulate specifically what you need nor guide you to get it. If you think about support as being *cognitive, affective,* and *physical,* this conceptualization will help you assess and secure the support you need to work as a nurse.

Cognitive support helps you think intelligently about your job, decide how to approach problems, discover the how and why of doing things a certain way, and provides some criteria for doing your work. *Affective* support is the good feeling that accompanies open, direct communication with colleagues. The reassurance that teammates will consider your point of view and the comfort of freely expressing opinions augments your positive feelings about work. *Physical* support is concrete assistance given by people, computers, equipment, or spatial arrangements of the environment which make your nursing more streamlined.

One method of providing nurses cognitive support is through mentors (Kinsey, 1990). In a summary of the favorable incidents associated with mentorship, nurse leaders ranked career advice, scholarly stimulation, and professional role modeling as the top three influences. Coleman described a positive innovation for supporting and retaining nurses whereby the more experienced nurses were stimulated and challenged to advance their knowledge base and sharpen their consultative skills and then initiate changes on their units. Both receiving the counsel of mentoring and exploring new role options as experienced nurses provided immense satisfaction and strengthened nurse retention. One of the strategic plans some hospitals are implementing to attract and retain nurses is access to clinical specialists, nursing research support, staff development, staff orientation, and upward mobility (Corocoran, Meyer, & Magliaro, 1990, p. 27). These reports underline how nurses today want continued stimulation and chances for professional growth.

In the realm of affective support, nurses are demanding acknowledgment for the work they do. Charge nurses need continued support and confirmation of their important role in today's world, where nursing practices are changing, client acuity is higher, and nursing shortages are real (Franks & Hayden, 1990, p. 48). Respect, honor, and recognition of nurses and all employees by acknowledgment of positive performance is needed frequently, not merely at annual review (Spitzer-Lehmann, 1990, p. 67). Expressing gratitude and appreciation can create feelings of good will and nurturance among nurses that is a form of job gratification, making them feel better about their workplaces, clients, and colleagues (Geissler, 1990; Sanford, 1990). Callahan (1990) believes that burnout occurs when nurses realize that, no matter how developed their talents are, they aren't recognized. She urged hospitals to initiate a system of Positive Incident Reports that would be posted on the unit's bulletin board and then be included in the staff nurse's personnel file. A commendation for work well done might look like this example: "I'd like to commend Sheila Jersey, RN, for the empathy she showed the client in 1039 on the night of 10/12/90. Her words cut through his pain and delirium, grounding him in reality and allowing him to rest without further medication. She has a special ability to say just what the client needs to hear" (p. 64).

Hospital employers are realizing that one of the goals of recruitment and retention strategies must be to promote a work environment in which nurses at the bedside have the opportunity to have a say in administrative and clinical decisions affecting client care and to be recognized for their contribution (Doering, 1990; Ligon, 1990). The way one hospital fulfilled its dedication to listening to and involving nurses was to incorporate input and approval from nurses in the development and implementation of a dynamic, professional practice model (Huttner, 1990). Professional autonomy and inclusion in policy development and decision making, as well as quality assurance programs, is one of the key elements of a successful work place for attracting and retaining nursing staff (Corocoran, Meyer, & Magliaro, 1990).

The recent nursing literature abounds with articles related to cognitive and affective support for nurses in the workplace. Staffing requirements, an essential aspect of physical support, are discussed in the abundance of articles on retention. In this era it is believed that the provision of adequate cognitive and affective support will attract nurses to work and continue employment in agencies. The requirements for supplies, equipment, and environmental conveniences have likely been secured in most nursing work places through the efforts of technology, computerization, and stringent occupational hazard and safety regulations.

As nurses, we need to be assertive about securing the support necessary to function comfortably and confidently at work. The clearer we are about what support we need to do our job, the more likely we are to secure it. We spend a lot of energy attempting to improve the health status of our clients. Getting the support we need to do our work can help us maintain our health and enhance how we feel about our both work and co-workers.

Conceptualizing *cognitive, affective,* and *physical* components of support provides you with an organizing framework for your individual support assessment. The first step in your systematic approach is to determine whether you are satisfied with the quality and quantity of support for each facet. Quality refers to the nature or characteristics of the support; quantity refers to the amount of support.

Please look at the checklist entitled Credits and Debits in Your Support System at Work or School. Take a pencil and check off the pluses and minuses in your support system.

After you have completed this checklist, take note of those areas where you do have the support you need at work or school. It is easy enough to take for granted the support we do have, and noticing the benefits makes us more appreciative.

Next have a look at those areas where you indicated that the support you would like is not available. Answer the following questions about those instances where you are not satisfied with the quantity or quality of the support you receive:

1. What exactly dissatisfies me about the quantity or quality of support?
2. If I had a choice, how would I change things to ensure I receive the support I need?

Be as specific as possible when answering these questions. The clearer and more detailed you can be about the gaps in your support system at work or school, the greater your chances of rectifying the situation. What you are doing in answering these questions is indicating your desired outcome.

MAKING REQUESTS FOR THE SUPPORT YOU NEED AT WORK OR SCHOOL

The first step is to identify your needs for support. The next step is to decide if you wish to pursue acquiring this support. Can you manage without it, or would the presence of that support really enhance your working situation? Once you have decided to go after the support, your next step is to design your strategy. You need to answer the following questions:

• Who is the best person to ask for this support?
• What is the best way to seek this support?
• How can I present my case in a way to increase the probability of securing the support I want at work or school?

Let us take an example from each of the cognitive, affective, and physical domains and demonstrate effective and ineffective methods of seeking support.

Making a Request for Cognitive Support

You are a student nurse in a 2-year nursing diploma course in a rural area. On several occasions you have not been able to get important reference material for your nursing papers and projects. The nursing school's library is not stocked with several of the important and current nursing journals. To get the up-to-date information you need to make your written assignments scholarly, you have had to drive 60 miles to the university library. Since you do not have library take-out privileges at the uni-

CREDITS AND DEBITS IN YOUR SUPPORT SYSTEM AT WORK OR SCHOOL

For each cognitive, affective, or physical support item ask yourself:
1) Am I satisfied with the quality of support I get to do my job?
2) Am I satisfied with the quantity of support I get to do my job?

	Satisfied with:			
	Quality		Quantity	
	Yes	No	Yes	No
Cognitive Support				
1. **Inspiration:** You work with people whose knowledge and skill level shows how you can improve your nursing care.	—	—	—	—
2. **Information:** Written material (books, procedure manuals, memoranda) are available to provide clear information or instruction about relevant nursing procedures.	—	—	—	—
3. **Advice:** Colleagues offer expertise and willingness to help guide and/or direct you.	—	—	—	—
4. **Challenge:** Colleagues intellectually stimulate you by encouraging you to examine, question, and critique your nursing care.	—	—	—	—
5. **Direction:** Colleagues exhibit or freely share their philosophy and beliefs about nursing in a way that is helpful to you.	—	—	—	—
Affective Support				
6. **Empathy:** Colleagues show interest in you, listen to you, and you feel respected and understood.	—	—	—	—
7. **Recognition:** Colleagues acknowledge the knowledge and skills you possess, and you are able to make independent decisions and use your talents properly.	—	—	—	—
8. **Praise:** Colleagues express admiration for your work and compliment you or show attention and genuine interest in your nursing.	—	—	—	—
9. **Reassurance:** Forgiveness for imperfections of omission or commission is offered with acceptance and encouragement for you to continue to do your best nursing.	—	—	—	—

Continued.

CREDITS AND DEBITS IN YOUR SUPPORT SYSTEM AT WORK OR SCHOOL*—cont'd.

10. **Concern:** Colleagues show warm, caring interest in you as a person and you get a sense that they look forward to working with you; they are concerned for your welfare as a person (not just as a nurse or student).   —   —   —   —

11. **Feedback:** Honest, forthright evaluation of your work is offered or is available to you when you ask for it; constructive criticism is given in a straightforward, clear manner and is worded in such a way that you can accept it.   —   —   —   —

12. **Cooperation:** Colleagues share ideas with you; there is little greedy competitiveness and nurses enjoy working together to improve client care.   —   —   —   —

13. **Enthusiasm:** Nurses and others are keen about what they are doing and the atmosphere is lively; creative ideas to improve nursing care are encouraged.   —   —   —   —

Physical Support

14. **Adequate personnel:** Staff with essential knowledge and skills are available to carry out the necessary nursing functions.   —   —   —   —

15. **Sharing:** When circumstances dictate, colleagues share the workload and help each other; rarely do colleagues avoid helping or refuse to pitch in and lend a hand.   —   —   —   —

16. **Supplies:** Sufficient nursing or administrative supplies are consistently available to smoothly carry out your work.   —   —   —   —

17. **Equipment:** Equipment on your unit is efficient, in working order, and easily accessible.   —   —   —   —

18. **Environment:** The physical layout and decoration of your working environment allows you to work without inconvenience, hassles, or unpleasant distractions.   —   —   —   —

*From: Smith (1984). Need support at work? Think CAPs! *The Canadian Nurse,* 81 (8), pp. 40-43.

versity, you must plow through many references in the library. Occasionally you have written away for material you need for a paper, but it has never arrived in time for your deadline.

In the area of cognitive support you need better access to information. You decide that it is essential for you and your classmates to have these journals conveniently available if you are going to process all pertinent information and draw sound conclusions about the nursing issues you are studying. You have complained to the librarian in your nursing school and he has been ineffective in changing the situation. If you are going to get any action on this important issue you must go to the director of your nursing school.

After making an appointment with the director, you begin to prepare your strategy. In the 20 minutes you have been allotted with your director, you must make her aware of the gaps in the nursing journals in the library, convince her that this situation is serious, and urge her to rectify things so that you and your colleagues will have the support you need.

You secure a list of the journals the library has and find out from the librarian which journals are rarely used by the students. Next, you survey your classmates to compile a list of journals which they would like to have in the school library. You also get some specific information from your colleagues about how often they have had to seek information from another library or have submitted an incomplete assignment because the information was unavailable.

Armed with this information, you next prepare yourself for the interview with your director. You envision yourself looking relaxed and calm as you talk to her. In your mind's eye you see yourself presenting your arguments in a clear, straightforward, assertive manner. You notice how your director is paying attention to what you are saying; she is even taking notes. You visualize her saying that she will personally make sure that the deficits will be remedied, and students will be provided with the information support they need.

Here is an example of how your interview with your director might go if you were assertive:

An Assertive Approach

Assertive You: "Thank you for seeing me, Mrs. King. I want to talk to you about the library resources for the students in the program. Although our library has an excellent selection of the most recent textbooks in nursing, it is lacking some of the most current and frequently used nursing journals."

Mrs. King: "Oh? Is that the case? Can you tell me any more about the situation?"

Assertive You: "Yes, I can. I have talked to my classmates and made a list of those journals we would like to have available in the library. I have made a copy which you may keep [hands director a well-organized list]. The asterisks indicate the number of times students have wanted access to articles in these journals. As you can see, they are in demand frequently. When we don't have the information from these journals our knowledge base is incomplete. We feel like we are missing important information.

"I've checked with the librarian, and he has pointed out that there are some journals that our students never use from one year to the next. These journals are listed on the bottom of the sheet. I would like to request that the school purchase the journals we students are needing and stop our subscription to those journals which are not being used. We've tried going to the university library or writing away for this information but both these methods are inconvenient. It would save a lot of time and aggravation if we could have the journals on the list."

Mrs. King: "I can't argue with your facts. You have certainly done your homework. Your suggestion sounds like a good solution to the situation. I certainly want our students to have access to the most current information. I assure you that I will bring the matter up with the librarian and the teachers, and I'll get back to you within a week about the matter. Thank you for bringing this important matter to my attention."

Your assertive approach worked! By thanking Mrs. King for seeing you, you showed your respect for her busy timetable. You reinforced your awareness by getting right to the point of your visit with her. Your acknowledgment of the assets of your school library told Mrs. King that you were appreciative of the positive resources available, and not just complaining. You clearly outlined the situation, indicating why it is a problem, and respectfully offered a possible solution. Your research and approach to Mrs. King helped you secure the cognitive support you need.

In contrast to this assertive approach, you could have used an unassertive or aggressive approach with Mrs. King. Let us examine the consequences of both these less effective approaches.

An Unassertive Approach

When we act unassertively in any situation we come across as being unsure, undecided, and unconfident. These unassertive qualities give the message to another that we do not expect to receive what we are asking for. Messages of uncertainty work against us by putting doubts about our requests in the minds of potential providers. Here is an example of an unassertive approach:

Unassertive You: "I appreciate you seeing me, Mrs. King. It's about the library problem. Uh, ... did you know that we don't have some of the journals we need?"

Mrs. King: "What's this about a library problem? What journals are you referring to?"

Unassertive You: "Well, I'm not the only one who has had to go to the university library to get access to the journals I needed for my assignments. It's quite a problem you see . . . I mean, it takes a lot of time to get this information."

Mrs. King: "Yes, I know. Library research is very time consuming. Is there a problem with the journals being out?"

Unassertive You: "Well, no. You see, that's just the problem. Some of the journals aren't there in the first place. What I mean to say is, I think we need to get some new journals in the library."

Mrs. King: "Well I'm open to that suggestion. Just which journals do you think we should get?"

Unassertive You: "Well, last week I needed the *Journal of Emergency Room Nursing* and it wasn't available, for example. I'm sure there are others, too, from the way others complain."

Mrs. King: "If you want me to order new journals, you will have to be more specific about what you need. I'll be happy to look into this matter when you provide me with the information to do so."

When we are unassertive we are asking to have our requests for support ignored. In this example you were not armed with the information you needed to impress on Mrs. King the importance of the library situation. Your content was not delivered in an objective, forthright manner. On counts of style, delivery, and preparation, being unassertive lost your case.

Let us look at an aggressive approach.

An Aggressive Approach

When we are aggressive we go after what we want in a way upsetting, disrespectful, or threatening to the other person. When we attack another person in our endeavours to get what we want, it creates a gulf and bad feelings that take considerable energy and time to overcome.

Here is an example of what an aggressive approach might be like:

Aggressive You: "Thanks for seeing me, Mrs. King. You've just got to do something about this library situation. I'm fed up having to go 60 miles away to the university library to get the stuff I need to complete the assignments required for this program. It's got to change. It's unfair to students when we can't get the latest information. How would you like to hand in assignments based on half-baked ideas?"

Mrs. King: "I can see you are upset about the library situation, and it sounds quite important. When you have calmed down and can talk to me rationally about the problem, I'd be glad to meet with you."

Being aggressive did not get you what you were seeking. But it did create an unpleasant relationship between you and your director of nursing. Now there are two problems. When we are aggressive we are often out of control, and do not present our arguments in a logical, clear way. A rational, well planned, assertive approach is more likely to secure the needed support and maintain a good relationship.

Making a Request for Affective Support

You are a third-year nursing student in a 4-year baccalaureate nursing program. You have noticed that as each academic semester commences your colleagues are becoming more and more competitive about grades. When marks are posted students converge on the posting and hover around checking out how each student did. Some students are very upset or down in the dumps for days if they receive anything less than a B+.

There is less sharing of articles, ideas, and any material which would help colleagues do well on assignments. Students are starting to hoard materials, as if hoping that another person will not do well if the material is not easily accessible. Trying to get the academic edge is the name of the game and it has resulted in bickering, unfriendliness, and back-biting. You are aware of the loss of cooperation among your colleagues. This situation leaves you feeling isolated and bereft and you sense it makes others feel that way too.

You decide to try to rectify or reverse the situation. After giving the matter some thought, you decide that the best strategy is to get your closest colleagues together and raise your concerns. Having the whole group present would provide more influence than trying to reach each person individually. You decide to invite your group over for coffee, with the plan to bring up your agenda.

In preparation, you think through how you will approach the topic. You decide to allow some time for chitchat and for everyone to get re-acquainted. You plan to have coffee and some snacks to break the ice and get everyone mixing. You decide that the best way to broach the subject is to begin with your feelings of loss. Because the discussion could disintegrate into a gripe session if there is no plan put forth, you come up with several suggestions that the group could consider.

In addition to planning the content, you spend some time preparing yourself emotionally for the meeting with your fellow students. You envision yourself and your colleagues looking relaxed. You imagine that when you raise the issue of lack of cooperative support your classmates look interested and agree with your assessment of the situation. In your mind's eye others look eager to return to your more cooperative ways of relating to each other, and there are even suggestions from the group members.

When you are prepared, you carry out your plan. Following is what an assertive approach to your request for support might be like.

An Assertive Approach

After your colleagues have enjoyed getting re-acquainted, you bring up your issue in the following way:

> **Assertive You:** "I'm really enjoying seeing all of you again. It's like old times. Something I've noticed as we get further along in the program is that we are becoming more obsessed with grades. It's really bothering me that we don't share ideas and material the way we used to. It's like we are all operating in isolation—each student for herself. It's too cutthroat for me. I'd like to propose that we restart our weekly study group so that we can share our ideas and knowledge, and our books and articles too. I think we could really help each other, and it would make us feel more like we were in this thing together instead of in competition. What do you think?"

> **Colleague:** "I think it's a great idea. I've been feeling lonely for our shared times, but I guess I just assumed you guys were so 'nose to the grindstone' that you didn't need our group support. I'd love to start meeting again."

> **Another Colleague:** "I think it would be a good idea to make a list of what projects we are working on and circulate it. Then when we find articles on someone's topic we could let them know. It wouldn't take any more time, and it would really help us all out."

> **Another Colleague:** "I'm house sitting for my brother and he has a huge dining room table that we could use for our meetings . . . ."

Your assertive strategy worked! By putting effort into setting the scene and allowing the opportunity for people to realize how much they had missed each other, you furthered your cause immensely. By expressing your feelings, you avoided blaming anyone. Including a suggestion got the ball rolling and gave others a chance to put forth their ideas. It is likely that your strategy has got things in motion for securing the cooperative support you were after.

Consider how things might have gone if you had chosen an unassertive approach.

An Unassertive Approach

When we act unassertively, at some level we are conveying that we do not have much faith in ourselves or our ideas. If we are not able to convey that we believe strongly in what we are saying, then it is highly unlikely that we will convince anyone else. Behaving unassertively involves little advance preparation and little visualization of positive outcomes. When we act unassertively we look unsure and sound hesitant. Here is what your strategy might have been like if you had taken an unassertive approach:

You invite your colleagues over for coffee and sooner or later the conversation rolls around to school and grades. Soon every one is comparing how they are doing on their assignments and an uncomfortable atmosphere of competition surfaces. You attempt to intervene with:

Unassertive You: "Uh, . . . this is the kind of thing I find so disappointing . . . I mean, all we ever talk about any more is grades and who's got an A . . ."

A Colleague: "Well, it's only natural. That's what we are here for. Grades are the most important thing in our lives as students."

Unassertive You: "Well, they are important, I agree. But so is feeling good and sharing things with friends."

A Colleague: "Yes, but when we get good grades that's the thing that makes us feel good these days."

Unassertive You: "Well, I was wondering if we could help each other out more, like we used to do. Don't you ever long to get our study group together?"

A Colleague: "Those days were fun. But now we hardly take any of the same subjects. I'm afraid it would take more time and energy than I've got to get us together and make it time well spent."

Being unassertive got you nowhere except feeling more discouraged about the situation. By not presenting a positive, concrete solution to your complaints you missed an opportunity to influence your colleagues' outlook on the situation. You avoided emphasizing the benefits of sharing and consequently your colleagues swayed the argument to the negative aspects of meeting. Not only did you fail to get cooperation, but you are likely feeling disappointed in your lack of assertiveness.

Consider how the scene might change if you were aggressive.

An Aggressive Approach

Although we may get what we want when we are aggressive, we lose out on the good feelings between ourself and the other person. Sometimes the bad feelings generated by aggressiveness take extensive time to repair.

Here is one possible scenario if you were to use an aggressive approach:

Aggressive You: "Come on you guys, stop talking about school and grades. I've had enough of it. You've got your heads buried so deeply in the books that you can't even take time to have fun. I remember when you used to be a fun group to be with. Now I get the feeling that if anyone does well it's like stealing marks from each other. When are you going to wake up and realize that those little numbers on your papers aren't nearly as important as having some contact as people."

A Colleague: "Well, you may not care about grades, but I do. I might want to go to graduate school some day and my grades have to be good. You don't even take that into consideration."

Another Colleague: "If you can't even see how important school is to some of us, then there's no point in getting together. I think we're on different wavelengths."

By being aggressive you have further ostracized yourself from your source of support. Your demonstration of insensitivity about the value your friends put on school has cost you their cooperation. By not seeing things through their eyes you have lost your connection to a valuable source of support.

Making a Request for Physical Support

You are a nurse working on a surgical unit in a general hospital. About 6 months ago the head nurse asked all nursing personnel to complete a health history on newly admitted clients. Part of this history involves asking personal questions about, for example, drug use, religious beliefs, and sleeping habits. Any information which might be important for the nursing staff to know about clients who will be undergoing an anaesthetic is included. There is no place to interview clients in private on your unit, and you have felt uncomfortable asking clients some of these questions within the hearing range of other clients and staff on the unit. To complete these initial histories you need the physical support of adequate private space.

You have identified what dissatisfies you about the lack of private space; now you need to decide how you would like to see things changed. You know there is absolutely no possibility of getting a room designated for interviewing alone because of budget cutbacks. What would be satisfactory is a room that could be booked in advance for a private interview with clients and used for other purposes as well. There is a room on the unit which is designated for Dr. Gait, the physician in charge of the unit. She makes rounds each morning and occasionally uses her room then, but at other times it is not used by anyone. You decide to attempt to secure access to Dr. Gait's office for the purpose of completing the initial histories on clients. It is important to have the privacy and you feel certain that you can complete the histories more accurately if you had it.

Having decided to seek support, the next step is to determine how to go about acquiring it. The interpersonal style you use to make your request will greatly influence the outcome. A meek or indirect approach leaves you open to being misunderstood or ignored. An aggressive or overly confrontative presentation will put others on the defensive and likely result in rejection. A balance of speaking up for your rights for support without hurting others is what the situation requires.

You already know that the other nurses on the unit agree that a private room is necessary. The lines of communication on the unit dictate that you should make your request to the head nurse. You decide that she needs some advance notice about the issue, and you approach her with a request for a meeting time to discuss the issue. Your request for a meeting is simple, straightforward, and clear:

> **Assertive You:** "Miss Peters, I would like to make an appointment with you to discuss the need for some private space in which to conduct our initial histories. I'm on duty for the next 3 days. Do you have about 15 or 20 minutes during that time when I can discuss this matter with you?"

Once the meeting has been arranged, you need to plan your strategy for the meeting. You have asked for about 15 minutes during which time you must convince Miss Peters of the importance of having a private place to interview clients. You prepare for the meeting by itemizing all the reasons you and your colleagues have come up with for needing privacy. Because you are well aware that you will have more success at having your request granted if you can present a reasonable solution, you itemize the reasons for using Dr. Gait's office so that you can defend suggesting it as a solution to the problem.

Having secured your facts, you now ready yourself for your encounter with Miss Peters. You prepare by visualizing yourself talking to her in a relaxed, confident manner. In your mind's eye you envision her listening to you intently, nodding her head in agreement with the points you are making. You imagine yourself successfully counteracting any arguments she has against the use of Dr. Gait's office. All in all, your covert rehearsal of the meeting is successful, increasing your confidence.

Here is an example of how your meeting with your head nurse, Miss Peters, might go if you were assertive.

An Assertive Approach

> **Assertive You:** "Thank you for setting aside the time to meet with me, Miss Peters. As you know I wish to discuss the need for some private space to complete the initial health histories on our clients. I've talked to the other nurses and we all agree that the histories provide some important information about our clients

that increases their safety in undergoing anaesthesia. Also it gives us a chance to relax the clients and put them at ease. However, there is one major problem we have encountered. Because there is no designated space for us to talk to our clients, we end up interviewing them in the corridor, or their rooms, or in the sunroom; in all these locations what they say can be overheard by other clients and staff. We are concerned that some clients may hold back information about themselves that might be important because of the lack of confidentiality.

"We would like to have a room where we could take newly admitted clients and interview them in private. A little checking shows that Dr. Gait rarely uses her office in the afternoons. I and the other nurses suggest that Dr. Gait's office might be a place we could use. What do you think of this idea?"

Miss Peters: "I can see your point about the privacy. As you know I'm interested in having the histories completed, so I would like to push for a room if the privacy will mean the histories will be more accurately completed. In the past Dr. Gait has wanted her office off limits to nurses because she has done her dictating and teaching to her residents in there. But from what you are saying she doesn't use the office for those purposes any more. I will talk to her about making her office available to our nursing staff in the afternoons. Thank you for your interest and your suggestions."

Your assertive strategy worked! By starting off stating that you and your colleagues supported the histories, you avoided putting your head nurse on the defensive and you invited her to listen. Your reasons for needing a private room were sound on two counts: client safety and client respect. Your astute inclusion of the data about the vacancy of Dr. Gait's office added credibility to your suggestion. You ended your suggestion by respectfully inviting the head nurse's opinion. Your delivery was forthright. Never once did you beat around the bush or sound hesitant. And you did not have to rush since you had pre-booked the time with your head nurse.

Here are some examples of ineffective ways to make the same request for a private room.

An Unassertive Approach

When we behave unassertively we do not give full credit to our needs. We act shyly, or make light of factors that are really important to us. When we avoid expressing ourselves clearly and forthrightly, we waive control over our legitimate rights. Behaving unassertively invites others to walk all over us.

In this situation an unassertive nurse would not likely book time with her head nurse, but probably she would chance that she could catch the head nurse's attention without advance notice. Unassertive nurses would not likely plan an effective strategy in advance, and would not likely envision themselves being successful. Verbally unassertive approaches are limp, unclear, and do not convey confidence or conviction. Here is an example of an unassertive approach:

Unassertive You: "Uh, Miss Peters, do you have a few minutes?"

Miss Peters has no idea what you want to talk to her about, nor how long it will take. If she is a typically busy head nurse, she will probably have other things planned for that moment.

Miss Peters: "I can see you briefly. What is it about?"

Unassertive You: "Well, it's about those histories you want us to do on the new clients. I think it's rather hard . . . I mean, sometimes there are so many people around. It's hard to talk to the clients when there's no privacy, do you know what I mean? Something's really got to be done, I think."

It is possible that this approach may put Miss Peters on the defensive. You have given the impression that completing the histories is difficult by not finishing your sentence. You have provided no rationale for the idea that privacy is essential. By not clearly explaining your points you are ensuring that Miss Peters will not understand, and then she will not be sympathetic to your cause.

Miss Peters: "Well, I realize that it might be difficult to do the histories, but it's essential that the information be collected. Client safety in the O.R. depends on this information."

Unassertive You: "Uh, yes . . . it is important. It's just that, you know, it's hard to talk to the clients when there are other people around. Isn't there a quiet place we could go to? How about Dr. Gait's office?"

Miss Peters: "Well, you know that she needs her office to be available to her. You can always use a quiet corner of the sunroom, or even ask the other clients to leave the room if you want to have a private interview."

Unassertive You: "Yeah . . . I guess so. I haven't tried that yet. Maybe that'll work. . . . I hate to ask a client to leave, . . . but I'll give it a try."

You have lost your case! By not being clear about what you wanted, and not articulately defending your suggestion to your head nurse, you have permitted your head nurse to overlook your suggestion and to force you to continue the way you have been. Had you better prepared your defence and your speech you may have secured the support you were requesting.

An Aggressive Approach

When we behave aggressively we forget to give due respect to the other person's rights. We become so intent on getting what we want that we tend to bulldoze the other person. Here is an example of an aggressive approach to trying to secure a private place for interviewing:

> **Aggressive You:** "Miss Peters, I need to see you as soon as possible about the initial histories. When can you see me? Today?"

This rush on Miss Peters does not give her much breathing space. You have indicated there is an urgency about your need to see her which is out of proportion to the truth. In no way have you respected her own timetable or any agenda she may wish to complete. Already she is probably on the defensive.

When you get to see Miss Peters you begin with:

> **Aggressive You:** "You've got to do something about getting us a quiet place to do these initial histories you want done on all the clients. It's impossible to do them when everyone can hear what you are saying. How would you like to spill your guts about your sex life or pills you take when every client and staff member around can hear? If you don't get us a quiet place then they just won't be done right. Why can't we use Dr. Gait's office? We nurses don't have any private space and this one doctor has a whole office to herself."

> **Miss Peters:** "It's not up to you to dictate how the office space will be assigned on the unit. When you've learned proper etiquette and protocol I'd be glad to re-discuss this issue with you. In the meantime, do the best you can. That'll be all for today."

You have made your dissatisfaction very clear. However, in the process of doing so you have put your head nurse on the defensive and created a rift between you. There are now two problems to be solved: the lack of privacy and the discord between the two of you. When we attack another person, they are likely to divert energy to their injured feelings instead of the issue for which you are fighting. Using an aggressive approach like this diminishes the chances that you will secure the physical support you were hoping to get.

The Importance of Planning an Assertive Strategy for Making Requests

The examples above illustrate the importance of planning and implementing an assertive strategy for seeking cognitive, affective, or physical support. If it is important for you to have the support you have identified, then it is important to invest the time and energy in securing it. As a nurse, you spend considerable energy trying to meet your clients' needs for support. If you can secure the support you need at work or school, then it is more likely that you will have the energy to extend support to your clients and colleagues. Nurses who keep on giving without adequate cognitive, affective, or physical support are probably draining their own reserves. We spend a lot of time trying to get our clients to take care of their health; securing the support we need as nurses provides them with an example to follow.

Just because you use an assertive approach does not mean that you will get the support you are after. Sometimes support is not forthcoming, no matter what strategy is used. On occasion your colleagues may not have the interest or skills to support you. Other times there may not be the money or time to provide you with the support you are seeking. At those times you must decide whether you can continue to work in the system without the support. If you cannot secure the support you need from others at work or school, you may be able to get some support from friends or family to see you through. Only *you* can decide whether the support is adequate. Since you are the seeker and receiver, it is your perception of the support that is important.

Providing Support at Work and School

The CAPS (Cognitive, Affective, Physical Support) framework is helpful for articulating exactly what support you need at work and school. It can also be a guideline to help you determine your colleagues' need for support. Support is one of those nebulous concepts and breaking it down into cognitive, affective, and physical components helps you to decipher your colleagues' needs for support. One way to get support is to offer it to others. In so doing a bond is built between you which encourages both parties to give and take.

Whether in the classroom or on the wards, the work of nursing can be stressful. The literature has indicated that efforts to counteract this stress have been effective. Several authors have described how structured group support meetings may relieve the negative impact on nurses working in intensive care areas (Skinner, 1980; Scully, 1981). The absence of pathological symptoms in palliative care nurses was attributed to the availability of a support group (Quenneville, Falardeau & Rochette, 1981-1982). Another study reported that it was the ongoing day-to-day support that made hospice nurses feel energetic and cared for at work (Smith & Varoglu, 1983).

Contributing to the effort to build up a solid support system at work and school will contribute to your feelings of confidence and competence. It is worth the effort to learn the assertive way to make requests for the support you need.

PRACTICING MAKING REQUESTS FOR SUPPORT

Exercise 1. In relation to a unit where you are working, or to school, complete the Credits and Debits in Your Support System at Work or School. Answer the two questions:

1. What exactly dissatisfies me about the quality or quantity of support?
2. If I had a choice, how would I change things to ensure that I would get the support I need?

Take one area where you would like more support and plan an assertive strategy for securing it. Think about who is the best person to approach to get this support. If more than one person is involved, is it better to see them individually or in a group? What is the best approach to take? Consider whether you should provide advance notice in the form of a memo or whether your request would be better made spontaneously. Think about what data you will need to defend your need for this support. If you need information from others, make sure you give them adequate time to prepare it for you. If it would be helpful for your potential supporter to have access to any information, make sure you bring a copy for him or her. Consider your timing carefully. Good timing can facilitate the meeting of your request, and bad timing can ensure that your needs for support will go to the bottom of the list.

It may be helpful for you to write down your desired outcome and the strategy you intend to use. This act will formalize your intent and force you to think through your strategy. As you proceed you will have something concrete to refer to.

Once you are satisfied with your strategy, then carry it out. Attempt to be assertive in your approach, and avoid being unassertive or aggressive.

As soon as possible after the event, review what went well and what you would like to have done differently. If you were successful in securing the support you were after, jot down what made your request so successful. Conversely, if you did not secure the support you were after, what factors contributed to this disappointment? Examine whether your success or failure was because of your strategy and approach or some other factors.

After you have carried out this exercise on your own, compare notes with your colleagues. In general, what factors contribute to the success of securing the support you need?

To gain competence in making requests in an assertive way, practice this exercise again for some of the other gaps in your cognitive, affective, or physical support system.

Exercise 2. For this exercise work in threes. One person will request support from another in your group. The third person will give feedback on how assertively the requester sought support. When you are the requester, choose one of the cognitive, affective, or physical supports that you would like to secure. Explain to the person roleplaying the provider of this support some details of her role (she is a teacher or a colleague, etc.).

When you are clear about your roles, act out a scene where you are requesting support. After you have completed your request, seek feedback from the person providing the support and the feedback giver on how assertive you were in making your request.

What have you learned about your ability to be assertive in requesting support? Where do you excel in being assertive? What suggestions do you have for improving your ability to be assertive?

Switch roles so that each of you has the opportunity to roleplay the requester, the provider, and the feedback giver.

After you have done this exercise in your small groups, join your colleagues in the rest of your class and compare what you have learned about requesting support.

REFERENCES

Baider, L. & Porath, S. (1981). Uncovering fear: Group experience of nurses in a cancer ward. *International Journal of Nursing Studies, 18,* 47-52.

Callahan, M. (1990). Applauding the artistry of nursing. *Nursing 90, 20* (10), 63-64.

Cobb, S. (1976). Social support as a moderator of life stress. *Psychosomatic Medicine, 38* (5), pp. 300-314.

Coleman, B. (1990). Advanced nursing apprenticeship program: A strategy for retention of experienced critical care nurses. *Heart & Lung, 19* (3), 236-242.

Corcoran, N.M., Meyer, L.A., Magliaro, B.L. (1990). Retention: The key to the 21st century for health care institutions. *Nursing Administration Quarterly, 14* (4), 23-31.

Deming, A.L. (1984). Personal effectiveness groups: A new approach to faculty development. *Journal of College Student Personnel,* January, 54-60.

Diminno, M., & Thompson, E. (1980). An interactional support group for graduate nursing students: A report. *Journal of Nursing Education, 19* (3), pp. 16-22.

Dimond, M., & Jones, S.L. (1983). Social support: A review and theoretical integration. In P.L. Chinn (Ed.), *Advances in Nursing Theory Development,* (pp. 235-249). Rockville, Md.: An Aspen Publication.

Doering, L. (1990). Recruitment and retention: Successful strategies in critical care. *Heart & Lung, 19* (3), 220-224.

Franks, J.C., & Hayden, M.J. (1990). Establishing a permanent charge nurse support group. *Nursing Management, 21* (6), 46-48.

Geissler, E.M. (1990). Nurturance flows two ways. *American Journal of Nursing, 90* (4), 72-74.

Goetzel, R.Z., Shelov, S., & Croen, L.G. (1983). Evaluating medical student self-help support groups: A general systems model. *Small Group Behavior, 14,* (3), 337-352.

Gottlieb, B.H. (1983). *Social support strategies: Guidelines for mental health practice.* (Volume 7, Sage studies in community mental health.) Beverly Hills, Calif.: Sage Publications.

Gray-Toft, P., & Anderson, J.G. (1983). A hospital staff support program: Design and evaluation. *International Journal of Nursing Studies, 20* (3), 137-147.

Hay, D. & Oken, D. (1972). The psychological stresses of Intensive Care Unit nursing. *Psychosomatic Medicine, 4* (2), 109-118.

Huttner, C.A. (1990). Strategies for recruitment and retention of critical care nurses: A cardiovascular program experience. *Heart & Lung, 19* (3), 230-236.

Jacobs, R. (1982). Nurses matter too. *Nursing Mirror,* February, 27-29.

Kinsey, D.C. (1990). Mentorship and influence in nursing. *Nursing Management, 21* (5), 45-46.

Ligon, R. (1990). A blueprint for involving staff in policy development. *Nursing Management, 21* (7), 30.

Lin, N., Ensel, W., Simeone, R., & Kwo, W. (1979). Social support, stressful life events, and illness: a model and an empirical test. *Journal of Health and Social Behavior,* 20, pp. 108-119.

McDermott, B. (1983). A preventive approach to staff stress. *Canadian Nurse, 79* (2), 27-29.

Mueller, D.P. (1980). Social networks: A promising direction for research on the relationship of social environment to psychiatric disorder. *Social Sciences and Medicine, 14A,* 147-161.

Pilisuk, M., & Froland, C. (1978). Kinship, social networks, social support and health. *Social Sciences and Medicine,* 12B, pp. 273-280.

Quenneville, Y., Falardeau, M., & Rochette, D. (1981-82). Evaluation of staff support system in a palliative care unit. *OMEGA, 12* (4), pp. 355-358.

Sanford, K. (1990). Nurses, let's support each other more. *Nursing 90, 20* (1), 109-118.

Scully, R. (1981). Staff support groups: helping nurses to help themselves. *The Journal of Nursing Administration, 11* (3), pp. 48-51.

Skinner, K. (1980). Support group for ICU nurses. *Nursing Outlook,* May, pp. 296-299.

Smith, S.P. (1984). Need support at work? Think CAPs. *Canadian Nurse, 81* (8), pp. 40-43.

Smith, S.P., & Varoglu, G. (1983). Support for Hospice nurses. In K.A. Mitchell (Ed.), *Proceedings of the first annual Pacific Health Forum '83,* pp. 101-111. UBC, Vancouver, B.C.: University of British Columbia Health Care & Epidemiology Alumni Association.

Smith, S.P. (1986). Support for nurses working in extended-care. University of Victoria, Victoria, B.C., Unpublished masters thesis.

Spitzer-Lehmann, R. (1990). Recruitment and retention of our greatext asset. *Nursing Administrative Quarterly, 14* (4), 66-69.

Taerk, G. (1983). Psychological support of oncology nurses: A role for the liaison psychiatrist. *Canadian Journal of Psychiatry, 28,* 532-535.

Webster, S., Kelly, L.A., Johst, B., Weber, R., & Wickes, L. (1982). A method of stress management: The support group. *Nursing Management, 13* (9), 26-30.

Weiner, M.F., & Caldwell, T. (1983). The process and impact of an ICU nurse support group. *International Journal of Psychiatry in Medicine, 13* (1), 47-55.

White, S.K. (1990). Symposium on successful recruitment and retention strategies in critical care: Overview. *Heart & Lung, 19* (3), 219-220.

SUGGESTIONS FOR FURTHER READING

Flanagan, L. (1990). *Survival skills in the workplace: What every nurse should know.* Kansas City, Mo.: American Nurses' Association.

This booklet guides nurses get the support they need to make the most of their skills and abilities in the workplace of the 1990s, with more complex healthcare services, scarcer financial resources, increasing ethical dilemmas, and personnel shortages.

Wilson, G.L., Hantz, A.M., & Hanna, M.S. (1985). *Interpersonal growth through communication.* Dubuque, Iowa: Wm. C. Brown Publishers.

Chapter 8, Defending and Supporting, delineates defensive and supportive communication for nurse readers and provides ways to help nurses choose to remain supportive.

PART 2

POSITIVE COMMUNICATION AFFECT

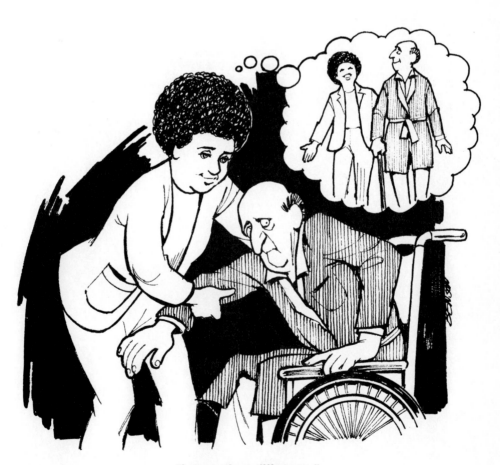

"I can make a difference."

INTRODUCTION TO PART 2: POSITIVE COMMUNICATION AFFECT

After studying Part One you understand the essential communication behaviors for relating to clients and colleagues in assertive and responsible ways. Part Two will increase your desire to communicate assertively and responsibly.

You can understand all there is to know about the essential communication behaviors but until you feel comfortable and self-assured your skill level will not grow to its full potential of excellence. The next four chapters will teach you ways to increase your confidence and comfort in communicating assertively and responsibly.

There are several factors which interfere with nurses' ability to communicate assertively and responsibly. You may never have been exposed to, or reinforced for, communicating assertively and responsibly; worse, you may have been discouraged or punished in some way for your attempts. Chapter 15, Feedback, teaches you how to seek and accept feedback on the way you communicate so that you can shape your method of relating to clients and colleagues in a positive way. As you see your improvement, your desire to communicate effectively will grow.

There are some myths that prevent nurses from communicating assertively and responsibly. You may think you have to perfect the interpersonal communication behaviors you learned in Part One before using them with clients and colleagues. Or you may believe that if you try to communicate assertively and responsibly you will fail. Beliefs like these prevent you from becoming a skilled communicator. By using the methods you will learn in Part.Two you can surmount these negative traps. Relaxation (chapter 16), Imagery (chapter 17), and Positive Self-Talk (chapter 18) present you with techniques for remaining calm, rationally assessing your skill level, keeping yourself focused on your strengths, and envisioning yourself communicating successfully. You will learn to overcome your fear of making a mistake and being overwhelmed if your communication is not perfect.

An enhanced positive communication affect, combined with your communication competence, will prepare you for Part Three, where you will augment your communication skill level.

CHAPTER 15

Feedback

*"Show me the man who insists that he
welcomes criticism if only it is 'constructive'
and I will show you a man who does not
want to hear any criticism at all."*

Harold L. Ickes

OBJECTIVES

The ability to give and receive feedback is one that you will use time and time again, in both your personal and professional lives. By the end of this chapter you will be able to explain the meaning of feedback and articulate why it is important in developing your interpersonal communication skill level.

The exercises at the end of most of the chapters in this book provide chances for you to practise seeking, receiving, and giving feedback. You are encouraged to take the opportunity to experience delivering feedback that is receivable. It is hoped that you will become more comfortable seeking and receiving feedback.

THE IMPORTANCE OF FEEDBACK

Unraveling the meaning of feedback is best done by breaking it down into its two components—"feed" and "back." In one sense of the word, "feed" implies to nourish, even comfort, or to meet another's needs. "Back" in this context is to return something to another. Combining these two notions, feedback means the returning of nourishment to another person. In this sense, feedback is something positive—a gift for the other person. The gift that is given is one person's thoughts and feelings about another's behavior.

■The author gratefully acknowledges Dr. Vance Peavy's work on feedback.

Feedback helps us see our behavior from another's perspective. This reflection tells us how someone else is reacting to our communication. This picture helps us decide whether to continue acting in the same way or to change. Viewed this way, feedback is a springboard for self-growth. Feeling happy with ourselves is one of the most joyous experiences in life. This contentment is an acknowledgement of what we like about ourselves and it solidifies our self-concept. Contemplating a change in our way of behaving is really envisioning a new self-concept. Feedback has the potential for expanding our development as human beings.

There is a difference between giving feedback and giving advice. Giving feedback is merely a reflection about how another's behavior has affected us, not advice about how a person should change. After receiving our feedback, clients or colleagues may wish to make changes in their behavior. One thing we might be asked is: "What do you think I should do to change?" Often we will have some advice, but a note of caution is in order.

To avoid hurting the feelings of receivers, and to ensure we are being respectful, these options should be made as suggestions for their consideration. We can never know what changes will be comfortable or suitable for another person, because each of us must decide what suits our personal style and priorities. Our suggestions will be more readily received if they are offered tentatively, such as:

"Something I've tried is this. . . ." "Perhaps adding this change will help you." Or "When I was trying to change in the same way, my sister-in-law suggested I do this. . . . It worked for me and maybe it will work for you."

These examples allow the receiver the final option of accepting or rejecting.

For feedback to be integrated it must be delivered in a way that is receivable and the receiver must be open to considering the feedback. Here are some steps you can follow to increase the probability that your feedback will be accepted.

How to Give Feedback
Check Your Agenda for Wanting to Give Feedback

What is motivating you to give feedback? What do you hope to accomplish by delivering feedback? Any reasons based on the belief that your feedback will benefit the other person by increasing the opportunities for self-growth are acceptable to the intention of feedback. There are many reasons for giving feedback that are unacceptable in a caring, therapeutic relationship. Feeling irritable and wanting to lash out at another as a way of getting revenge, wanting to display our superior knowledge to "show up" another, or wanting to rigidly control the behavior of clients or colleagues because of intolerance are not good reasons for giving feedback.

Gain Permission to Give Feedback

The next step is to gain permission from your client or colleague to give feedback. Requesting permission may be done verbally by simply asking if the other person would like the feedback. Or the request can be made through a nonverbal checking out.

The following example includes verbal and nonverbal ways of getting permission to give feedback.

You have been teaching a new father to bathe his newborn and he has given a return demonstration.

> "I noticed how securely you have been holding your baby daughter—I'm sure it makes her feel safe and secure. It looks like she's enjoying the bath you are giving her and especially how you are talking to her. I'd like to point out one suggestion for improvement."

Here you pause and look at the father who nods his approval for you to continue.

> "When you allow your daughter's umbilical cord to get wet it increases the chance that she'll get an infection. I've got some suggestions, if you'd like to hear them, for how you could keep her cord dry."

Again you make eye contact with the father and do not proceed until he conveys his interest in your information.

> "Some ways to keep the cord dry are to fill the tub with less water and hold her at about a 45-degree angle. Also you can squeeze out the washcloth so that water doesn't accidentally drip on her cord. What do you think of these suggestions?"

Be Specific

Giving feedback to clients or colleagues is not your chance to bombard them with everything about their behavior that you like or dislike. To give your feedback impact you must focus on specific, observable behavior. The following situation between two nurse colleagues illustrates how to be specific when giving feedback.

You are on the evening shift and are still relatively new to the procedures on the unit. Before the night shift comes on you always have last minute charting and tying together of loose ends for your report. For the past 4 nights one of the night nurses has come on duty ½ hour early and tried to engage you in a social conversation. Your hints that you don't have time to talk at that moment have been ignored and she has persisted in bending your ear about her date or how she slept that day. You approach her with:

"Rhonda, I'd like to talk to you about how your coming on early and talking to me is affecting me."

At this point you wait until she's agreeable to discuss the issue and proceed with:

"I'd love to talk with you, but when you try to capture my attention at the end of my shift it agitates me because I'm trying to tie up so many loose ends and get things in order for the night shift. I find myself getting so tense that I can't pay enough attention to what you are trying to tell me and I don't get my work completed the way I'd like to. Do you understand what I'm saying?"

Here you must pause and give Rhonda a chance to respond. You might proceed with:

"I've got a suggestion that will allow me to get my last-minute work done and still give us a chance to visit before I leave. Want to hear it?"

Keeping your feedback to observable behavior prevents you from blurting out something cruel like: "Can't you wait till your shift starts to talk my ear off?" Or "I can't stand you bugging me like this!" Being specific helps you keep feedback realistic and acceptable.

Convey Your Perspective

When you give feedback you must remind yourself that you are reporting your view of things. Nothing is innately or objectively right or wrong about your perspective; it is simply how you see the world. However, since every relationship you have with colleagues and clients has importance and influence for both parties, your reactions are important to others.

When looking in the mirror after getting your hair cut in a new style, you might smile with approval, blush with embarrassment, or refuse to pay for such an outrageous coiffure! The hairdresser might glow with pleasure at your sophisticated new image and your friends may look ambivalent about the new you. Any of these reactions is legitimate and none is better than the other. Each reaction is feedback based on the viewer's frame of reference. You need to keep in mind when you are giving feedback that, important as your views are, the receiver may not agree with your perspective.

To ensure that you give feedback respectfully, you can couch your comments with phrases like these:

"As I see it . . ."
"I felt happy (sad) when you clapped (did not applaud)."
"From my perspective . . ."
"The way I see things is . . ."

Using the first person to convey your thoughts and feelings prevents you from accusing or labeling the other person's behavior.

Invite Comments from the Receiver

Since the feedback you give is from your perspective, it is important to keep in mind your client's or colleague's feelings about receiving your comments. One way to do this is to check out their reactions with phrases like: "What do you think about my comments to you?" or, "Could you tell me your reactions to what I've just told you . . .?" Giving feedback requires consideration. You never know how a client or colleague will respond to your feedback and you must allow them to express their reactions. People need time to grasp what you are saying, mull it over, ask for more information, and express their feelings and thoughts about what you have said.

Be Genuine

It warrants saying that the giver of feedback should be honest when expressing his views. If you do not mean it, do not say it! When you are sincere in giving feedback you build trust. If you are verbalizing something positive, but the frown on your face indicates displeasure, then the receiver of your feedback will get a mixed message. It is important to keep your verbal and nonverbal behavior congruent.

Check Out How Your Feedback Is Being Received

If you can honestly say that the feedback was given in the best interests of the receiver, if you gained permission before proceeding with your feedback, and if you were specific in your comments and gave them tentatively, then you know within yourself that you have given feedback in a caring way.

In addition to your self-assessment, you can also pick up clues from your clients or colleagues about whether your way of giving feedback is acceptable. If they indicate that they understand what you are saying, and verbally and nonverbally indicate that they would like you to continue, then you know that your manner of giving feedback is respectful. If they become embarrassed, angry, or move away from you, they may be indicating that they are not yet ready to receive any feedback from you, or at least not in the dosage you are administering. When you pick up clues that your clients or colleagues are becoming defensive about your comments it is important that you pause and check with them on how to proceed. You might stop altogether or choose gentler and more receivable words.

How to Receive Feedback

Because feedback is an opportunity for self-growth it is worthwhile knowing how to get the most out of the experience. Clearly, giving feedback requires risking another's feelings and the relationship you have. Knowing about that risk has implications for how you can act when one of your clients or colleagues takes the chance to give you feedback.

Center

It is important to center when receiving feedback. Centering means not thinking or worrying about some other issue but attending to the feedback and respectfully listening.

Arrange to Have Enough Time to Receive the Feedback

Being unrushed at the time feedback is being given is also important. If you know you are hurried, then convey to your client or colleague that you value receiving his ideas and you would like to schedule another time to hear them. Making another appointment is important because it indicates that you respect his opinions and intend to follow through. You could say:

> "I am touched that you have gone to the effort of preparing some feedback for me on the inservice I gave. Could we schedule a convenient time to go over your views? I want to hear what you have to say when I'm not so pressed for time as I am today, so I can take it all in."

Make Sure You Understand the Feedback

Let the feedback giver have the floor long enough to clearly state his views and then ask questions about anything that was unclear.

After your nursing instructor has given you feedback on your sterile technique you might respond with:

> "I think I understand your comments. You noticed I opened the tray before washing my hands and then I left the tray exposed to the air while I washed them. And I had the client's furniture placed in my way so I had to lean over the sterile field and I almost contaminated it. I think those were the main points where I need to improve, weren't they?"

It is not only respectful to repeat the feedback to ensure that you understood but it is a way of once more outlining the points as a reminder for yourself.

Request Some Guidance on How to Change

If you would like to make changes in your behavior because of the feedback, then ask for some directions for change *if* you genuinely want to hear them. Consider this example:

Your student nurse colleague has given you some feedback about your leadership style during your first week as team leader. Most of her comments were positive, but she also indicated that she occasionally felt slighted or put down when you unilaterally made decisions about the nursing care for her clients.

You feel a bit shocked to hear about her reaction because you had assumed that it was up to you as team leader to completely take charge, but you feel badly that your style of not consulting your team members may cause them to feel unimportant or left out. Because you want to change to a more respectful leadership style you could ask your colleague:

> "Thank you for your comments. I'm pleased with where I seem to be doing well but I really want to overcome being so autocratic. What could I do differently as team leader to make you feel more included in the decision making for your clients?"

Show Appreciation for the Feedback

Thank your client or colleague for his feedback. Even if you are not going to change, it has likely been of benefit to hear another's point of view about your behavior, and for this information you can express your gratitude. Here is an example:

One of your nursing instructors tells you that she fears your habit of only taking half of the allotted time for lunch will wear you out, and she worries about your health. You respond with:

> "Thanks for your concern, Mrs. Brown. I find that the physical nursing care on this medical floor demands much more of me than the E.N.T. floor I just came from, where I had more than enough time. I'm slowly getting more accustomed to the pace in the 9 days I've been here, and I'm sure I'll soon be organized and relaxed enough to take the full break at lunch time."

Think about the Feedback You Receive

It is you who will benefit from thinking over any feedback you have been given. Take the opportunity to consider the implications of feedback given to you. Here is an example:

One of your patients, uncomfortable because of her pain, often lashes out at others. As you start her bath one morning she snarls at you:

> "Oh! It's you! Miss Sugary Sweet Nancy Nurse! Your smile is sickening and your cheeriness is just too much to take this morning! Go away and find someone else to gush over!"

Your first reaction may be one of hurt. Or you may brush off her comments and rationalize that she spoke them out of her pain and did not really mean them. As time passes you might find yourself recalling her words and starting to wonder if you are too cheery and bubbly with your clients to the point that you keep your distance and do not allow yourself to reach out to their sadness or worries. To be fair to yourself you should really check out the answer to your concern about your possible insensitivity.

By re-evaluating your ability to be warm and compassionate with your clients you will learn about your strong points and areas where you could be connecting more humanly with your clients. If you can make use of the feedback you receive it can provide you with directions for your personal and professional growth and development.

About Seeking Feedback

As you get comfortable with receiving feedback you may wish to seek out feedback from others before they offer it. To seek out feedback is to publicly announce that you are ready for self-growth; it implies that you have the confidence to look at your strengths and areas where you could make improvements.

Be Sure You Are Ready to Receive Feedback

Before seeking feedback check to see that you are really ready to receive it. When you are not fully open to receiving feedback you will convey that message either verbally or nonverbally. Verbally you may become angry, get defensive, or make excuses to rationalize your behavior. Nonverbally you may physically tune out feedback by losing eye contact, turning your body away, or folding your arms to create a barrier against the penetration of the feedback. Both these verbal and nonverbal responses are disrespectful to the person from whom you are asking feedback.

There are times when we are simply not ready to hear feedback. In those cases we should protect ourselves and not seek out other's reactions until we are confident enough to examine them. Receiving feedback with implications for change when we feel shaky or unconfident may only serve to make us feel worse about ourselves. It is a risk to ask for feedback; when we are ready to receive feedback it then has great potential for self-growth.

Be Specific in Your Request for Feedback

Clarify which aspects of your behavior you want feedback about. Delineating those areas will help your clients and colleagues focus and ensure that you receive the information you want to hear.

For example, after you complete a preoperative teaching session with your surgical client you ask him:

"What did you think about the session?"

This request for feedback is vague and would not help your client to focus on any particular area.

The following request would help your client to focus his comments:

"I included these diagrams because I hoped it would make you familiar with some of the equipment you'll see in the recovery room and in the unit. Did the pictures help to clarify things for you?"

Feedback and Caring Communication

If you follow the guidelines for giving, receiving, and seeking feedback outlined above, your feedback behavior will be assertive. Clearly, feedback is a responsible process because it allows participants to make use of all the information available. In your interpersonal communication skills development, feedback is a crucial factor.

PRACTICING FEEDBACK

Exercise 1. Find a partner in the class. One of you takes the listener role and the other the speaker role. The speaker will choose any topic and talk about it for 5 minutes. The listener will convey interest in the speaker's topic and use the communication behaviors she learned in Part One.

At the end of 5 minutes the listener will make a specific request to the speaker for feedback on her listening skills. The speaker will respond by giving feedback on the specific points requested by the listener. If appropriate the speaker will offer to give additional feedback on the abilities of the listener. The listener will respond to the feedback given by the speaker.

After you have finished this exercise take a few minutes to answer these questions.

As the speaker:
1. Was the listener's request for feedback specific?
2. Did the listener look like she was open to receiving feedback from you?

As the listener:
1. How specific was your request for feedback on your listening skills to your speaker?
2. How openly did you respond to your colleague's feedback?
3. Was the speaker's feedback to you specific, clear, and tentative?

After you have answered these questions, switch roles and repeat the exercise.

This exercise provides you with the chance to seek, receive, and give feedback. What have you learned about feedback from completing this exercise? Get together with the rest of the class and compare your notes about the important and delicate communication behavior of feedback.

Exercise 2. Over the next week pay attention to how others give you feedback. What do they do to make you feel comfortable about receiving their feedback? What could they do differently to make their feedback more receivable?

At the end of the week you may wish to get together with your colleagues and compare notes on your observations about effective and ineffective ways of giving feedback.

Exercise 3. Over the next few days keep track of how often you seek out feedback from others. What factors make it comfortable for you to seek feedback? Observe how you receive feedback. What is your assessment of your ability to receive feedback from others?

After you have completed this exercise, in the class as a whole pool your ideas about what factors increase the possibility that people will seek out feedback, and what increases the possibility that they will receive it openly.

Exercise 4. Now that you know how to seek and receive feedback, take every opportunity to get feedback on your interpersonal communication skills. Ask your classmates or instructors to observe you when you are interacting with clients. Or tape record your dialogue with a client and replay it for feedback. Taking the time to get their opinions and suggestions for improvement will enhance your ability to communicate in a caring way.

REFERENCE

Peavy, R.V. (1982). *Counselor training: Concepts and procedures for instructors and supervisors.* Unpublished manuscript. Department of Psychological Foundations in Education, University of Victoria, Victoria, B.C.

SUGGESTIONS FOR FURTHER READING

Brooks, W.D., & Emmert, P. (1980). *Interpersonal communication* (2nd ed.). Dubuque, Iowa: Wm. C. Brown Company Publishers.
  Chapter 7, Listening and Feedback, is divided into two parts. The first section discusses listening as a way of receiving feedback. The latter part of the chapter is devoted to a discussion of feedback. Definitions, types, problems, and effects of feedback are discussed.
Parsons, V., & Sanford, N. (1979). *Interpersonal interaction in nursing: Basic concepts in nurse-patient communication.* Menlo Park, Calif.: Addison-Wesley Publishing Company.
  Chapter 6 is all about feedback. Students will learn about different kinds of feedback and criteria for effective feedback. The chapter invites active reader participation with a pre-test, exercises, and post-test.
Weaver, R.L. (1981). *Understanding interpersonal communication* (2nd ed.). Glenview, Ill.: Scott, Foresman and Company.
  The importance of feedback is emphasized in chapter 4. Styles of positive feedback are explained and the importance of feedback in interpersonal communication is defended.

CHAPTER 16

Relaxation

*"One of the greatest necessities in
America is to discover creative solitude."*

Carl Sandburg

OBJECTIVES

As a student in the professional program of nursing, juggling a full life in
addition to your academic responsibilities, it is likely you have experienced some of the unwanted effects of stress. This chapter is designed to
encourage you to take charge of your reactions to stressful interpersonal
situations in the workplace and develop a habit of daily relaxation to
eliminate some of the negative buildup of stress in your body.

THE IMPORTANCE OF RELAXING YOUR BODY

Chapter 17, Imagery, and chapter 18, Positive Self-talk, will help you
prepare your mind for communicating effectively in your interpersonal
encounters with clients and colleagues. This chapter focuses on preparing
your body to relax during your workplace interactions. As a student in
nursing, you know that the communication between the mind and body is
interactive and messages from one affect the other. If your mind is worried about something, then your mental stewing can trigger tension in
your muscles, resulting in soreness, headaches, or digestive upsets. In
turn, bodily tension is an aggravating signal to your mind that you are
not at peace and something is "eating away at you." If you allow these
physical symptoms of stress to build up, you are in danger of eventually
damaging your body.

Carrying around tightened muscles, tension headaches, or digestive
disturbances reflects your "dis-ease" and registers diminished well being.
Built-up stress reactions steal valuable energy and put you at risk of
holding back or closing off in interpersonal relationships with clients and
colleagues. You can see that it is assertive to learn to minimize your ten-

sion and expand your relaxation response in the workplace. There are benefits for you and your clients (or colleagues) when you are more relaxed.

NURSING IS A STRESSFUL OCCUPATION

The literature abounds with documentation of the stressfulness of nursing as a profession. Calhoun (1980) cited four main events responsible for workplace stress and conflict: multiple levels of authority, heterogeneity of personnel, work interdependence, and specialization. All four criteria apply to the nursing profession. As nurses, you navigate several organizational structures to ensure client well-being: the nursing hierarchy, the medical association, and the agency's bureaucracy. To survive this organizational maze, you need effective interpersonal communication techniques and efficient management skills.

Not only do nurses require a sound knowledge in their own area of expertise but, in order to be effective in helping clients, you need to know the role and functions of other health care professionals, how to communicate clearly to other members of the health care team, and be able to coordinate work efforts of all these disciplines. The changing exposure to different personnel demands that you quickly size up how to relate to colleagues effectively, adding one more stress to an already complex working environment.

One of the most frequently cited sources of stress in nursing is the excessive workload demand, giving nurses the feeling that they are "in a race against time" (Nicholson, 1990). These factors are overlaid by nurses' day-to-day encounters with distressing and anxiety-provoking situations, and insufficient resources in these times of health care restraint.

Overriding all of these specific sources of stress is the well documented strain of being a helping professional (Freudenberger, 1983; Burke, 1985). As helping professionals each of you has a vision of what your workplace, colleagues, and clients will be like, and these images may not prepare you for the reality you encounter.

In the nursing literature of the 1970s and 1980s claims were made from all sectors of nursing about the stressfulness of each area.* The conclusion is that each area of nursing practice has its unique sources of stress related to differences in the quantity and quality of the nursing tasks.

The nursing literature of the 1990s attends to what health care workplaces have done or must do to recruit and retain nurses (Barigar & Sheafor, 1990; Coleman, 1990; Corcoran, Meyer, & Magliaro, 1990; Doering, 1990; Huttner, 1990; Spitzer-Lehmann, 1990; Werkema, 1990;

---

*(Vreeland & Ellis, 1969; Kornfeld, 1971; Hay & Oken, 1972; Cassem & Hackett, 1975; West, 1975; Oskins, 1980; Taerk, 1983; Baider & Porath, 1981; Chiriboga, Jenkins & Bailey, 1983; Stehle, 1981; Keane, Ducette, & Adler, 1985; Gentry, Foster, & Froehling, 1972; Maloney & Bartz, 1983).

White, 1990). Retention programs acknowledge the stressfulness of nursing as a career and promote organizational reforms to minimize some of the stressfulness of the nursing workplace.

Whatever agencies employing nurses can do to support nurses is welcome. As individual nurses we can, and must, complement these organizational reforms with our own methods of stress reduction. This chapter invites you to empower yourself by taking charge of your individual resourcefulness for increasing your relaxation response.

Part of your health teaching with any client is reviewing the basics of health promotion such as eating nutritiously, exercising regularly, securing adequate sleep, engaging in supportive social encounters, and making time for solitude and/or spiritual contemplation. Your knowledge of the benefits of taking care of oneself physically, emotionally, socially, and spiritually is sound. With the investment you have in health, you likely try to incorporate these health behaviors in your own daily life. The return on your investment is an enhanced feeling of well-being and a readiness to handle the stress of working as a nurse. This chapter invites you to add two practices to help you relax and prepare for stress in your interpersonal relationships with clients and colleagues: daily meditation and on-the-spot relaxation exercises. Both these techniques are designed to relax your body, putting it in a state where the fight-or-flight response or the defense-alarm syndrome of arousal is greatly diminished or eliminated, freeing your energy for communicating effectively (Pelletier, 1977).

MEDITATION AS A WAY TO AUGMENT YOUR RELAXATION RESPONSE

Meditation is an experiental exercise involving your actual attention, not your belief system or other cognitive processes. Meditation is a highly individualized and personal practice, and effective meditation does not in any way require you to adhere to rigid group norms or abdicate your life to a spiritual or secular leader. Meditation is something you do by yourself and for yourself in order to benefit from the subjective sense of deep relaxation and unstressing of the body's musculature; also, you possibly come to know yourself more fully. Meditation is psychologically and physically refreshing and energy-restoring (Pelletier, 1977).

It has been empirically verified that the meditative process relieves nervous system stress more efficiently than either dreaming or sleeping. Marked physiological alterations have been proved to accompany meditation: reduction of the metabolic rate; reduction of the breathing rate to four to six breaths per minute; an increase in the amount of the alpha waves of eight to twelve cycles in the brain; the appearance of theta waves of five to eight cycles in the brain; and a 20% reduction in the blood pressure of hypertensive patients (Pelletier, 1977, pp. 212-213).

The regenerating effects of meditation are experienced during the meditation itself and they have a carry-over effect into your daily activities (Pelletier, 1977, p. 200). Once you have learned the low arousal effect during the meditation practice you can maintain this state of neurophysiological functioning in response to stressful situations to minimize stress activity. It is impossible to be relaxed and tense at the same time, and your enhanced ability to maintain relaxation during the day in the face of stressful interpersonal situations is what will help to minimize the stress effects on you. With practice you will be able to call upon your low arousal state as needed during your working day. By itself this mechanism is helpful, and your heightened feelings of being able to cope with pressures of everyday life will augment your good feelings (Pelletier, 1977, p. 201). When you learn to diminish your reaction to stressors you are freeing yourself to deal with aspects of the interpersonal situation more worthy of your energy. Being able to shift focus from being tight or nervous to feeling calm and in charge allows you to communicate more effectively with your clients and colleagues.

Concentration is essential in all systems of meditation. Meditation will teach you to fix your attention firmly upon a given task for increasingly protracted periods of time, overcoming your usual habit of flitting from one subject to another. When the incessant activity of your mind is stilled you will experience that aspect of your being which is prior to and distinct from both your thoughts and attention itself. It is this state which has been described as transcendental awareness, cosmic consciousness, or *satori* (Pelletier, 1977, p. 225).

"This goal may seem deceptively simple. Once you have tried truly to quiet your mind, or to allow images to run through it without letting any particular one become distracting, you will understand why practice and perseverance are necessary if you are to be successful. Mental activity is a wayward and not easily controlled phenomenon. At first it seems to have a life of its own. When you exert will or volition and attempt to become quiet, it is very likely that you will be perversely and regularly disobeyed. Your mind jumps unbidden from one thought or concern to another despite your efforts to concentrate on eliminating such activity. With practice and experimentation to determine the best approach for you personally, you can gradually increase your ability to regulate your attention and reduce or rectify the mind's overwhelming tendency to generate incessant activity and distractions. At this point the subtle benefits of meditation become more pronounced" (Pelletier, 1977, pp. 193-194).

GUIDELINES FOR BEGINNING TO PRACTICE MEDITATION

This chapter provides some beginning guidelines to begin practicing meditation on your own. The meditation procedure described here is adapted from the standard clinical meditation (Cormier & Cormier, 1991). There are other forms of meditation and you may wish to read or even take a course or individualized instruction in meditation.

Make Time to Meditate

To experience benefits from meditation you need to meditate for 15 to 30 minutes at least once a day. This commitment means setting aside that time consistently. "Many individuals say that they have an extremely busy schedule and simply do not have the opportunity to sit for such a long period of time each day. Very often a realistic examination of a person's schedule indicates that in fact there is sufficient time if the individual is conscientious and serious in his efforts. To some extent, the minor life reorientation necessitated by meditative practice may be responsible for its success. It involves a reordering of life priorities and behavioral patterns" (Pelletier, 1977, p. 224).

Set the Climate to Meditate

Find a quiet place to meditate where you will not be disturbed. Silence the ringer on your phone and engage your answering machine for the time you are meditating. Tell others that you do not wish to be disturbed for a specified length of time and assure them that you will be available after your meditation. Taking these precautions frees you to relax instead of tensing at sounds in your environment. Many people find it best to meditate first thing in the morning when their home is quiet and the world has not yet started to intrude. For nurses doing shift work other arrangements can be made. Some people choose a quiet place outside their home such as the hospital chapel.

Secure a Comfortable Position for Meditation

Find a position that is truly comfortable for you where you are supported by minimal muscular work. Support your back and feet if necessary. Adjust the room temperature so that you are comfortable. If you are warm enough you are more likely to stay relaxed and not be distracted.

Develop a Passive Attitude

Reassure yourself that you are not being tested on how well you meditate and put aside worrying about your technique. Distracting thoughts are likely to occur during your meditation, especially at first when you are learning to focus. Let these thoughts pass without becoming worried about their intrusion or your ability.

Select a Mental Device

To help you shift your thoughts away from logical, externally oriented thoughts, select a mental device—a phrase, a word, or a sound that you can repeat while you meditate. Repetition of this sound, called a *mantra,* assists in breaking the stream of distracting thoughts. Some suggestions for a mental device are single-syllable sounds of words such as "in," "out," "one," or "zum" that can be repeated silently or in a low tone while meditating. Select a mantra that is not emotionally charged and is soothing to you. Make up a word if you like (Cormier & Cormier, 1991).

Relax Your Body

When you are ready to begin your meditation, start by relaxing your body. Start with the muscle groups in the head and work to the feet. Say to yourself: "Relax your face; now allow your neck muscles to thaw; let your head relax; take the tension out of your shoulders; let your chest muscles loosen; allow your abdomen to soften; let your back muscles unfreeze; take the tension out of your thigh muscles; let your calves melt; and, allow your feet to rest comfortably supported." As you tune into the difference between relaxation and tension in your muscles you will be able to quickly release tightness in your body in preparation for your meditation times. Wearing comfortable, loose fitting clothing will help you assume a posture that is relaxing.

Focus on Your Breathing

Breathe through your nose and focus on, or become aware of, your breathing. This awareness will help you relax. Breathe easily and naturally, allowing the air to come to you on each inhalation (Cormier & Cormier, 1991). Exhale slowly, allowing all the air out of the lungs. You will find this focus on your breathing very peaceful. When you are stressed your breathing is quicker, and just slowing your breathing down and appreciating its rhythm begins to relieve tension. Remember not to control your breathing and become light-headed. Just breathe easily and naturally.

While you are focusing on your breathing you can repeat your mental device silently on inhalation and exhalation, keeping your attention on your breathing and your mental device.

Meditate for 10 Minutes

Start off with meditating for 10 minutes, increasing the time to 15 or 20 minutes as you gain experience in being still. Close your eyes during your meditation if this helps to keep you focused on your breathing and your mantra. Do not think things over or problem solve during this quiet time. Your meditation time is time out from running your life, managing time, controlling events, and performing as an adult in our hectic world. In this quiet time, for 10 to 20 minutes, you are free to just sit and breathe. Don't expend energy judging your thoughts or critizing any distractions; simply let them pass by and remain focused on the present, on your breathing and on your mental device.

Allow your images and thoughts to flow freely. Your mantra will come back to you. While you are meditating you do not need to expend a great effort or concentrate. Enjoy this quiet, peaceful experience. If you need to open your eyes to check the time, arrange to have a clock in view so that moving is unnecessary.

Experience Your Unique Meditation

There are no rules or "shoulds" for what you will experience in your meditations. Enjoy the peaceful hiatus in which you can unwind and experience the sensation of relaxation. You may discover sensations in your body that you were previously too busy to notice. It may happen that in addition to your peacefulness, you achieve a level of stillness in which you might be pervaded with the overwhelming and joyous knowledge that all of existence is a unity and that you are at one with it. Pelletier describes this powerful feeling as dissolving all fear, including the fear of death, and an inundation of warmth, joy, and harmony (1977, p. 226).

End Your Meditation Peacefully

When it is time to end your meditation, take a pause before standing up and moving. It may be soothing to sit for a brief moment with your eyes closed before slowly opening them. Don't rush away; rather, gently leave your meditation and enter your world refreshed and relaxed.

ON-THE-SPOT RELAXATION EXERCISES AS A WAY TO RELIEVE YOUR BODILY TENSION IN THE FACE OF AN INTERPERSONAL STRESSOR

Meditating on a daily basis will make you more relaxed and vital at work or school. Even with this new peacefulness there will be times when a distraught client, an enraged family member, or an agitated colleague can raise your tension level. It would be ideal, but probably impractical, if you could leave the unit for some quiet time when clients and colleagues upset your peacefulness. What can help are some on-the-spot ways to regain your relaxation response. This chapter gives you some creative techniques that you can call upon to cool you down when the heat is on. So when the unit is understaffed, client census is overloaded, and you are encountering interpersonal stress, here is what you can do to relax your body.

STRATEGIES FOR RELAXING YOUR BODY WHEN YOUR STRESSOR IS IMMEDIATE

There are some stressful situations that provide no warning. It helps to have in your repertoire on-the-spot methods for relaxing your body and preventing it from seizing up in a stressful encounter. Here are some suggestions for relaxing your body the moment you are faced with unexpected interpersonal stress. Each of these brief relaxation exercises can be done on a moment's notice with no need for privacy or special equipment. They can be done as you walk down the corridor, ride on the elevator, or stand up to face the person who is stressing you.

An Unexpected Stressful Interpersonal Encounter

It is noon on the orthopedic unit where you are in your third week of clinical work. The lunches have not arrived and the clients are hungry. You are hungry. A physician strides out of the elevator, spies you, and heads in your direction. Her forceful walk, scowl, furrowed brow, and finger pointed in your direction give you clues that she is irate about something and, since you are the only nurse in the vicinity, it is likely you will bear the brunt of her aggression.

Here are some ideas of what you can do to relax your body before tension seizes up your muscles in a fright-flight response. These techniques can be done in-the-moment while you are awaiting the approach of the irate physician (your stressor) and even while you are communicating assertively in the face of this threat.

Sprinkling Shower

The spray from the imaginary shower nozzle is right above your head and you can feel the water trickling through your hair and warming your shoulder muscles on its way down your back. Your hunched shoulders sag with relief under the warmth. You feel the warm soapy water slushing over your body, caressing your muscles and heating your skin a shade of red. The soapy lather massages your skin as it flows over you, warming your legs and feet before it disappears down the drain. As you lift your face up to the nozzle you are pelted with a clear stream of fresh water. Someone has adjusted the nozzle; you sense a firm staccato pressure on your face and over your neck and shoulders. You notice that this beating of water is simultaneously comforting and invigorating. You feel regenerated. The comforting relief you experience from the water surrounding your body makes you sigh deeply. The pressure of the water eases up to a refreshing sprinkle. As the shower turns off you are suddenly dry, and you feel warm and refreshed. As you relax, say to yourself: "This is relaxation. This is how it feels to be loose. This is what I want."

Sunbeam

Picture a radiant ball of light situated just above your head, creating a field of bright rays vibrating in a protective pyramid around your body. Feel its protective glow encircling your body to a diameter of 4 feet. Notice that the light feels warm and, as it envelops you, you are comforted by its penetrating rays. You find yourself stopping what you are doing and raising your face to bask in the heat of the radiant sun above your head. You can actually feel the light infiltrate your body, permeating your cells. This experience is comforting, and to your surprise you can actually feel the warmth from the light circulating from your head to your toes. Now you notice that the light is twinkling and, as it touches your skin, you feel unusually invigorated. The sparkling sunbeams dance over your skin, dissipating any tension you were feeling. Your energy opens up in response to the warmth and tingling. As you relax your muscles are overwhelmed to the core of your being with a feeling of profound comfort and safety in the rays of your own special sunbeam. As you relax, say to yourself: "This is relaxation. This is how it feels to be loose. This is what I want."

Safety Shield

Picture a clear plexiglass shield that rises up to surround you when you sense danger. Your protective shield is about 2 feet away from your body, and it allows you to move freely while it protects you on all sides. You can see quite clearly into the outside world, just as if the shield were invisible. Inside your shield, the air is fresh and tingles your skin as it circulates around your body. This is your personal air supply and when you breathe it in you notice it penetrates your lungs with a fresh cool air which you can feel invigorating your cells as it circulates throughout your body. You feel energized and nourished by this special supply of air in your protected space. You also notice that you feel calm and well defended inside your shield, because you realize that the shield deflects tension away from you. You are relaxed and free from any tensions outside your shield and you feel this assurance in your body. You notice your breathing slowing with the nourishing air, and your muscles are loose and fluidly mobile. You relax because you know you are safe. As you relax, say to yourself: "This is relaxation. This is how it feels to be loose. This is what I want."

Sweeper

A magic broom comes out of nowhere to sweep the tension from your body. It rakes through your hair, leaving your scalp tingling as the circulation is invigorated. Your head feels warm and tension-free after this stimulation. You notice your neck is mobile and relaxed instead of stiff. As it sweeps the stress from your shoulders, they relax and feel lighter. You stand less rigidly and notice your back is free from any tension. This broom is powerful and thorough in its ability to brush the stress off and away from your body. You can feel its bristles brush away the tension from your abdomen and the front and backs of your legs. When your feet are swept you feel lighter and more mobile; this sensation is energizing. You know you are tension free and you feel safe when the stress is swept into a pan and thrown far away from your body. Without the encumbrance of stress and tension you feel ready to handle anything. The sweeping has regenerated your batteries and renewed your energy. Your feet are moving with renewed energy and you're tempted to get up and dance on the balls of your feet. You feel alive and free! As you relax, say to yourself: "This is relaxation. This is how it feels to be loose. This is what I want."

Massage

A pair of powerful hands comes out of nowhere and lay themselves across your shoulders. These large but gentle hands are unusually warm and radiate a heat to your upper back. The motion is soothing and heat penetrates deep inside. You rotate your shoulders easily after these comforting hands have massaged out the tension. There is no effort to stand or move. You are very relaxed. The hands move up to knead the knots in your neck muscles. The touch is magical, as if by merely being there the hands can dissipate tightness from built up tension. Before moving on, the hands shake out the tension away from your body so that it is removed far from you and no longer a threat. Next the hands move to your lower back and massage the tightness out of your spine. The pressure is firm, and with each small circular stroke you notice your breathing gets more relaxed; it slows down and you are totally soothed by the comfort and compassion emanating from the hands. You can feel the muscles in your neck, shoulders, and back filling with blood, getting warm and supple under the gifted touch of the hands as they massage away fear and tightness. You feel release and a sense of freedom. You feel warm and protected. As you relax, say to yourself: "This is relaxation. This is how it feels to be loose. This is what I want."

Advantages of On-the-Spot Relaxation Exercises

Each of these brief but powerful relaxation strategies takes about a minute to experience. In that short time you can shift from tightness and fear to relaxation and a feeling of competence to cope with what is threatening you. Using these calming strategies will give you inner self-confidence. As you get sensitive to knowing when your body is relaxed, not tense, you will be even more skilled at relaxing your body in the face of tension. Relaxation is a skill, a coordination of mind and muscles, and it can be learned by anyone who wants to do so and is willing to spend the time and effort (Percival, Percival, & Taylor, 1977).

STRETCHING YOUR BODY TO RELAXATION IN PREPARATION FOR A STRESSFUL INTERPERSONAL ENCOUNTER

When you have more warning about a stressful interpersonal encounter, you can add some stretching to relax your body to augment the benefits of meditation and the on-the-spot exercises. Before encountering a stressor, or at any time during your hectic day, break away from the busy pace of the unit and find a quiet place in which to relax your muscles for a minute or so. Find some privacy in the washroom, an empty office, an unused stairwell, or the linen cupboard. Here are some stretches you can do that take little space, and you can do them from the standing position without any equipment.

These exercises involve tensing and relaxing the muscles until you feel the difference between the two sensations and learn to consciously relax any tense muscle. As your muscles learn the difference, they themselves will develop a relaxation response (Percival, Percival, & Taylor, 1977).

High Stretch and Relax

Stand erect and stack your hands on top of your head. While taking a deep breath reach high overhead, lifting your chest and moving your head back slightly. Stretch slowly until you have your hands as high as they will go. Hold for 3 seconds. Now exhale, letting the air out with a long, easy sigh, while dropping your arms slowly to your sides. Let your shoulders sag, your head fall forward, and your knees go loose and slightly bent. Remain in this relaxed position for 3 to 5 seconds. Allow all the tension to seep out of your neck, arms, shoulders, and your chest muscles. Repeat a few times before returning to work (Percival, Percival, & Taylor, 1977, p. 88).

Shoulder Rotation

This stretch improves shoulder flexibility and relaxation of you shoulder girdle. Stand with your feet comfortably apart. Raise your elbows to shoulder height, allowing your forearms and hands to dangle loosely. Rotate elbows forward in large circles at a medium pace, keeping your hands and arms loose throughout. Move the shoulders in as large an arc as possible for about 20 rotations (Percival, Percival, & Taylor, 1977, p. 94).

Shoulder Shrug and Relax

This relaxation exercise can even be done while you are talking on the phone. Stand with your feet comfortably apart. As you take a deep breath, shrug your shoulders up to your ears and moderately tighten the muscles throughout your body. Hold for 3 to 5 seconds. Now exhale with a long deep sigh, letting your shoulders drop down and your muscles go loose so that your knees bend slightly and your head drops forward to your chest. Repeat a few times (Percival, Percival, & Taylor, 1977, p. 95).

Arms Out, Up, and Relax

Stand erect with your feet comfortably apart. Lift your arms out to your sides and up over you head, simultaneously pulling your stomach in and lifting your chest. When you've reached as high as you can, let your arms drop loosely down. Allow your head to sag so your chin touches your chest and your knees go "soft." Try to get as loose and limp as you can. Feel the tension drain out. Repeat several times before returning to work (Percival, Percival, & Taylor, 1977, p. 96).

With practice you will be able to call on your relaxation response at any moment. Being able to relax gives you the power to release tension in your muscles, reclaiming that energy for dealing with interpersonal stressors in your life as a nurse. In the next few chapters, you will learn ways to prepare your *mindset* to handle difficult situations in your relationships with clients and colleagues.

PRACTICING RELAXATION

Exercise 1. During the next week practice meditating for 10 minutes twice a day, perhaps once in the morning and later in the afternoon. After each of your meditations, keep notes of what the experience was like for you. Here are some questions to think about (but do not be limited by them). How does the experience of meditating make a difference to you? How does your mantra (sound) work for you? What thoughts or images occur? Are you able to let distracting thoughts float by and return to focusing on your breathing and mantra?

Make an opportunity to talk about the practice of meditating with your classmates. Although meditation is a private event, you may feel comfortable exchanging ideas about how to make the process of meditation work more effectively so that it contributes to expanding your feelings of relaxation.

Exercise 2. Give the on-the-spot relaxation visions a try over the next few days. Focus on trying to stay with the relaxation feeling your vision creates in your body. Note when you get distracted and design a way of refocusing on your soothing internal technique. Note when you are able to distinguish the change from tension in your muscles to letting go in a relaxation response. As you practice you will get more and more astute at recognizing the difference, and soon it will be within your power to quickly and simply allow the tension to escape from your body.

Exercise 3. The next time you are on one of your clinical units take a moment away from the hectic pace to try out one of the relaxing stretch-release exercises. Time yourself to see how long it took to find a spot and complete a few relaxing stretch-releases. You will likely be surprised at how little time it takes. Just breaking away from the unit with the anticipation and intention of doing something good for yourself is beneficial, and the stretching and releasing reminds your body to relax. Note how refreshed you feel when you return to the unit.

Make a time in your class to talk about creative ways to incorporate a stretch-release exercise into your work day.

REFERENCES

Baider, L., & Porath, S. (1981). Uncovering fear: Group experience of nurses in a cancer ward. *International Journal of Nursing Studies, 18,* 47-52.

Barigar, D.L., & Sheafor, M.L. (1990). Recruiting staff nurses: A marketing approach. *Nursing Management, 21*(1), 27-29.

Burke, R.J. (1985). *Stress and burnout in organizations: Implications for personnel and human resource management.* Unpublished manuscript. York, Ontario, Canada: York University, Faculty of Administrative Studies.

Calhoun, G.L. (1980). Hospitals are high-stress employers. *Hospitals,* June.

Cassem, N.H., & Hackett, T.P. (1975). Stress on the nurse and therapist in the intensive-care unit and the coronary-care unit. *Heart & Lung, 4*(2), 252-259.

Chiriboga, D.A., Jenkins, G., Bailey, J. (1983). Stress and coping among Hospice nurses: Test of an analytic model. *Nursing Research, 32*(5), 294-299.

Coleman, B. (1990). Advanced nursing apprenticeship program: A strategy for retention of experienced critical care nurses. *Heart & Lung, 19*(3), 236-242.

Cormier, W.H., & Cormier, L.S. (1991). *Interviewing strategies for helpers: Fundamental skills and cognitive behavioral interventions* (3rd ed.). Pacific Grove, Calif.: Brooks/Cole Publishing Company.

Corcoran, N.M., Meyer, L.A., & Magliaro, B.L. (1990). Retention: The key to the 21st century for health care institutions. *Nursing Administrative Quarterly, 14*(4), 23-31.

Doering, L. (1990). Recruitment and retention: Successful strategies in critical care. *Heart & Lung, 19*(3), 220-223.

Freudenberger, H.J. (1983). Burnout: Contemporary issues, trends, and concerns. In B.A. Farber, (Ed.), *Stress and burnout in the human service professions* (pp. 23-28). New York: Pergamon Press.

Gentry, N.D., Foster, S.B., & Froehling, S. (1972). Psychological response to situational stress in intensive and non-intensive nursing. *Heart & Lung,* Nov.-Dec., 793-796.

Hay, D., & Oken, D. (1972). The psychological stresses of Intensive Care Unit nursing. *Psychosomatic Medicine, 4*(2), 109-118.

Huttner, C.A. (1990). Strategies for recruitment and retention of critical care nurses: A cardiovascular program experience. *Heart & Lung, 19*(3), 230-235.

Keane, A., Ducette, J., & Adler, D.C. (1985). Stress in ICU and non-ICU nurses. *Nursing Research, 34*(4), 231-236.

Kornfeld, D.S. (1971). Psychiatric problems of an Intensive Care Unit. *Medical Clinics of North America, 55*(5), 1353-1364.

Maloney, J.P., & Bartz, C. (1983). Stress-tolerant people: Intensive care nurses compared with non-intensive care nurses. *Heart & Lung, 12*(2), 27-29.

Nicholson, L.G. (1990). Stress management in nursing. *Nursing Management,* April, 53-55.

Oskins, S.L. (1980). Identification of situational stressors and coping methods by intensive care nurses. *Heart & Lung, 8*(5), 953-960.

Pelletier, K.R. (1977). *Mind as healer, mind as slayer: A holistic approach to preventing stress disorders.* New York: Dell Publishing Company.

Percival, J., Percival, L., Taylor, J. (1977). *The complete guide to total fitness.* Scarborough, Ontario, Canada: Prentice-Hall of Canada, Ltd.

Spitzer-Lehmann, R. (1990). Recruitment and retention of our greatest asset. *Nursing Administrative Quarterly, 14*(4), 66-69.

Stehle, J.L. (1981). Critical care nursing stress: The findings revisited. *Nursing Research, 30*(3), 182-186.

Taerk, G. (1983). Psychological support of oncology nurses: A role for the liaison psychiatrist. *Canadian Journal of Psychiatry, 28,* 532-535.

Vreeland, R., & Ellis, G.L. (1969). Stresses on the nurse in an Intensive-Care Unit. *Journal of the American Medical Association, 208*(2), 332-334.

Werkema, J.A. (1990). Opening a new critical care nursing unit during a nursing shortage: Recruitment and retention strategies. *Heart & Lung, 19*(3), 224-229.

West, N.D. (1975). Stress associated with ICUs affect patients, families, staff. *Hospitals, 49,* 62-63.

White, S.K. (1990). Overview: Symposium on successful recruitment and retention strategies in critical care. *Heart & Lung, 19*(3), 219-220.

SUGGESTIONS FOR FURTHER READING

American Nurses' Association. (1990). *Survival skills in the workplace: What every nurse should know*. Kansas City, Mo.: Author.

This booklet, written by Lyndia Flanagan, provides nurses with a complete overview of the current issues creating stress in the workplace and lends practical strategies for coping with them. Strategies include enhanced self-awareness, finely tuned communication skills, and organizational know-how.

Breakwell, G.M. (1990). Are you stressed out? *American Journal of Nursing, 90*(8), 31-33.

In this brief article Breakwell outlines the negative effects of stress and includes a test for checking your stress level. Salient advice is offered for controlling workplace stress.

Hanson, P.G. (1989). *Stress for Success: Thriving on stress at work*. Toronto, Ontario, Canada: Collins Publishers.

This comprehensive text advises readers on how to handle all types of stress in the workplace. It explains how to deal with the most stressful work related challenges. It is full of good ideas which nurses can readily apply and is written in a concise, readable way.

Hardin, S.B. (1990). Nursing occupational distress. In J.M. McCloskey & H.K. Grace (Eds.) *Current issues in nursing,* (pp. 490-494). St. Louis: Mosby–Year Book.

In this overview, Hardin outlines the roles of individual nurses and organizations in contributing to, and relieving, work related stress.

Purtilo, R. (1990). *Health professional and patient interaction*. Philadelphia: W.B. Saunders Company.

Chapter 1 focuses on what it is like to be a health professional student, describing some of the anxieties most students experience. It is comforting for nurse students to know that the stress they experience is a part of being a professional. The chapter ends with encouragement to persevere through stressful times. Chapter 3 will help nurse readers identify some reasons why nurses and other health professionals may fail to take precautions to safeguard their own health. The benefits of solitude are encouraged.

Wilson, G.L., Hantz, A.M., Hanna, M.S. (1985). *Interpersonal growth through communication*. Dubuque, Iowa: Wm. C. Brown Publishers.

Chapter 9 provides nurse readers with an overview of the negative consequences of stress upon both the individual and the organization. The plan included in this chapter is a systematic tool for taking charge of stress in one's life.

CHAPTER 17

Imagery

*"Each man is the
architect of his own fate."*

Appius Caecus

OBJECTIVES

Your imagination is active most of your waking hours. The purpose of this chapter is to make you more aware of how creating images in your mind's eye can help you be a more effective communicator. You will learn the meaning of imagery and become more knowledgeable about how you can visualize to improve your performance as a communicator. The exercises at the end of the chapter provide you with an opportunity to practice imagery and experience how imagery can increase your feelings of confidence and competence in your communication.

WHAT IS IMAGERY?

Imagery is defined in the *World Book Dictionary* as descriptions and figures of speech that help the mind form forceful or beautiful pictures (Barnhart, 1975, p. 1042). The term *visualize* or *visualization* is interchangeable with the term *imagery*. Visualize is defined as follows: to form a mental picture of something invisible, absent, or abstract (Barnhart, 1975, p. 2324).

Imagery or visualization is a process of mentally picturing an event we wish to occur in the present or future. It is a process of actually experiencing a picture that we hold in our mind's eye. In visualizing our picture we may incorporate our senses to taste it, smell it, feel it, and imagine the sounds and emotions associated with it. For example, when we visualize a freshly baked apple pie we can actually smell it, taste the apples, and visualize eating the pie. When we visualize ourselves communi-

---

■This chapter was written by Sharon G. Allen Duncan, R.N., B.S.N.

cating such as by listening actively, we can hear ourselves articulating empathic words, feel ourselves being warm, genuine and natural, and enjoy observing a positive interaction between ourselves and our clients or colleagues.

Imagery is a process similar to daydreaming; however, imagery is combined with a conscious purpose. It is much more than mere fantasy. The key to successful visualization is to be clear about what you want and then commit to that course of action in your imagery. This is a crucial step for producing successful results with your imagery. Let your mind's eye create what you want with no concern about constraints or limitations (Mayer, 1984, p. 32).

In this chapter the focus will be on how you can use imagery to positively influence your interpersonal communication. You will learn the steps required to formulate a clear image of how you want to communicate with your clients or colleagues. You can then use that visualization to help you actualize your vision in reality.

Imagery has been used in physical healing for a long time. You may be interested in the history of visualization in medicine.

History of Imagery

Imagery may be the oldest healing technique used by humans. Early records of these techniques have been found on cuneiform tablets in Babylonia and Sumeria. Greek, Egyptian, Oriental, and ancient Indian civilizations used visualization. Even today Navaho Indians and Canadian Eskimos practice imagery for healing purposes (Samuels, 1975, pp. 209-213).

In all these cultures the disease was seen as a demonic force that had incorporated itself into the ill person's being. The shaman or physician-priest would heal through rituals or ceremonies by confronting the disease-causing demon with a positive force and exorcising the demon from the patient. The shaman derived his power from visualizing a higher authority, god, or spirit. At that time medicine was controlled by religion, mysticism, and magic (Samuels, 1975, p. 215).

Paracelsus, a Renaissance physician, is known as the father of scientific medicine and modern drug therapy. A man opposed to the notion of separating the healing process from the spirit, he said: "The spirit is the master, imagination the tool, and the body the plastic material. The power of the imagination is a great factor in medicine. It may produce diseases in man and in animals, and it may cure them. . . . Ills of the body may be cured by the physical remedies or by the power of the spirit acting through the soul" (Hartmann, 1973, p. 112). His views differed from the early shamanistic views because he believed people's own thoughts, as well as gods and spirits, could heal them. (Samuels, 1975, p. 218).

It was during the Renaissance that the mind-body dichotomy occurred. Rene Descartes assisted in establishing the split in his attempts to free scientific questions from arguments concerning God. Scientists could then be concerned about the body without theological debate and the philosophers and theologians were left to study the spirit and mind (Flynn, 1980, p. 42).

Since the Renaissance, techniques of healing divided into two systems: scientific and religious. Our Western society has adopted scientific healing—surgery and drug therapy. With increasing scientific investigation and medical specialization, the mind-body-spirit split continued into the twentieth century. However, by 1900 a number of medical scientists began investigating how the mind affects the body and healing (Samuels, 1975, p. 218).

Physiologist Edmund Jacobson, searching for effective methods of relaxation, showed that the imagery we use in thought processes produces a muscular reactivity that resembles what occurs during the actual performing of the act. That is, if we imagine ourselves in our mind's eye as running, the muscles we normally use when we run will contract slightly (Jacobson, 1942).

Many scientists and the medical profession have continued to accept that the autonomic nervous system is unconscious, automatic, and not within conscious control. In the late 1960s physiologists Dr. Leo DiCara and Dr. Neal Miller demonstrated that parts of the autonomic nervous system can be conditioned and controlled. Using animals, they determined that rats could learn how to alter their stomach acidity, brain wave patterns, blood pressure, and blood flow (Miller, 1969, pp. 434-445). Furthermore, in their work with humans, scientists have verified the ability yogis have to control specific processes of the body such as metabolic rate and heart rate (Lauria, 1968, pp. 140-143).

Groundwork laid by these scientists and others has been revolutionary in the current shift away from the body-mind-spirit split to body-mind integration. The implications of these findings for nursing and medicine are extraordinary and exciting!

Application of Imagery in Health Care

A contemporary example of a body-mind integration system is Autogenic Therapy. This is a psychophysiological technique developed by Dr. J.H. Schultz that works successfully with both specific and general visualization methods. When a specific autogenic technique is used, a specific physiological process or organ may be affected. For example, a client with excessive gastric secretions was asked to gaze at the dryness and texture of blotting paper while imagining absorbent dryness. Tests indicated that after 10 days of doing these visualizations the client's excessive secretions normalized (Luthe, 1969, p. 16).

Dr. O. Carl Simonton, an oncologist and radiologist who has specialized since 1965 in the treatment of cancer using visualization, was impressed by some of his terminally ill patients who had spontaneous remissions and recovered from cancer against all odds. Simonton observed in these clients a consistent, positive attitude about life and about the possibility of recovering from cancer (Samuels, 1975, p. 226).

His theory is that we all have cancer many times in our life and that normally a person's immune system destroys the cancer cells. Based on his own work and work of fellow researchers, Simonton uses a mind-body model to suggest that psychological stress, depression, and despair received by the limbic system via the hypothalamus causes suppression within the immune system and leaves the body open to developing cancer. Furthermore, the hypothalamus responds to stress by triggering the pituitary gland and producing a hormonal imbalance. This is significant since it has been shown that an imbalance in our adrenal hormones creates a greater susceptibility to carcinogens. Hormonal imbalance can result in the body producing an increased number of abnormal cells. With a weakened immune system there is an inability of the body systems to combat these cells. These physiological changes create optimal conditions for the growth of cancer (Simonton, 1980, pp. 78-80).

With this model in mind Simonton suggests that the cancer development cycle can be reversed. The first and crucial step in assisting cancer clients toward recovery involves strengthening their beliefs in the power of their body defenses and the effectiveness of their medical treatment. It should be stressed here that Simonton acknowledges the value of medical intervention in treating cancer. According to his mind-body model medical treatment, irradiation, chemotherapy, or surgery serves to destroy existing cancer cells, while psychological intervention is an ally that reverses the cycle of cancer growth (Simonton, 1980, p. 82).

Once this notion is accepted by the client, feelings of hope and anticipation are recorded by the limbic system in place of the hopelessness and despair. The hypothalamus receives the new message of an increased will to live and in turn reverses the suppression of the immune system and restores the body's defenses against abnormal cells. The body's hormonal balance is restored and fewer abnormal cells are produced. With the immune system functioning normally and the decrease in the number of abnormal cells, optimal conditions are created for cancer regression (Simonton, 1980, pp. 80-82).

Simonton designed techniques that would affect his client's attitude about life and curing cancer. These techniques include forms of both relaxation and visualization. When relaxed, the client is asked to visualize a natural, peaceful scene. He is then asked to see his cancer in his mind's eye as being weak and confused cells. Next the client is instructed to picture his white blood cells as a vast army, strong and aggressive, coming into the cancer area and devouring the abnormal cells; to see the cancer shrinking and picture it being flushed out of the body via the urine and stool. When the cancer has disappeared in the client's imagery, he is asked to see himself as well and full of energy, reaching goals and feeling fulfilled in life (Simonton, 1980, pp. 121-122).

Simonton has established that all clients who are enthusiastic about feeling better, and who implicitly follow instructions, show dramatic relief of their symptoms and marked improvement in their condition (Bolen, 1973, p. 21).

These findings suggest that imagery plays a basic role in causing disease and in facilitating its cure. There is evidence that visualization can influence a person's heart rate, blood flow, immune response, and total physiology. Knowing this, what then are the implications of imagery?

Implications of Imagery

How does the knowledge that it is possible for us to voluntarily affect our autonomic nervous system using visualization influence us in our nursing care? First the nurse must adopt a holistic philosophy of mind, body, and spirit integration. A holistic perspective emphasizes the interrelationship of the parts that make up the whole person. It acknowledges that the mind affects the body and vice versa. Accepting this notion of interdependence the nurse understands the power there is within our whole mind-body-spirit being to heal ourselves. This internal power can be used to maintain and increase our level of wellness, either alone or in conjunction with an external source of healing (Samuels, 1974, p. 61).

Imagery is also gaining increasing acceptance in the areas of corporation finance and sports. Psychologist Steven Devore, along with researchers at the University of California, Harvard, Yale and Stanford, discovered a frequent characteristic of executives of major U.S. corporations. "These people knew what they wanted out of life," says DeVore. "They could see it, taste it, smell it, and imagine the sounds and emotions associated with it. They prelived it before they had it. And that sharp, sensory vision became a powerful driving force in their lives" (Mayer, 1984, p. 32).

Dr. Alan Richardson at the University of Western Australia conducted an experiment with two basketball teams. One group practiced 20 minutes longer a day and the other group used their 20 minutes to imagine that they were playing the game and mentally corrected themselves each time they missed a basket. After a period of weeks the group that physically practiced the game improved 24%, and the group visualizing themselves as practicing improved 23%! (Mayer, 1984, p. 48).

Jack Nicklaus uses visualization to improve the muscle memory and motor skills involved in golf. He has stated that good golf requires one half mental rehearsal and one half physical coordination. He never hits a shot without first seeing a sharp, clear picture of that shot in his mind's eye (Mayer, 1984, p. 48).

Imagery has been used in medicine, athletics, and business. It is a process that can be used by people in various walks of life to achieve success in whatever they value. We will now look at how imagery can be used by nurses to improve their interpersonal communication skills.

The Relationship Between Imagery and Interpersonal Communication

If we are clear about what is important to us, and if we are committed to creating what we value, imagery is an invaluable tool for self-direction (Mayer, 1984, p. 32). This idea is the key to how imagery can be used by nurses to improve their interpersonal communication skills. If you are clear that it is important to be an effective nurse communicator, and you are committed to creating that outcome, then imagery can help you achieve that goal.

As a professional nurse you will want to implement the interpersonal communication skills you will be learning in this book in a way that is beneficial to your clients, your colleagues, and yourself. Imagery will grant you a visualization of yourself implementing these skills in a helpful and effective way. It will provide you with a picture of yourself as a nurse who can handle a variety of interpersonal situations confidently and competently. These images will act like a beacon, beckoning you to achieve the goal of being a competent nurse communicator.

As you read about each of the interpersonal communication behaviors, you will learn the correct way to implement each one with your clients and colleagues. You will develop a vision of yourself executing the communication behavior you are studying. This perception may be fuzzy and vague at first. It is essential that you work at making this image of yourself as clear as possible. You need to create an image that envisions you communicating in a positive, effective, and competent manner. The more detailed and specific you can make your visualization, the more effective it will be to guide your actual communication.

Imagining yourself being successful operates like a rehearsal. This mental dry run helps cement an image of yourself carrying out the skill correctly. When the "dress" rehearsal goes well, it gives you confidence that your live performance will also be positive. Amazingly, the actual visualization process may take you 1 minute or less. The more you use this process the more proficient you will become.

Seeing yourself perform the way you want to is just one more step toward successfully carrying out your performance in public. Having a visualization of yourself communicating well makes the future reality a viable possibility. Imagery helps you become familiar with your desired outcome so that you start accepting the notion that achieving your ideal is possible and forthcoming. Imagery makes you believe that you can achieve your goals.

Imagery can be influential in helping us communicate in a way that is in keeping with our goals as a nurse. If physical health, basketball, golf scores, and management strategies can be improved through visualization, so can nurses' interpersonal communication skills.

How to Use Imagery to Improve Your Ability to Communicate

Here are some of the essential points of effective imagery. First of all, imagery requires *discipline;* that is, the willingness to briefly stop what you are doing and proceed with the visualization process. Imagery is most effective when you are relaxed, so begin your imagery with three deep breaths to facilitate *relaxation.* (Also refer to chapter 16 for a relaxation exercise.) Relaxation will assist you with letting go of the thoughts swimming around in your head. This enables you to *focus* on *becoming clear* about what you want to create with your imagery. Once you are clear about your goal or purpose, *commit to creating* it with no reservations and *with complete faith* that your goal or purpose will be attained. Using all your *senses,* allow yourself to *feel the experience* of your goal being attained as though it were happening at the very moment of your visualization.

Although this may sound complex to you at the outset, with a little practice you will be able to go through these steps quickly and effectively.

You might think that the practice of visualization is quite abstract since it occurs unseen inside your head. On the contrary, there are some concrete and specific steps you can take to ensure that your visualization influences your future performance in the way you intend. Here are some systematic steps you can take to make sure that your visualization has the desired results:

• Be clear about your desired outcome

Before you envision how you will communicate you must be clear about what it is you are trying to achieve. Is it your aim to be warm and comforting? Do you want to get some specific information from your client or colleague? Is it your intention to get a point across? Whatever your purpose is in communicating, you must be crystal clear about what you want to happen. The more tailored your mental rehearsal is to reality the more positive influence it will have on your subsequent performance.

It might be helpful for you to compare a poorly articulated goal and a clearer, more detailed one.

> Barb and Jane are both nurses working on a burn unit. Both nurses are concerned about Mrs. Charter, who has become withdrawn and weepy in the last 48 hours. Each nurse decides on her own desired outcome for this unhappy client situation.
>
> Barb makes it her goal to help Mrs. Charter overcome her blue mood. This goal is not as clear as it might be because it does not provide Barb with many clues about how to proceed. Not only is it not specific, but it is unlikely that it is a logical place to begin without more data.
>
> Jane's aim is to find out if Mrs. Charter is aware of what might be causing her mood change and to discuss with her if there is anything that can be done to lift her mood. Her aim is to put Mrs.

Charter at ease so that she can talk more freely about her feelings. This clearer desired outcome provides Jane with some guidelines on how to proceed.

• Mentally outline from beginning to end the whole interaction you will be having with your client or colleague

You will feel more prepared for your interaction if you complete this step in your mental imagery. For instance, if you are going to be teaching a client to care for his colostomy do not limit your visualization to the time when you will be talking. Bring into your vision your preparation time, post-session time, and the direct teaching time. When you visualize your preparation you will anticipate all the equipment you will need and consequently have it ready. You might become aware that you fear embarrassment discussing the hygiene and sexual aspects of colostomy care with your male client. This awareness will prompt you to talk over your concerns with a more experienced colleague before the session so that when you do your teaching you will feel less uncomfortable.

When imagining the actual teaching session, consider the beginning, middle, and termination. Find out how much time you have and imagine yourself using the time effectively and productively for both you and your client. Envision the termination: will you want time to debrief and discuss things with a colleague afterward? Is it likely that you will have follow-up assignments after the session for which you must allow time such as making referrals, writing records or securing information for the client? By mentally going through the whole encounter you will be much better prepared.

• Concentrate on visualizing as many details as possible about your face-to-face encounter with your client or colleague

Envision the most ideal environment for your encounter and take in all its details. In reality try to approximate this location in terms of privacy, lighting, warmth, accessibility to equipment, or whatever other criteria are important.

Visualize how you would like to be dressed for your interaction. If it is a play session with the children on the pediatric medical unit you will likely envision yourself in a brightly colored pant suit uniform. If you are mentally preparing yourself for your job performance interview with your head nurse envision yourself wearing a uniform in which you feel your best.

Pay attention to your posture and facial expressions. If you want to be businesslike with a serious middle-aged client, then picture how you will move to convey your intentions. If you wish to appear relaxed and confident as you present your case at your first nursing rounds, mentally see and feel yourself carrying off this composure.

As you direct yourself in your visions to create a positive impression, notice in your mind's eye that others are responding favorably. For example, you may observe that you are being listened to and taken seriously and that your client or colleague seems interested in what you have to say.

In addition to your visual imagery use your other senses. For instance, listen to what you are saying and how you are saying it. If what you are saying does not come across in the way you intended it, then roll back the reel and replay it. On the rerun visualize yourself communicating more closely in line with how you would ideally like to do. The beauty of mentally rehearsing is that you can repeat it as many times as you like until you get it right! Tune into your words and the way you are saying them striving to hear the content and quality you desire.

Envision how you want to feel during your communication and be sure to concentrate on the positive. Engender feelings of calmness, confidence, competence, or compassion—or however you want to be feeling in reality. It is important to pause and actually experience these good feelings in your rehearsal, so you will be more likely to recognize them and allow them to surface in the real situation. Also visualize your client or colleague having feelings that are appropriate for the situation.

Using your wide-angle lens, see the whole interaction going as you planned. For example, with your encouragement your adolescent client looks eager to try wearing designer jeans over his ileostomy bag; your bereaved colleague feels relieved to have shed a few tears with you after the death of her long-term client; your skeptical supervisor seems positively impressed with your suggestion for a new staffing schedule; and your once worried client is able to drop off to sleep after your reassuring preoperative teaching session.

• Envision the best and plan for the unexpected

There are times when we are concerned about an interaction with a client or colleague for fear we will not be able to communicate in the way we want. Envisioning a positive rehearsal helps relieve some of that worry. To augment your confidence, it is a wise plan to envision some of the unexpected turns of events you might possibly encounter in reality, and practice how to cope with them. For example, if it is your first time to teach prenatal classes and you are afraid that there might be questions about labor and delivery that you cannot answer, it would be wise to imagine a scene where you are asked one of these questions and then rehearse the best way to respond. You may gain comfort with saying "I don't know . . . but I'll find out for you" if you visualize it in advance. Or an angry co-worker might unnerve you with her hostility. If you visualize her attack in advance you can covertly prepare yourself for some effective ways to cope with the anger.

Practicing this way expands your repertoire and prepares you for many contingencies. If you have prepared yourself for several versions of what to expect, and rehearsed for several options, you will feel a lot more confident handling yourself in the real situation.

• Rehearse repeatedly where necessary

Each of us has interpersonal situations in which we feel unconfident. Some of us shudder at having to interact with angry hostile people, whereas others remain calm and empathic with volatile clients and colleagues. Some of us dread taking charge of teaching sessions, whereas others love that opportunity. Some of us feel we relate better on a one-to-one basis, and others prefer groups. For those interpersonal situations in which you feel uncomfortable it is a wise plan to repeat your positive visualization several times. Repeatedly go over the picture of yourself performing successfully in your difficult area. A one-shot visualization may not allow you to register all the things you must do to make your communication successful. Seeing yourself handling things well in many visualizations will more thoroughly prepare you for the event. Repeating the scene in your mind's eye prevents you from feeling shocked in the actual event—you will be able to act instead of react.

When we are concerned about a situation we can lapse into forecasting the worst or we can choose to concentrate on seeing a positive picture. A positive visualization attracts like a magnet, getting you closer to your goal. If you repeat your positive visualization enough times it will help you perform well in reality.

• Review your live performance and update your visualization

After you have completed the interaction with your client or colleague, it is a good idea to take time to evaluate how it went. If there were parts of your interaction that you are less than pleased with, think positively about how you could improve your next exchange and visualize that happening. For example, envision how you could rephrase your words, set the room up differently, or include gestures such as touch. This rehearsal will prepare you for the next time.

Do not put yourself down for your errors of omission or commission. Instead, give yourself credit for your improvements. Remember that you are learning and consider that each practice will get you closer to the way you want to communicate to clients and colleagues. Think back to your rehearsal and notice where you met or even surpassed your ideals. Visualize patting yourself on the back and congratulating yourself on your successes. Taking time to commend yourself will augment your self-confidence.

PRACTICING IMAGERY

Exercise 1. In your everyday life take the opportunity to use imagery to help you communicate more effectively with others. For example, if you would like to invite a classmate to go shopping with you, visualize how you would like to extend the invitation and envision her enthusiastic response. Prepare yourself for a refusal by hearing her extend her regrets, and watch yourself respond smoothly. Or you may have an upcoming test of your nursing care practice. Take time to see yourself successfully completing each part of the test, and imagine your instructor giving you top grades.

After a few days of trying to use imagery take stock of the ways in which it has helped you. What personal adaptations to the process of imagery have you made that might be useful for your colleagues to apply? In the class as a whole compare reflections on the benefits of imagery.

Visualizing Yourself as Successful!

As you practice imagery you will discover it is a skill that requires discipline and concentration. It is self-constructive to develop the power of concentration in order to visualize yourself communicating in an effective way. If we want to be self-destructive, we can let our thoughts take control of us by allowing visions of making mistakes, embarrassing ourselves, or failing to communicate effectively to dominate our visions. If we permit negative and unproductive thoughts to worry and plague us we might fall into the trap of acting out the failure. On the other hand, our chances for success are augmented by mentally rehearsing a positive outcome. If you have seen yourself succeeding in your mind's eye, it is but one more step to perform in reality.

As you practice you will discover that imagery does not require much time and can be done anywhere. In the shower, on the bus, as you walk to your meeting, at the nurses' station—you can visualize anywhere because your imagination is always active. What imagery emphasizes is taking control of your thinking so that you create positive, self-enhancing pictures of yourself which facilitate more hopeful and confident feelings. Because imagery can be done conveniently, you can repeatedly bring into your awareness the image of the successful you.

As you learn each of the communication behaviors in this book, practice a positive visualization of yourself using them correctly. Rehearsing with the valuable assistance of imagery will help you feel confident and facilitate the integration of the skill into your communications repertoire.

REFERENCES

Ardell, D.B. (1977). *High level wellness*. Emmaus, Penn.: Rodale Press.
Barnhart, C.L. (Ed.) (1975). *World Book Dictionary*. Chicago: Doubleday & Co. Inc.
Bolen, J. (1973, July). Meditation and psychotherapy in the treatment of cancer. *Psychic*, p. 20.
Flynn, P. (1980). *Holistic health: The art and science of care*. Bowie, Md.: Robert J. Brady Co.
Hartmann, F. (1973). *Paracelsus: Life and prophecies*. Blauvelt, N.Y.: Rudolf Steiner Publications.
Jacobson, E. (1942). *Progressive relaxation*. Chicago: University of Chicago Press.
Lauria, A. (1968). *The mind of a mnemonist*. New York: Basic Books Inc.
Luthe, W. (1969). *Autogenic Therapy: Vol. II*. New York: Grune and Stratton.
Mayer, A.J. (1984, January). Visualization. *en Route*, pp. 30-32, 48, 50.
Miller, N. (1969). Learning and visceral and glandular responses. *Science, 163*, pp. 434-445.
Samuels, M., & Bennett, H.Z. (1974). *Be well*. Toronto, Canada: Random House Inc.
Samuels, M., & Samuels, N. (1975). *Seeing with the mind's eye*. New York: Random House Inc.
Simonton, O.C., Matthews-Simonton, S., & Creighton, L. (1980). *Getting well again*. New York: Bantam Books Inc.

SUGGESTIONS FOR FURTHER READING

Cormier, W.H., & Cormier, L.S. (1991). *Interviewing strategies for helpers: Fundamental skills and cognitive behavioral interventions* (3rd ed.). Pacific Grove, Calif.: Brooks/Cole Publishing Company.

The authors provide an up-to-date review of the therapeutic applications of imagery. The currency and comprehensiveness of Cormier and Cormier's work make this reference a useful source of information about imagery. In the chapter entitled "Emotive Imagery and Covert Modelling," the authors demonstrate through inclusion of dialogue how to use the client's imagination for modelling and rehearsal. Steps for assessing the client's imagery potential and for practing imagery with clients are included.

Samuels, M., Samuels, N. (1975). *Seeing with the mind's eye: The history techniques and uses of visualization.* New York, New York: Random House, Incorporated; Berkeley, Calif.: The Book Works.

Although this text is an older publication, its coverage of the topic of imagery is comprehensive for interested readers. In addition to unravelling the history of imagery in religion, healing and psychology, it provides readers with visualization techniques, and demonstrates the application of imagery in all aspects of our lives, including healing.

Siegel, B.S. (1989). *Peace, love and healing: Bodymind communication and the path to self healing: An exploration.* New York: Harper & Row Incorporated.

For readers wanting to learn more about imagery, Bernie Siegel discusses the use of imagery and visualization as it applies to health and health care. Nurse readers can transfer this information to using imagery and visualization for improved communication with clients and colleagues.

CHAPTER 18

Positive
Self-talk

*"Man is disturbed not by things
but the views he takes of them."*

Epictetus

OBJECTIVES

This chapter will make you aware of how much your thoughts influence
your communication and all your nursing actions. You will learn to control your thinking so that it influences your interactions with clients and
colleagues in a positive way. Practicing positive self-talk will develop confidence in your communication and nursing practice in general.

WHAT IS SELF-TALK?

Self-talk is not unlike the conversation that occurs between two people.
Meichenbaum (1977) suggests that we have an ongoing internal dialogue—we speak to ourselves and we listen to ourselves. Self-talk is
called by other names in the literature: self-verbalization, inner thought,
inner speech, self-instruction, or that "little voice" in your head that
forms a self-communication system.

Cognitive-behaviorists have learned about the powerful influence this
internal dialogue has on our behavior. Our thoughts are our interpretations of the world, our judgments about our own behavior, and our assumptions about others' reactions to us. Our feelings are directly influenced by our thoughts, and how we construe our world provides the
blueprint for our actions. It is not what is happening to us that is so significant, but how we interpret what is happening to us and what we do
under the influence of these thoughts.

For any situation or interpersonal encounter we have, our self-talk
determines the following:

- Our attitude towards the situation
- What we see, hear and attend to
- How we interpret what we take in
- What we think the outcome will be
- How we act (including what we feel, say and do)
- How we appraise the consequences of our actions

It is important that our internal dialogue be in our own best interests because it is a continuous and powerful influence on our well-being and performance. Cognitive-behaviorists believe our internal dialogue causes problems when it is irrational, unrealistic, or ineffective (Meichenbaum, 1977).

Our internal dialogue can be constructive or destructive. Here are examples of positive and negative self-talk. As you read the examples think about their possible effects on the nurses in the situation.

Tanya and Deirdre are nursing students in their first year. As they anticipate their forthcoming clinical placements these thoughts go through their minds:

> **Tanya:** "I've heard the head nurse is a real battle-axe. I hate people like that. They have miserable dispositions that grate on my nerves. I just know I'm not going to like this unit. I'll be on pins and needles the whole time. She's sure to pick on me, and knowing me I'll probably make some blunder that'll be a red flag for her to show me up. And we have to go there for 3 long weeks. I'll be glad when it's over."

Tanya has set herself up for an unhappy and unfruitful clinical placement. Her negative thoughts about the placement have entrenched the notion that she will be miserable there. This negative self-talk is destructive. Thinking the way she does, Tanya will likely act defensively and be so on edge that she *will* make a mistake. Her attitude will probably isolate her from friendly sources of support on the unit.

> **Deirdre:** "I've heard the head nurse is a real stickler for good nursing care and demands a lot from her staff. It's neat that I get to go to a unit where the nursing care is so good. I'm sure I'll learn a lot. I'm looking forward to trying out some of the procedures I've been practicing in the classroom where I can get some feedback and pointers. I'm also nervous because I'm so inexperienced, but I know I'll have the best teachers and get a lot out of the experience. Too bad it's only for 3 weeks."

Deirdre has mentally prepared herself for a happy and rewarding clinical experience. Her interpretation of the excellence of the nursing care makes her keen to observe the nurses and reap the benefits of their experience. Her positive self-talk sets her up to risk interacting with the staff and getting the most out of the experience.

Our self-talk goes on continuously in our heads and is so automatic that we have to stop and listen to hear whether it is exerting a negative or positive influence on our feelings and behavior. If we want to have control of this habitual process we need to stop and listen to our thoughts, decide how we want to change, and systematically convert our thinking so that it influences our behavior in the intended direction.

Here is an example of a typical situation many student nurses encounter in the clinical area. As you read the scenario put yourself in the position of the student nurse and write down your reactions.

You are a nursing student just entering your second year after your summer vacation. To date, your clinical experience has been on the specialty units of your hospital: ophthalmology, gynecology, and the diabetic unit. As a first-year student you were only assigned three clients at the most. Now that you are a second-year student you are going to the large medical unit in your hospital and you will be expected to handle a full client load and complete all treatment procedures for this assignment. You are unaccustomed to managing a large case load. It is late August and some of the regular staff nurses on the unit are on vacation and are not being replaced because of budget cutbacks. You know the unit has a full census of clients. Your clinical instructor told you the staff is looking forward to your arrival because they need an extra pair of hands on the unit.

After you have written your reactions, put the list aside for the moment and review the following example of Suzanne's negative self-talk as she encounters the same situation.

> **Suzanne:** "I'll never cope! I wish this nursing school had organized my clinical experiences better so I'd be prepared to take on a full client load at this point. I'm nervous already thinking about it. Why did I ever come into nursing? I wish it were winter; then the unit wouldn't be short staffed and they wouldn't be counting on me so much. I've never had to do the treatments and all the care for a full load of clients; I know I can't move that fast. I'll be throwing a wash cloth at one and rushing to do a dressing on another. I can see it now. I'll be feeling panicky the whole time. I'll probably be on the unit till 6 every day trying to get caught up on my charting. How can I give good nursing care and be rushing around like a chicken without its head?"

Suzanne's self-talk is destructive. It is escalating her anxiety and focusing on all the things that could possibly go wrong. Suzanne is drowning in a flood of doomsday thinking. With a mind set like hers she will be tuned into anything negative and may force a self-fulfilling prophecy. Her self-talk dismisses any self-confidence and makes her anxious before, and likely during, the experience.

Take a moment to write down a constructive internal dialogue that Suzanne could use in the same situation.

Here is an example of positive self-talk for Suzanne. Compare your suggestions with this example.

Suzanne: "This is going to be difficult. I'm going to have to learn to move quickly and be super organized to manage a large client load and all the treatments. I know I can do it. And I know the experienced nurses on the floor will help me. I find it hard to keep a lot of things in my head and have a lot of clients, but it is something I need to learn to do in nursing. Here is a good opportunity to increase my efficiency. The staff nurses know that I'm a student and will not expect miracles from me. They will be glad for the contribution I can make to the unit. I must find out more about the unit from Betty so that I can prepare myself as much as possible for the experience."

This self-talk is constructive. Suzanne's internal dialogue in this example is realistic and hopeful. By acknowledging her assets Suzanne will go onto the unit feeling confident. She is likely to approach the staff in a friendly way and seek tips from them on how to organize herself better. Thinking about her situation as a challenge provides Suzanne with a positive goal for her career as a nurse. By deciding to seek out information beforehand she is increasing her chances of success.

Now go back to your own internal dialogue you generated earlier in this exercise. Determine whether it is positive or negative. Would your self-talk facilitate your best interests, or is it potentially destructive?

Positive Self-talk is Assertive and Responsible

The previous examples demonstrate how self-talk can be harmful or helpful to us. Positive self-talk is helpful because it emphasizes our strengths and our ability to handle the situations confronting us. This mental preparation makes us feel hopeful and confident. We have the right to feel good about how we handle situations we encounter, and positive self-talk is one technique we can use to ensure that our rights are realized. It is assertive to keep our internal dialogue positive.

Positive self-talk is not unrealistic or wishful thinking. It involves an accurate assessment of our abilities and the situation we are facing. Not having the knowledge or skills to effectively handle an interpersonal situation is no reason to think less of ourselves or put ourselves down. Admitting our lack of experience, and acknowledging our willingness and ability to learn, realistically prepares us to tackle the situation. This positive kind of mental assessment is responsible because it takes into account the facts of the situation. Mentally putting ourselves down or discrediting our abilities is not responsible thinking.

Butler (1981) warns us that when our self-talk is negative we are carrying around a toxic environment for ourselves everywhere we go. Negative self-talk is harsh and judgmental, demanding superhero achievements, chastising us for failing, and generally making us feel tense and dissatisfied with ourselves. Butler (1981) encourages us to develop a positive, supportive way of talking to ourselves to cushion us from negative events.

Becoming aware of our self-talk is the first step to discovering if it is in our best interests. Learning how to change our self-talk starts with such an assessment. Butler (1981) suggests we ask ourselves the following questions to assess our self-talk:

1. What am I telling myself?
2. What negative thoughts am I generating that are destructive to me?
3. What positive thoughts am I generating that are constructive for me?
4. Is my self-talk helping me?

The answers to these questions will point out where our thinking is serviceable or nonbeneficial. This assessment alerts us to whether we need to change our self-talk.

The next step is to specify how we need to change our internal dialogue so that it is more positive. At first this planning will require considerable effort, until it becomes part of our awareness to tune into our internal dialogue and adjust it quickly. Later in this chapter you will get experience in reformulating self-talk.

The Relationship Between Self-talk and Interpersonal Communication

In Part One you learned about behaviors that are essential for caring communication. Parts of your self-talk will be about your ability to implement these behaviors with your clients and colleagues. How you construct your internal dialogue can enhance or diminish your skill level.

Here are samples in relation to the communication behaviors of empathy and confrontation.

Example 1: Self-talk about Empathy

Here is what one nurse said to herself about empathy:

"I can't be empathic and sound natural."

"I'll trip over my words."

"If I try using empathy I'll sound artificial."

"My colleagues will laugh at me if I change my style and try to be empathic."

"I don't think I can think up an empathic response fast enough in a 'real' conversation to make it sound sincere."

"I'll look and feel awkward trying to be empathic."

Examine this nurse's self-talk

1. **What is she telling herself?** She is telling herself that she will feel uncomfortable, silly, and unnatural if she attempts to be empathic.

She is convincing herself that her friends will not admire her attempts and that she will lose their respect.

2. **What negative thoughts is she generating that are destructive?** She is convincing herself that she will not be effective in her employment of empathy. She expects that she should be perfect the first time she is empathic. She is not permitting any failure, nor is she hopeful that her colleagues will support her.

3. **What positive thoughts is she generating?** This nurse is not generating one positive thought that might give her the hope and encouragement to try being more empathic.

4. **Is her self-talk helping her?** This self-talk will likely stop her from including empathy in her communication strategies. These thoughts will make her feel badly on two counts: she will miss providing the benefits of empathy to others and she will feel disappointed in her lack of willingness to try. She is left feeling convinced that neither she nor her colleagues have confidence in her ability. Her thoughts are unassertive and irresponsible and not in any way helpful to her.

5. **How can she change her self-talk so that it is more positive?** Here are examples of how her self-talk could be more positive.

"I'm going to try to use empathy even if I am a little stilted and awkward at first."

"I am convinced of the importance of empathy and know that my colleagues and clients will appreciate my efforts to show them that I understand, even if I am not perfect in my attempts."

"Some of my colleagues may teasingly comment on the change when I try to be more empathic; I will not let their put-downs deter me from including empathy in my communication."

"It may take me a while to find the right words to express myself empathically but that's okay. It will likely seem longer to me than to the other person."

"I really want to improve my communication and I know that something new takes time to learn. I can be patient with myself until empathy comes more naturally in my interactions with others."

This positive self-talk is assertive and responsible. It underlies the importance this nurse places on being empathic and gives her encouragement to try being more understanding. It is not a glib dialogue, but rather it realistically assesses her ability to weather the struggle of trying something new until it becomes a natural part of her communication. This positive self-talk is helpful because it boosts confidence and facilitates the incorporation of a new skill into her repertoire.

Example 2: Self-talk about Confrontation

Here is one nurse's self-talk about confrontation:

> "I think it's better to keep peace by not saying anything to the boss about his abrasive manner to me these past few days."

> "If I confront him he'll think I'm one of those feminists on a soapbox and he'll be wary of me hereafter."

> "He'll pull rank on me and get angry if I confront him."

> "The more I think about it the crazier it seems for me to be upset about his manner; he's probably got something on his mind and doesn't realize he's taking it out on me."

> "What if I get all upset and mix up my words? I'd really look like a fool then."

Examine this nurse's self-talk

1. **What is she telling herself?** She is convincing herself that she would be better off not to confront her boss about an issue important to her. She is arguing that her feelings are not as important as those of her boss.
2. **What negative thoughts is she generating which are destructive?** This nurse is denying her own feelings by deceiving herself that it might be better to let this episode pass. This self-deception undermines her judgment. She is creating bad feelings about herself by suggesting that being a "feminist" is undesirable. She attempts to frighten herself with the assumption that her boss will get angry and, furthermore, that she would not be able to handle his anger. She imagines the worst scenario and tries to convince herself that she is likely to fail.
3. **What positive thoughts is she generating?** This nurse's self-talk is entirely negative and contains nothing positive for her.
4. **Is her self-talk helping her?** This negative self-talk would only deter her from standing up for something which is important to her: her desire to be treated with respect. This approach makes her doubt her ability to confront and to handle one possible consequence of a confrontation: her boss' possible anger. Her negative self-talk is unassertive and irresponsible and is in no way helpful to her.
5. **How can she change her self-talk to make it more positive?** Here are examples of how her self-talk could be more positive.

> "I don't like to confront my boss, but I don't like to be treated disrespectfully, so I will confront him."

> "I know I can make my points clear to him without being aggressive or hurting his feelings."

> "My boss may become angry or hostile when I confront him, but I can handle this reaction without backing off or becoming defensive."

"I have practiced confrontation and feel confident that I can carry it off."

"If my confrontation isn't perfect, it doesn't matter; that I make my point as clearly as possible is what counts."

"Just because he's my boss is no reason to treat me so badly. I have the right to be treated with respect."

This positive self-talk is assertive and responsible. It encourages the nurse to stand up for herself and it takes into account her ability to handle several possible outcomes. It is encouraging and supportive and would set this nurse up with the comfort and confidence to carry out her confrontation.

In Part Three of this book you will learn how to communicate assertively and responsibly in the following situations where nurses are known to have difficulty:

- When clients or colleagues are distressed
- When clients or colleagues are aggressive
- When there is team conflict
- When evaluation anxiety is experienced
- When encountering unpopular clients

In all these situations *positive* self-talk is important. Here are examples of self-talk in two of the above situations.

Example 3: Self-talk When Colleagues Are Distressed

Here is one nurse's self-talk when encountering a colleague who is distressed and crying:

"I hate it when colleagues cry; I mean, with clients it's okay, I expect them to be upset. I don't know what to do when staff at work cry."

"Whenever anyone at work cries my lacrimals overflow, too, and I'm useless to them."

"If anyone cries I don't know what I'll do. I just can't cope when grown people cry."

"I don't know what to do to make her feel better. What if she won't stop crying?"

"If I can't help her to calm down then I'm not much good."

Examine this nurse's self-talk

1. **What is she telling herself?** This nurse is telling herself that staff members do not have the same feelings and reactions as clients. She is telling herself that a lot is expected of her and that if she does not perform adequately by calming down her upset colleague then she is not

an effective person. She is convinced that if she cries too it will be detrimental to her colleague.

2. **What negative thoughts is she generating that are destructive?**
   She is putting considerable pressure on herself to perform in the only way that she thinks is acceptable. She is assuming that she will not be helpful to her colleague and gives no credit to herself. Her denial of a normal range of feelings in her colleagues prevents her compassion from surfacing in a way that would be helpful. Her impending sense of failure if she does not perform perfectly is likely making her tense.

3. **What positive thoughts is she generating?** This nurse is not saying anything comforting or encouraging to herself.

4. **Is her self-talk helpful?** Her self-talk is unassertive because it downplays her potential to be helpful. It is not responsible because it distorts reality. Her self-talk would hinder her ability to reach out to her colleague and communicate in a helpful way. The restrictions imposed by this negative thinking would leave her feeling inadequate.

5. **How can she change her self-talk so that it is more positive?** Here are examples of how her self-talk could be more positive.

   "Everybody gets upset and staff are no exception."

   "I may not be able to stop her from crying but I think I can comfort her."

   "I always cry when any other staff member cries; but that's okay. It just shows how compassionate I am. My crying doesn't interfere with my ability to be helpful."

   "She may not respond to my efforts to calm her down but that doesn't mean I'm a bad nurse. Each of us has someone special we can relate to when we are upset."

   "I don't have to do a lot to be helpful. No weird and wonderful heroics are expected. Just staying close by is often enough."

These inner thoughts are reassuring and confidence-building. They are responsible because they do not distort the reality of the situation. They are assertive because they acknowledge the nurse's desire and ability to help. This positive self-talk is helpful.

Example 4: Self-talk When There is Team Conflict

Here is a sample of one nurse's thinking about the conflict situation on her nursing unit.

"All I want is a peaceful place to work. Wherever I go there are power struggles and I hate it."

"I just know this conflict is going to drag on; I wish I worked on Unit One. They never have any conflicts there."

"Maybe I should transfer to another unit; I can't do anything about the conflicts on our team."

"I thought we had dealt with this conflict once and for all; I just hate these drawn-out disagreements."

"Whenever we discuss that upsetting issue my stomach gets in a knot and I feel like exploding; I don't know how much more I can take."

"I'm useless when there's conflict. I just let it tear me apart and that's no good."

"I'm afraid I'm going to give the team leader a piece of my mind. She should get this conflict under control."

Examine this nurse's self-talk

1. **What is she telling herself?** This nurse has the erroneous notion that conflict is brief, easily resolved, and nonrecurring. The false expectation that there are some places where conflict does not occur is self-defeating. She is trying to convince herself that there is little she can do about the conflict. She feels that the team leader should magically control the conflict.

2. **What negative thoughts is she generating that are destructive?** Her unrealistic ideas about the nature of conflict are causing her grief. Her image of herself as someone with little control in conflict situations makes her feel hopeless and ineffective. Her anticipation of unpleasant physical signs and symptoms in conflict situations initiates her anxiety at the slightest indication of conflict.

3. **What positive thoughts is she generating?** There is nothing reassuring and hopeful about her thinking.

4. **Is her self-talk helpful?** Her self-talk is unassertive because it does not grant her any power to contribute to the resolution of the conflict. Her distorted perception about her lack of influence to affect change is irresponsible. These thoughts are not helpful because they immobilize her and increase her tension about the conflict.

5. **How can she change her self-talk so that it is more positive?** Here are examples of how her self-talk could be more positive.

"Every unit has conflict; it is an unavoidable part of working with others."

"Sometimes creative and effective ways of handling situations can come out of conflict. Maybe there are some positive benefits to this conflict."

"I can keep my cool to express my feelings about the conflict on our unit. My ideas will have more impact if I remain calm."

"Each thing I do to diminish the conflict goes a long way to resolving our problems. No one person can eliminate the conflict alone, but each contribution is significant."

"I get anxious when there's conflict on the unit but it is not over-whelming. I can keep it under control."

This positive self-talk is assertive and responsible. Admitting that conflict is a normal part of working with others removes the shock of dis-agreement and makes her more apt to tackle the problem. Believing that whatever steps she takes to manage the conflict are significant promotes positive action on her part. Putting her anxiety in perspective allows her to function without being ashamed or overwhelmed. She is responsible in her assessment of the situation and her ability. This positive internal di-alogue is assertive in its acknowledgment of her desire to handle situa-tions effectively.

In his book *Pulling Your Own Strings* Dyer (1978) challenges us by suggesting that several ideas we take for granted do not exist in reality (p. 187). Some examples are "disasters," "a good boy," "a stupid person," and "a perfect person." Each of these concepts represents a judgment about reality. Negative self-talk about our ability to communicate or han-dle interpersonal situations is our destructive and self-defeating judg-ment. Dyer advises us not to be victimized and encourages us to subscribe to thoughts that are reality based and self-enhancing. If we can apply this advice to our *intrapersonal* communication it will stand us in good stead for our *interpersonal* encounters with clients and colleagues. Talking to ourselves in encouraging, realistic ways increases our ability to commu-nicate with others in assertive and responsible ways.

Bach and Torbet (1983) purport that we have two voices in our inner life: our "inner enemy" and our "inner ally." Our inner enemy keeps a running inventory of our weaknesses, maintains a certain misery level and keeps all joyless, negative information on file, and can display it at a moment's notice. Our inner ally is interested in action, growth, and change and prevents us from getting bogged down in doubts and fears. Our ally reassures us of the benefits and rewards of success and the plea-sures of trying, encouraging us to take risks that will help get us where we want to go. When we make mistakes it is our inner ally that comforts us and helps us view our mistakes in perspective.

As you practice enhancing and augmenting your interpersonal com-munication skills, focus on what your inner ally tells you. Allow comfort-ing and realistic thoughts to support and encourage you while learning.

Using Positive Self-talk to Enhance Your Interpersonal Communication

Positive self-talk can help you at three phases of interpersonal communi-cation: before, during, and after.

• **Before** your interaction with a client or colleague you can take con-trol of your thoughts and focus on realistic and encouraging inner dia-logue that will make you feel more confident about your forthcoming en-counter. This preparation makes you focus on your strengths rather than worrying about potential catastrophes. When you feel prepared you will likely act more competently.

For some encounters you have hours or days to prepare your positive self-talk. At other times you get little preparation time. However, even for surprise encounters you can quickly tune into your internal dialogue (it is continuously active) and talk to yourself in encouraging ways.

For example, as you are walking down to answer the bell of a client who is yelling, "Nurse! Where in the heck are you? NURSE!!" you can be saying these words to yourself:

> **Positive You:** "He's impatient and angry, and it could get me upset. But I will stay calm and collected. Slow down, relax your breathing, and loosen up your shoulders. You will find out what is troubling him and be able to handle it. Haste makes waste, so just remain steady and pay attention to each thing that you are doing. Here's his room now, just relax and focus. Tune in."

This preparation will prime you to handle this aggressive client situation calmly and effectively.

• **During** your conversation you can tune into your inner voice and concentrate on supportive dialogue. For example, if your client's face is turning red, his voice is getting louder, and his language is getting more hostile, you can say to yourself:

> **Positive You:** "He's getting angry. That's okay. I can handle his outburst. I will remain calm and find out what is so upsetting for him. My breathing is regular, my posture is relaxed, and I will keep my voice steady. There's no point in getting upset."

This positive self-talk will remind you to stay in control and handle the situation effectively. The comfort provided by your own supportive thoughts helps you to act the way you want.

• **After** an encounter you can use positive self-talk to constructively review your performance. Noting your successes and your areas where improvement is needed are both important. This example of a constructive review would be helpful:

> **Positive You:** "I thought I controlled my fear of his hostility really well. I actually remained calm and kept my voice tone on an even pitch. I think what I said to him helped to calm him down but next time I'd like to achieve a relaxed body posture. My fists were clenched and my shoulders were pretty tight and I could feel that my knees were locked. When I can relax my body that will be one more positive message going out that I am in control and confident."

Positive self-talk is a tool you carry with you and is available at a moment's notice. When you have yourself on your side you are never alone and you always have an encouraging supporter on whom to call.

PRACTICING POSITIVE SELF-TALK

Exercise 1. As you attempt to use each of the communication behaviors in Part One in real life, or as part of the exercises at the end of each chapter, try using positive self-talk to enhance your skill level.

Exercise 2. Any time you encounter a difficult interpersonal situation, whether in practice or real life, try talking positively with yourself to augment your ability to communicate assertively and responsibly.

Exercise 3. As a class compare your experiences with employing positive self-talk after you have practiced using it as suggested in the above exercises. What difficulties did you encounter in employing positive self-talk? What successes did you have by keeping your internal dialogue positive?

Exercise 4. For this exercise work in threes. One will be the nurse interviewer, another the client, and the third the feedback giver. The client and nurse will determine the purpose of their interview in advance. It is important to be clear about your roles in advance and to keep the roleplay situation simple. After 5 minutes of interaction the feedback giver will comment on the nurse's communication skills.

Before each person begins the roleplay stop and tune into your self-talk. Ask yourself if your self-talk is helping you. Change any negative thoughts into constructive ones. During the roleplay try to focus on the voice inside your head and generate encouraging thoughts about your role performance (of nurse, client, or giver of feedback).

After the interaction pause and listen to the voice in your head. If you hear negative or destructive thoughts about your role performance, then make your internal dialogue more supportive.

After you have completed this exercise pool together your reflections about employing positive self-talk. What have you learned about your own self-talk? How does your self-talk influence your performance?

REFERENCES AND SUGGESTIONS FOR FURTHER READING

The following references provide enjoyable reading to the nurse reader who is interested in learning more about positive self-talk.

Butler, P.E. (1981). *Talking to yourself*. New York: Stein and Day, Publishers.

Bach, G., & Torbet, L. (1983). The everyday slow torture of self-hate. *New Woman*. Palm Beach, Fla.: New Woman, Incorporated, Publishers.

Dyer, W.W. (1978). *Pulling your own strings*. New York: A Funk & Wagnalls Book, Published by Thomas Y. Cromwell Company.

The following two references are for the reader who desires an in-depth review of the research and theoretical approaches of cognitive-behavior modification.

Cormier, W.H., & Cormier, L.S. (1991). *Interviewing strategies for helpers: Fundamental skills and cognitive behavioral interventions* (3rd ed.). Pacific Grove, Calif. Brooks/Cole Publishing Company.

Chapter 16, "Cognitive restructuring, reframing, and stress inoculation," is written to explain the theoretical underpinnings of these therapies and provides guidelines for practitioners to use these approaches in practice.

Meichenbaum, D. (1977). *Cognitive-behavior modification: An integrative approach*. New York: Plenum Press.

PART 3

COMMUNICATION SKILL

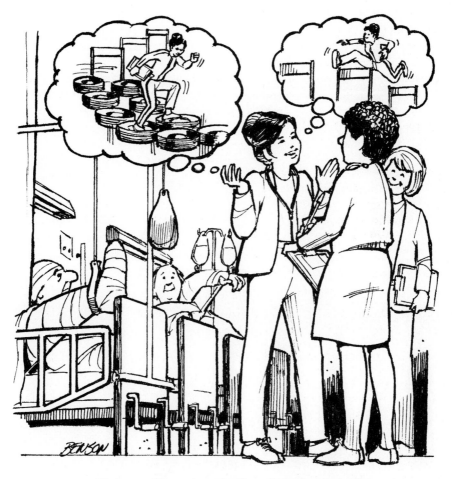

"Fit to run the communication obstacle course."

INTRODUCTION TO PART 3: COMMUNICATION SKILL

You know there are three important factors that contribute to producing effective nurse communicators:

- A sound knowledge of the essential communication behaviors *(communication competence)*
- Liking and wanting to produce these appropriate communication behaviors *(positive communication affect)*
- The ability to produce these essential communication behaviors *(communication skill)*

In Part One you augmented your understanding of the basic communication behaviors and in Part Two you developed some techniques for increasing the likelihood that you will feel positive about communicating assertively and responsibly. In Part Three you will get practice communicating effectively in those situations where nurses have most difficulty.

In his extensive literature review of health professionals' interpersonal skills Gerrard (1978) discovered that their communication skills are weak in situations involving:

- **Evaluation anxiety:** when they fear making a mistake or being negatively evaluated
- **Distressed clients:** clients who are upset, sad, depressed, and crying
- **Aggressive clients:** clients who are abusive, angry, rejecting, or manipulative
- **Unpopular clients:** clients who lack verbal or social skills and do not meet standards for "good" client behavior
- **Team conflict:** when there is conflict between health professionals

Part Three of this textbook is devoted to assisting you in handling these five difficult interpersonal situations in assertive and responsible ways. Step by step guidelines are suggested for handling evaluation anxiety. You get feedback on your choices of the most assertive and responsible ways to relate to distressed and aggressive clients and colleagues. Some concrete ways for maximizing your compassion with unpopular clients are proffered. You will learn assertive and responsible ways to manage team conflict.

REFERENCE

Gerrard, B. (1978). *Interpersonal skills for health professionals: A review of the literature.* Unpublished manuscript. McMaster University, Hamilton, Ontario, Canada.

CHAPTER 19

Overcoming
Evaluation Anxiety

*"You gain strength, courage and confidence
by every experience in which you really stop
to look fear in the face."*

Eleanor Roosevelt

OBJECTIVES

At some time you may have experienced how debilitating evaluation anxiety can be. This chapter provides you with techniques for controlling and overcoming evaluation anxiety. Applying the ideas you glean from this chapter will help you feel better prepared for performance appraisals, examinations, and informal evaluations.

WHAT IS EVALUATION ANXIETY?

Even though we easily toss off the old saying "to err is human," most of us prefer that someone else be the one to err! In our competitive North American culture we idolize excellence in personal performance, products, and services. Advertisements bombard us from billboards, radio, and TV about "better" or "improved" products. We spend years in an educational system that makes judgments about our physical and psychological abilities through a variety of examinations and elaborate grading systems. Making mistakes is the antithesis of our cultural standard for excellence. Our preoccupation with perfection makes it difficult to accept that making mistakes is a normal part of human endeavor.

Evaluation anxiety occurs when we are upset about having our performance judged and are intimidated by the evaluation process. One form of evaluation anxiety is test anxiety, which has negative effects on academic performance. For nursing students, test anxiety could manifest in

252

both written examinations and evaluations of clinical proficiency. Instead of focusing on relevant parts of the task students with high test anxiety worry about their performance and how well others are doing, and they ruminate about alternatives (Meichenbaum, 1972). High test anxiety is associated with intrusion of irrelevant thoughts such as preoccupation with feelings of inadequacy, anticipation of punishment, and loss of status and esteem (p. 370).

Accompanying these cognitive aspects of test anxiety is emotionality, the autonomic arousal aspect of anxiety, and a variety of physical symptoms including increased heart rate, muscular tension, gastrointestinal changes, changes in breathing, and dietary and sleep pattern disturbances (Meichenbaum, 1972, p. 370). These physiological symptoms are distressing and need to be abated just as much as the negative thought processes. Learning to relax and deescalate the unpleasant symptoms helps diminish their negative effects.

Gerrard's (1978) review of the literature unearthed that one of the most significant and recurring problems experienced by health professionals is a fear of making a mistake and being negatively evaluated. Clinicians in practice revealed fears about committing errors in diagnosis or treatment. In a study to identify specific clinical situations that were anxiety-producing for junior and senior nursing students, Kleehammer, Hart, and Keck (1990) discovered that the highest anxiety-producing situation for both groups was the fear of making mistakes (p. 186). Examples of other nursing situations that engendered anxiety in the students in this study were the initial clinical experience on a unit, nursing procedures, hospital equipment, evaluation by faculty, being observed by instructors, being late, and talking with physicians (p. 184).

The two major factors underlying evaluation anxiety in nurses are concern for client safety and concern for our own security.

Concern for client safety: Nursing involves caring for the health of fellow human beings. Health is a precious commodity, making the stakes high if a nursing error detracts from the client's health or pushes him into illness. This responsibility underlies our anxiety about making an error in our nursing practice.

Concern for our own security: Clients are becoming more knowledgeable and critical about health care. No longer content to passively submit to treatment, consumers of health care are demanding to know the rationale for regimens and to have access to a second opinion. In extreme cases clients are suing physicians and other health care professionals, including nurses, for ineffective health care. This potential threat from clients hovers as a powerful source of disapproval, with implications for career advancement and public embarrassment. Today, nurses are aware of our accountability for the nursing care we deliver and our vulnerability to investigations of these actions through a legal process.

Evaluation anxiety is an unpleasant, ever-lurking phenomenon that, as two decades of literature reports, has threatened nurses and other health professionals. As nurses we are committed to making a positive difference for our clients, yet today's work environments are loaded with potential deterrents to this goal: inadequate staffing, higher acuity clients, technological advancements, and information overload. In its mildest form evaluation anxiety can detract from enjoyment in the workplace and, when strong, it can be overwhelming, interfering with our ability to perform competently as nurses.

As students in nursing, or as practicing registered nurses, we need to develop ways to minimize evaluation anxiety so that we can confidently handle clinical or written examinations, job performance appraisals, and everyday criticisms—all naturally recurring events in the professional life of nurses.

Characteristics of Evaluation Anxiety

People who suffer from evaluation anxiety exhibit ways of thinking that make them feel uneasy and interfere with their ability to perform in adaptive ways. The following characteristics of those experiencing evaluation anxiety have been reported in the literature (Dweck & Wortman, 1982; Wine, 1982).

- **Self-focus versus task-focus.** These people spend more time thinking about their performance than they devote to the task. Attention to their performance detracts from the necessary attention needed to do the task adequately.
- **Self-focused thoughts are negative and self-devaluing, and they lead to self-doubt.** Not only does a focus on self versus task detract from task performance but the focus on negative aspects of one's performance engenders feelings of anxiety.
- **Self-blame.** Some people with evaluation anxiety tend to blame themselves for their poor performance more than they do circumstances or other external factors.
- **Worry and concern about evaluation.** People with high evaluation anxiety tend to place a lot of emphasis on how they are doing in comparison to others and how the examiner is evaluating them.

Those with low evaluation anxiety react to performance evaluation with an external, situational, task-oriented focus. For those with high evaluation anxiety failure has self-evaluative meaning, signifying a lack of ability. Those with low evaluation anxiety generate thoughts about the task or situation that encourage solutions or completion of the task, whereas those with high anxiety give up and see themselves as the main reason for failure.

Options such as trying different strategies, or looking for an external causative factor, are not fully explored, leaving high anxiety types with feelings of failure and uneasiness. Mistakes are interpreted as failures, not as stepping stones in the process of discovering the final solution. People with high performance anxiety tend to attribute success to factors other than their own ability yet they readily assume failure is their doing. This view leads them to feel pressured in every new achievement situation (Dweck & Wortman, 1982; Wine, 1982).

In our culture it is easy to berate ourselves when we make a mistake. In addition to our self-chastisement we sometimes invent or exaggerate disapproval from others. How we internally evaluate ourselves can be constructive or destructive.

Here is an example of constructive and destructive thoughts in relation to being evaluated.

CONSTRUCTIVE THOUGHTS	DESTRUCTIVE THOUGHTS
"I'm doing a good job. I can't do everything I'd like to for my clients today because we're short staffed, but I'll make sure I do the most important things."	"I've got to do everything for my clients or I'll feel like a failure."
	"If I don't do everything just perfectly I'll be letting down my clients and the rest of the team."
"I've done the important things I can for the clients on the unit. Now I'll prepare a concise report for the evening staff."	"How can I possibly explain to the evening staff that I didn't get everything done on the day shift? They'll think I'm incompetent and disorganized."
"One thing I didn't make arrangements for was an extra load of linen for the evening staff. Now that I know you have to put your order in before 1:00 PM I won't forget in the future."	"They're going to crucify me for not arranging for an extra load of linen. They'll be mad at me for days for that 'boo boo'."
"I can go home knowing I did the best I could today. It was super busy and we were short staffed, but we gave our clients the best care we could under the circumstances."	"What a day! All I can think about is what still needs to be done. I'll be miserable all evening mulling over how I could have done things better."

How to Gain Control Over Your Evaluation Anxiety

Since evaluation anxiety affects cognitive, affective, and psychomotor dimensions, a multifaceted approach is needed to help overcome it.

You can use positive self-talk (see chapter 18) to overcome your self-defeating internal dialogue. Making sure that your inner voice is reassuring will comfort you in your day-to-day activities and at times when you are having an examination or a performance appraisal.

Relaxation (see chapter 16) will help you focus on the task and act more efficiently. You will feel more relaxed and overcome the negative physiological effects of evaluation anxiety when you relax.

Imagery (see chapter 17) will help you picture yourself performing in a way that makes you feel good about yourself. Your positive visualizations will keep you focused on performing your best and will engender positive feelings that will overpower the uneasiness generated by your anxiety.

Learning how to make use of feedback (see chapter 15) from others will help you prepare yourself for situations in which your performance is evaluated. Practice sessions with helpful colleagues can boost your confidence.

In addition to these four approaches, avoiding errors requires thinking before acting. Using the nursing process on a consistent basis helps to ensure that your nursing actions will be safe, ethical, and helpful.

Handling Job Performance Appraisals Assertively

At many points in our nursing careers we receive both formal and informal evaluations of our performance. For us, the purpose of these evaluations is to learn what we are doing well so that we can continue to do it, and where we need to improve our work performance. For the employer evaluations serve as a check on whether or not employees are fulfilling the expectations of the work contract.

Evaluations are helpful to both parties and should occur regularly. As the employee you can take an assertive approach to evaluations, which will help ease your anxiety. Here are some assertive steps you can take to prepare for an evaluation. This example is for a nurse employed in service. As a student nurse, apply the same preparatory procedures for evaluations at your school of nursing.

Before Your Evaluation

1. Find out what the schedule is for evaluations in your agency. Many agencies offer an evaluation for new employees after 3 to 6 months of probationary employment and yearly thereafter.
2. Find out in advance the criteria by which your employer will be evaluating you. Having this information gives you the chance to make notes about how you think you have met the standards expected of someone in your position.
3. If your employer does not have a standard criteria for evaluation, suggest that one be instituted soon. Request that your job description or the standards of nursing care prepared by your professional nursing association be used as the reference for determining your performance level.
4. Review what you and your colleagues in similar nursing positions actually do in the workplace. Compare this time and task allotment with what your job description outlines. At your evaluation point out any of these discrepancies to your employer. If job descriptions are not updated you may find that a significant part of your daily work is not being acknowledged.
5. Prepare your own evaluation of your work performance before meeting with your employer. Go to your appointment armed with specific examples of how you have met the requirements of your job description. Be aware of where you need to improve and what support you will need from your head nurse to make the necessary changes.
6. Develop goals you would like to work towards. Be as clear, realistic, and specific as possible in the preparation of these work objec-

tives so that you can articulate them clearly in your performance evaluation.

7. If the date when your evaluation should have occurred passes, then request an evaluation from your employer. Evaluations protect you by providing guidelines for maintaining or changing your professional behavior. You need feedback to know if your nursing care is within the legal and qualitative expectations of your agency.

8. Prepare mentally for your evaluation interview by ensuring that your self-talk is encouraging and visualize yourself looking and feeling calm and confident during your interview.

During Your Evaluation

1. Inform your employer that you wish to discuss your goals some time during the interview.

2. Allow your employer uninterrupted time to deliver his comments about your work.

3. Ask for clarification of any points that are not understandable. Request evidence of your employer's points so that he is forced to back up his comments with examples. These illustrations will clarify for you the kind of behavior your employer expects.

4. Your employer may have suggestions about ways in which you can improve your performance. Agree only to those changes that are realistic given your time and potential and support available in the workplace.

5. Share your performance goals with your employer and engage his support for the achievement of your career plans. Ask your employer for a list of goals he would like you to work towards.

6. Do not sign your evaluation until you are fully satisfied that it records an accurate and fair assessment of how you do your job.

7. Thank your employer for his efforts.

8. Come to an agreement about the date for your next evaluation.

After Your Job Appraisal Interview

1. Take time to reflect on how you handled the evaluation. Praise yourself for the ways you handled yourself assertively. Make note of things you would like to do differently in your next evaluation interview.

2. Follow up on the goals you and your employer set. Take some time to develop your strategy to achieve your objectives and set intermediate and final deadlines. Think about people and resources you can tap to help develop your talents.

3. Keep a diary of your work performance in preparation for your next performance evaluation.

4. Mackay (1990, p. 37) offers a suggestion to every job holder to ensure that they keep their jobs. His motto "deliver more than you promise" is his sure fire way to get you and your work noticed. Mackay urges employees: "Don't try to meet your quotas. Exceed them. Do what it takes

to set yourself apart from the pack. Make them need you." Nurses putting this attitude into practice would likely not feel anxious at job appraisal time.

Assessing the Validity and Reliability of an Employer's Appraisal System

The performance appraisal process should provide nurses with an evaluative component, which rates your nursing behavior against established criteria, and a career developmental component, which seeks to improve your nursing performance through self-learning and growth (ANA, 1990, pp. 20-21). Many appraisal systems that fail to provide the necessary input/feedback to enhance employee performance do so for some, or all, of the following reasons:

- **The appraisal process is conducted by upper management rather than the nurse employee's immediate supervisor.**

Performance appraisal is best handled at the management level closest to the nurse employee, by supervisors who have firsthand knowledge of her performance.

- **A single appraisal tool is used to evaluate all employees.**

A nurse's job description should form the basis of any performance evaluation, anchoring the appraisal with a pertinent and appropriate focus.

- **Evaluation and assessment focuses on personal traits rather than work behavior.**

Using the referent of the nurse's job description focuses on observable, measurable behaviors.

- **Behaviors which are the subject of evaluation/assessment fail to reflect the major substance of a specific job.**

A job description spells out precise job content, including nursing duties, nursing activities to be performed, nursing responsibilities, and results expected by the nurse's employer.

- **The weighting of traits and behaviors does not reflect their significance in the performance of a specific job.**

Ideally a nurse employee and her supervisor develop the job description in concert so that both parties have a clear understanding of the job expectations at the outset.

- **Criteria for identifying an acceptable level of performance are vague, leaving it open to varying interpretations.**

Tasks included in a nurse's job description should be specific, comprehensive, and stated in action verbs, minimizing the likelihood that a nurse employee will be evaluated on insignificant job behavior or personal traits. Acceptable levels of nurse performance must be clearly defined. If rating scales are used, the meaning of each rating should be open to a single interpretation.

- **There is little or no informal feedback on job performance and formal evaluation occurs infrequently.**

The appraisal system should allow for sufficient interaction throughout the process. Nurse job performance appraisal should entail systematic assessment/evaluation thoughout the designated period. Feedback (employment counseling or "coaching") should be ongoing, including recommendations for improvement. The more frequent the evaluation of nurse job performance the more likely nurses are to see the evaluation in the light of guidance and thus find the appraisal less stressful (ANA, 1990, p. 21).

If you do your part to ensure that your job performance appraisals are objective, fair, and frequent, you will do much to minimize you own evaluation anxiety.

Coping With the Anxiety of Written Examinations

Taking examinations is part of student life. Even as a registered nurse you may find yourself preparing for an examination as part of a continuing education course or degree program. Your grade symbolizes the level of achievement you have secured at a given point in time. Because many examinations offer only one chance to demonstrate your knowledge or skill, you may feel anxious about performing well at the given time of the examination. Here are some assertive steps you can take to make you feel better prepared and less anxious about examinations.

Before Your Examination

1. Find out all you can about what content (or skill) will be tested on the examination. This knowledge will help you narrow down the material to study.
2. Review the objectives for the course and focus on content that directly relates to these objectives.
3. Find out the format of the examination (whether it is multiple choice or essay type). This information will determine your study approach.
4. If you need guidance on how to study, then go to your teachers, the counseling center, or a study guide.
5. Consider forming or joining a study group. Effective study groups can make preparations for examinations fun and fruitful.
6. Make a realistic timetable of study preparations for the examination and stick to it. Keeping pace with your schedule will help you integrate the material you are studying. If you are rushed, prioritize what is important to learn and cover it first.
7. Find out where the examination is being held and familiarize yourself with the room. Choose a seat where you will be comfortable to write your exam. Be sure you know the exact hour of the exam.
8. Make sure you have all the necessary tools to help you in the exam, such as a spare calculator battery, sharpened pencils, a watch, tissues, and your good luck charm!
9. Mentally prepare before the exam by visualizing yourself in the examination room looking calm and smiling as you read the questions

because you know the answers. As you study for the exam be sure that your self-talk is positive. Tell yourself that you are learning and that you are covering the material in a sensible way. Encourage yourself and do not allow self-defeating thoughts about failure or mistakes to take over your internal dialogue.

10. Put yourself through a dry run of the examination. If it is a written test, then obtain exams from previous years and write them in the specified time limits. If there are no old exams, then make up your own questions and answer them in a simulated exam situation. If you are being examined on your nursing technique, then do the procedure in front of a colleague. Have her evaluate you using the criteria that your instructor will use.

11. Plan a post-exam reward. This treat will give you something to look forward to and will prevent you from dwelling on the examination after it is over.

During Your Examination

1. Decide in advance what time you will be arriving at the place of the examination. If you are the type who likes to talk with colleagues before the exam, arrive early. If pre-exam cramming with colleagues raises your anxiety level, then time your arrival accordingly.

2. Take time to calm down before even looking at the exam. Sit calmly and do your deep breathing.

3. Maintain this focused calm thoughout the exam. If you are thinking about passing or failing, instead of staying focused on the examination questions, your concentration will slip. Just as athletes don't perform their all-time best when they are thinking about winning the gold or breaking a record during an event (Orlick, 1986), neither will you perform your best if you are thinking about anything other than the best response to the question in front of you. Thinking about anything else creates anxiety and interferes with your concentration on the questions.

4. If you are distracted by an external interference (like noise from other candidates or the proctors, or uncomfortable conditions in the room) that can be stopped, be assertive and ask the proctor to handle the situation. If nothing can be done about the external distractions, then tell yourself to refocus, giving all your attention to the question at hand.

5. Read over the entire exam before answering any questions. This way you will know what is expected of you and you can pace yourself throughout the allotted time.

6. Before answering any question be sure you understand what is expected so that your answers will be at the appropriate level. If you merely describe an issue when you are expected to critique it, then you will not secure full marks.

7. Tackle questions to which you know the answers first. This strategy will boost your confidence.

8. Decide how much time to spend on any one question (usually deter- mined by the marks allotted) and stick to your timetable so that you are not rushed at the end.
9. If you finish before the allotted time period, read over your answers be- fore submitting them. This review will assure you that you have an- swered all the questions and you may think of some points to add.

After Your Examination

1. Decide whether or not you wish to join your colleagues for a "post mor- tem." Sometimes going over an examination only serves to increase your anxiety.
2. Follow through with your plan for an after-exam celebration. Doing something fun will help clear your mind and relax you after all the hard work you did preparing and writing the examination.
3. After you get your results check to see where you did well and where you need to improve. Find out if you need to bone up on content or if you need more experience interpreting the questions. This information will help you prepare for future exams.

Tips for Dealing with Criticism

Many people feel anxious about receiving criticism. Here are some per- ceptions on criticism which shed a more positive light on the issue.
1. Think about criticism as a gift instead of bad news. Criticism offers you the chance to re-evaluate your performance. People who take time to criticize you are often interested in you or the job you are doing.
2. Seek more information from the person who is criticizing you. Adler (1977) suggests asking for specific facts about the particular behavior for which you are being criticized. This information will help you de- termine the validity of the criticism.
3. You are not obliged to agree with all criticism sent your way. Take time to review it, extract what fits your self-assessment, and discard what does not fit.
4. If you receive criticism you have heard before, take note of it. There is likely some truth to criticism you repeatedly hear.
5. Reply to unjust or aggressive criticism; do not let it pass without speaking up about it. You will feel better about yourself if you con- front or correct your criticizer. "The world is filled with people who criticize destructively and woundingly for the feeling of superiority and power it gives them. They pick at others' faults to elevate their own virtues. You don't have to let them do it. You can assert yourself" (Baer, 1976).
6. Realize that criticism does not mean there is something wrong with you (Baer, 1976). You may be criticized for doing something ineffectively or incorrectly, but that in no way means *you* are in- effective.

Assertively Handling Difficult Situations Occurring in Nursing Student Performance Evaluations

There are some situations which increase our evaluation anxiety. We need to prepare ourselves for uncomfortable situations, such as when an evaluator is aggressive, when we are given an evaluation without time to prepare, or when serious allegations are made without evidence. Here are several examples of difficult evaluation situations with suggestions for handling them assertively.

Example 1: Harshly Delivered Criticism

Your clinical instructor tells you that your charting is fine, and your treatments are carried out superbly, and she compliments you on your effective sterile technique. She also points out that your organization is poor. She notes that your rooms look dishevelled and cluttered. "How can you or your clients find things you need in that confusion? Half the time your beds aren't made until after noon, and it usually looks like a tornado struck in your rooms. Your sloppiness is a black mark against the nursing profession."

You know that these comments are legitimate, even though they are delivered in an aggressive way. You tend to be disorganized and messy at home as well. Here is an assertive reply to this evaluation:

> **Assertive You:** "Thank you for the feedback on my nursing skills. I don't know what to do about my organization. It's a bad habit I've had for years, even before I came into nursing. I always admire nurses who can do things well and keep their work space uncluttered at the same time. I don't know where to begin. Can you give me some suggestions about how I can improve?"

This reply acknowledges both the compliments and the criticisms from your instructor. Your openness to improve your organization is demonstrated by your request for help. If you really want to improve you will follow through with some of the suggestions your instructor provides.

Example 2: Unexpected Aggressive Criticism

You have been the senior nursing student on the surgical floor in a general hospital for the past 7 weeks. Because it is your last week on the unit you decide to stop at the head nurse's office to thank her for the help she has been to you during your practicum.

Without requesting it, the head nurse gives you this piece of advice: "I'm glad you enjoyed your time with us. Here's some advice I'd like to give you before you leave us: improve your charting. It's a mess to read. I spent 10 minutes trying to decipher one of your notes the other day. You'll never make a good nurse if you can't communicate to the rest of the world what you've done."

Assertive You: "I am aware that my charting is too long and difficult to read. Miss Jameson, my clinical instructor, has also pointed out my need to improve. Do you have any suggestions to help me learn how to improve my charting?"

This reply acknowledges the feedback from your head nurse. Although her feedback is aggressive, you maintained an assertive stance in your response. Your request for guidance invites her to contribute to your development in a more positive way.

Example 3: Allegations without Evidence

Your clinical instructor is giving you your final evaluation on your performance on the maternity unit where you have been for the past 3 weeks. She has made several negative comments about your handling of the babies and your interactions with the new mothers. However, she has given no examples to support her comments and she has never observed you directly. You believe that your performance is acceptable and that it meets the standards set out in the procedure manual. You reply in the following way:

Assertive You: "My own assessment of my handling of the babies and my interactions with the mothers is that I treat them both with respect and care. I would appreciate you providing me with more concrete evidence of any rough handling, as this charge has serious implications for my career. I have worked closely with Mrs. Green in the nursery and Mrs. Nuthers on the unit. Both these staff nurses could provide you with a thorough assessment of my performance. I would like to have a joint meeting with you and these nurses to discuss my performance. I will not sign this evaluation form until this meeting has taken place."

This assertive response lets your instructor know that you intend to protect your reputation. You have made a reasonable request for another evaluation. Your straightforward manner, which is neither insulting nor disrespectful to your instructor, increases the likelihood of having another evaluation.

PRACTICING OVERCOMING EVALUATION ANXIETY

Exercise 1. Your colleague in the school of nursing has an important physiology test coming up in 2 days. Over coffee in the cafeteria she says:

Nervous Nina: "I'm terrified about this exam. Everyone says Jones is such a hard marker. I did okay on the first test but the stuff we've taken since then is a lot more complicated. I can't fail 'cause it'll put my course selection out of sequence. I've put so much time into studying this stuff that I'd better pass. I'll be glad when it's over."

How would you intervene to help minimize your friend's evaluation anxiety? Prepare your suggested strategy individually, then work in groups of four to compare your suggestions.

Exercise 2. You are a staff nurse working in the operating room of a general hospital. A student doing her clinical practicum in the operating room is talking to you at coffee break. This is what she says:

> **Anxious Anita:** "Geez, tomorrow's the big day. It's a double-barreled whammy for me. I've got to scrub for Dr. Shark and I've seen how he yells at students if they don't do exactly what he wants. And to top it off, my clinical instructor chooses tomorrow to evaluate me! I'll be a wreck by 4 o'clock tomorrow."

How would you help this student nurse cope with her evaluation anxiety? Prepare your own response and then work in groups of four to compare and share strategies.

Exercise 3. You are a staff nurse working in a small rural hospital. It is time for your 3-month evaluation from the Director of Nursing. In preparation for your performance evaluation interview (which you had to ask for) you search for an evaluation form. You soon discover that there is no standard evaluation form because performance evaluations are rarely done in this hospital. You also discover that your job description, which was written 4 years ago, is one that was copied from a large hospital in the city 200 miles away, and is irrelevant to your position in a rural hospital.

How would you handle this situation to reduce your evaluation anxiety? Compare your ideas with those of your colleagues.

Exercise 4. Here are some questions posed by the American Nurses' Association as one means of assessing the validity and reliability of your employer's appraisal system (ANA, 1990, p. 21). To how many of these questions would you answer "yes" at your place of employment (or prospective place)?

1. Are employees actively involved in determining policies and procedures for the appraisal process?
2. Is more than one type of performance appraisal tool used to evaluate an employee's performance? Are different tools used to evaluate different types of job assignments?
3. Is job performance appraisal handled at the management level closest to the employee?
4. Does the appraiser routinely collect relevant data about job performance or depend on recall to meet a deadline for completing appraisal forms?
5. Is there any type of review of a supervisor's appraisal of employees by upper management?

6. Is there a standard time frame for formal evaluation (quarterly, bi-annually, and so on)?
7. Does the appraisal process include goal setting? Is there sufficient opportunity to review progress in achieving these goals during the appraisal period?
8. Are the categories delineated in the evaluation tools realistic?
9. Do the categories delineated in the evaluation tools complement the job description?
10. Are the behaviors to be evaluated measurable?
11. Do the formats of the appraisal tool provide space for recording supporting evidence/concrete illustrations?
12. Are the standards/criteria for judging levels of job performance clearly defined?
13. Do the evaluation tools weigh categories of employee behavior on the basis of their importance to the job?
14. Is there a clear understanding of the impact of performance appraisal on salary increments, job status, and so on?
15. Are there clear steps available for an employee who is dissatisfied with the outcome of a job performance appraisal?

What action would you recommend if your agency does not have a fair system of job performance appraisal, making you and other employees feel more anxious about the evaluation?

Exercise 5. How could nurse employees follow Mackay's advice to job holders to "deliver more than you promise"? How could nurses "exceed their quotas"? Think about this method separately then compare your views in the class as a whole.

REFERENCES

Adler, R.B. (1977). *Confidence in communication: A guide to assertive and social skills.* New York: Holt, Rinehart and Winston.

American Nurses Association. (1990). *Survival skills in the workplace.* Kansas City, Mo.: Author.

Baer, J. (1976). *How to be an assertive (not aggressive) woman in life, in love and on the job: A total guide to self-assertiveness.* New York: Rawson Associates Publishers, Inc.

Dweck, C.S., & Wortman, C.B. (1982). Learned helplessness, anxiety and achievement motivation. In H.W. Krohne & Laux, L. (Eds.), *Achievement, stress, and anxiety* (pp. 93-125). Washington, D.C.: Hemisphere Publishing Corporation (distributed outside the U.S. by McGraw-Hill International Book Company).

Gerrard, B. (1978). *Interpersonal skills for health professionals: A review of the literature.* Unpublished manuscript. McMaster University, Hamilton, Ontario, Canada.

Kleehammer, K., Hart, A.L., Keck, J.F. (1990). Nursing students' perceptions of anxiety-producing situations in the clinical setting. *Journal of Nursing Education, 29*(4), 183-187.

Mackay, H. (1990). *Beware the naked man who offers you his shirt.* New York: Ivy Books.

Meichenbaum, D.H. (1972). Cognitive modification of test anxious college students. *Journal of Cousulting and Clinical Psychology, 39*(3), 370-380.

Orlick, T. (1986). *Psyching for sport: Mental training for athletes.* Champaign, Ill.: Leisure Press, A Division of Human Kinetics Publishers, Inc.

Wine, J.D. (1982). Evaluation anxiety: A cognitive-attentional construct. In H.W. Krohne & Laux, L. (Eds.), *Achievement, stress, and anxiety* (pp. 207-219). Washington, D.C.: Hemisphere

Publishing Corporation (distributed outside the U.S. by McGraw-Hill International Book Company).

SUGGESTIONS FOR FURTHER READING

Ellis, D. (1985). *Becoming a master student* (5th ed.). Rapid City, S.D.: College Survival Inc.
This comprehensive, easy-to-read book is full of excellent ideas for surviving successfully as a student. In relation to test anxiety there are dozens of practical suggestions for how students can take charge of themselves in test situations.

CHAPTER 20

Communicating Assertively and Responsibly with Distressed Clients and Colleagues

*"I never ask the wounded person
how he feels; I myself become the
wounded person."*

Walt Whitman

OBJECTIVES

This chapter is designed to give you practice communicating assertively and responsibly with distressed clients and colleagues. Some of the reasons you may have trouble relating to distressed clients and colleagues will be explained so that you can work on overcoming them. You will receive feedback on your ability to correctly use the communication behaviors you learned—in Parts One and Two—with distressed people. Through the practice of correcting your interventions you will develop the critical ability to continually improve your communication with distressed clients and colleagues.

WHY DISTRESSED BEHAVIOR IS A PROBLEM FOR NURSES

When people are distressed they are showing us their mental pain. Verbally and nonverbally they convey their anguish. Their loss of composure is a signal that they are disturbed by what is bothering them.

Changes in health status, illness, and hospitalization are some sources of distress in clients. The work of nurses and allied health professionals is known to be stressful and ripe for causing distress. We encounter distressed behavior frequently in our clients and occasionally in our colleagues; therefore, we need to develop some way to relate to them that soothes their distress without upsetting us. Maintaining our sensitivity to others' distress, so that we can respond in a caring way without being overcome and losing our objectivity, is one of a nurse's most difficult feats.

Gerrard's (1978) review of the literature about interpersonal problems experienced by health professionals clearly reveals that our reactions to emotionally-laden situations interfere with our ability to act effectively. Untoward reactions can come from within ourselves (feeling unsure or inadequate about how to act), the situation (feeling overcome or impotent), or the distressed person (distress invades the health professional).

It has been suggested that nurses develop a protective barrier against others' pain, or become insensitive to the discomfort of others, because they encounter so much suffering in the course of their daily work. Also it has been hypothesized that nurses stop responding in helpful ways because there is a dearth of positive role models (Gerrard, 1978).

If we become too involved with others' distress we overload ourselves emotionally and become ineffective. If we avoid the distress of others by ignoring or belittling it, we are left with the feeling of not giving the attention and support that is expected. Some nurses feel helpless about how to be therapeutic with distressed persons. Others feel annoyed or irritated that distressed clients or colleagues cannot solve their own problems. Thoughts about our own inadequacies, or judgments about the appropriateness of others' behavior, prevent us from acting in the best interests of the distressed person.

Ideally we need to keep calm enough to be able to understand the reason for the person's distress, remain nonjudgmental so that we can convey appropriate compassion for his situation, and be clear-headed to act responsibly on behalf of the distressed person.

IMPROVING YOUR COMMUNICATION SKILL WITH DISTRESSED CLIENTS AND COLLEAGUES

In the rest of this chapter you will be given situations involving distressed clients and colleagues. Your task is to assess each situation, determine the request being made, and choose the most assertive and responsible communication strategy.

Appendix A contains a critique of all the response choices for each situation in the chapter. It is worthwhile reading the advantages and drawbacks of each option.

Communicating with Upset Clients
Step One: Assessment of the Data

1. Review the following situation and formulate your own assessment of the client's thoughts, feelings, and requests.

Mr. James is a 58-year-old avid outdoorsman who has been hunting in the woods near your rural hospital. While climbing in steep terrain he slipped and fell 50 feet down a ragged incline. In addition to suffering multiple bruises and scratches, he broke his glasses. Today he was admitted to your hospital for overnight observation. As you make your first round on the evening shift you go into his room to introduce yourself:

> **You:** "Good afternoon, Mr. James. Welcome to our hospital. I'm sorry you have to be here under such unfortunate circumstances. How are you. . . ."

> **Mr. James:** "How long am I going to be here? Can you get me the phone? I need to reach my wife. Somebody's got to bring me my extra glasses. I can't drive . . . I can't do anything without them. You can have your damn hospital. Just get me a phone so I can make arrangements to get out of here."

Mr. James raises his voice as he is talking and turns away from you. He squeezes the bed sheet in his hands and looks exasperated.

2. On a separate sheet of paper write down your assessment of Mr. James' thoughts and feelings. Indicate what request Mr. James is making of you, his evening nurse.

3. Compare your assessment with the assessment that follows:

Thoughts: Mr. James thinks that he cannot manage without his glasses. He is aware that he must reach his wife so that arrangements can be made to get his spare glasses.

Feelings: He is upset that he cannot read, write, or see to drive. He feels trapped in this remote rural hospital. He desperately wants to talk to his wife about arranging to get home.

Request: Mr. James wants you to understand how frustrating it is for him to be stuck in this unfamiliar hospital. He is trying to get you to comprehend how dependent and immobile he is without his glasses. He wants you to help him contact his wife. Indirectly, he may be asking to be comforted; that is, to be helped to feel more at home in this strange place.

4. Did your assessment reflect an accurate analysis of the facts as they were presented? If not, return to the original data presented in the vignette and reassess the cognitive and affective messages. If so, then proceed with step two.

Step Two: Communication Strategies and Desired Outcomes

5. You have determined that Mr. James needs understanding, action, and comfort. Take a piece of paper and identify what communication behaviors you would use to show Mr. James how you intend to respond to his request. Indicate the desired outcome(s) of your suggested strategy.

6. Compare your suggested strategy with this one:

It is appropriate to meet Mr. James' request for understanding and action. A warm, genuine, respectful manner will convey that you care about him. An empathic response will ensure that he knows you understand his predicament and it will reduce any embarrassment he might feel for displaying his upset feelings in such a volatile way. If his upset behavior agitates you, then you can calm yourself and focus on his distress, using positive self-talk and imagery to prepare yourself to communicate assertively and responsibly.

This proposed strategy would help Mr. James relax and feel accepted. He will likely look calmer and feel more patient with his circumstances. Your compliance with his requests contributes to the development of a trusting rapport.

Step Three: Implementing and Evaluating Your Communication Strategy

7. Now you must reply to Mr. James. Develop your own response and write it on a separate sheet of paper. Keep it handy so that you can refer to it later.
8. At this point you get the chance to compare your suggested response with several options listed below. Look over each of the response choices and turn to Appendix A to read a critique of each.

As you review the following response choices, look for those that are congruent with your assessment of Mr. James' requests and your desire to communicate in an assertive and responsible way.

CHOICE A "You should be grateful to be alive. If that farmer hadn't heard you yelling and got you out of the ravine you'd be out there freezing at this very minute. You don't need to snap at me. I can hear. I'll get you the phone."

CHOICE Z "It's hard to be in a strange place where nothing is familiar. I know that feeling. I'll bring you the phone."

CHOICE J You get red in the face, clench your fists, then turn on your heel and head down the hall to get the portable phone for Mr. James.

CHOICE S "I'm sure you're eager to talk to your wife and make arrangements to get your glasses and get home. I'll get our portable phone for you right away. I can imagine it must be frustrating to be without your glasses, so please let us know how we can help you manage until you get them."

9. After you have found the most satisfactory strategy and discovered why the other options are unsuitable, go back to the suggested response you generated earlier in this exercise. Evaluate yours in terms of its assertiveness and responsibleness.

Communicating with Upset Colleagues
Step One: Assessment of the Data

1. Review the following situation and formulate what you think are your colleague's thoughts and feelings. Indicate what you think your colleague is requesting from you.

Joe is the intern on the medical unit where you have been a student for the past 6 weeks. Because you are both students working on the unit at the same times, you have become good friends. This day Joe looks preoccupied and you have noticed that he is not his usual good-natured self. He snapped at you for not having your client ready for his physical examination, even though he had not warned you about his plans. Later he approaches you with:

> **Joe:** "Shirley, I'm sorry for snapping at you earlier. I'm just not myself. Dayle just found out she's pregnant and it's all I can think about. I just can't imagine being a father. I can barely cope with being a husband and an intern. It's been the only thing on my mind since I found out 2 days ago. I can't think straight. I can't sleep . . . I still can't believe it. I don't know what I'm going to do. We want kids, but why now?"

2. On a separate sheet of paper write down your assessment of Joe's thoughts and feelings. Indicate what you think Joe is requesting from you, his colleague.
3. Compare your assessment with the assessment that follows:

Thoughts: Joe knows his wife is pregnant and is aware that his preoccupation with this unexpected, and not yet welcome, news is causing him to be short-tempered with you. He wants to be a father but does not think the timing is good.

Feelings: He regrets that he snapped at you. Joe is shocked by the news of his wife's unexpected pregnancy and is worried about how he can cope with the added strain of being a father when he is having difficulty juggling the two roles of intern and husband. He likely is tired because he has not been sleeping, and he is upset that he cannot think straight.

Request: Joe is asking you to accept his apology for snapping at you, and he wants you to understand how the news about the pregnancy is turning his life upside down. Indirectly he may be asking for some comfort for his miserable predicament.

4. Did your assessment reflect an accurate analysis of the facts as they were presented? If not, return to the original data presented in the vignette and reassess the cognitive and affective messages. If so, then proceed with step two.

Step Two: Communication Strategies and Desired Outcomes

5. You have determined that Joe wants you both to demonstrate your understanding of the shock he is experiencing and to act by accepting his apology. Identify what communication behaviors you would use to meet these two reasonable requests. Indicate the desired outcome of your suggested strategy.
6. Compare your suggested strategy with this one:

Warmth would show that you feel kindly toward Joe and you do not hold a grudge. An empathic response would convey your understanding to Joe. A self-disclosure about adjusting to the news about your own pregnancy (or another major event) would provide him with hope that getting used to the idea comes in time.

It is appropriate to meet Joe's requests. This strategy would make Joe feel relieved that you understand the reason for his outburst and that you forgive him. The hope you might give him—that he will work things out in time—would be comforting.

Step Three: Implementing and Evaluating Your Communication Strategy

7. Now you must reply to Joe. Develop your own response to Joe and write it on a separate sheet of paper. Keep it handy so that you can refer to it later.
8. At this point you get the chance to compare your response with several options listed below. Look over each of the response choices and turn to Appendix A to read a critique of each option.

   As you review the following response choices, be looking for those that are congruent with your assessment of Joe's requests and your desire to communicate in an assertive and responsible way.

CHOICE T "It's okay, Joe. We all get upset at times."

CHOICE F "Joe, I forgive you (smiling). I can see that you are preoccupied and upset with the unexpected news of Dayle's pregnancy. It seems overwhelming right now to imagine trying to squeeze in being a father when you are busy enough being a husband and getting your career launched. I too felt shocked when I first found out I was pregnant, but after several weeks I began to accept the idea. By the end of term I was even looking forward to Sarah's birth."

CHOICE V "OK this time, Joe, but don't let it happen again. You really threw my whole schedule off this morning. That's great news about Dayle. So you're going to be a father, eh? I love being a parent and I know you will too once you get used to the idea. It just takes a few weeks to get over the initial shock and then you'll be fine."

CHOICE O "Apology accepted, Joe. It's easy to see that you're upset with your news. Things will turn out, Joe. You'll get used to the idea."

9. After you have found the most assertive and responsible choice, and checked out why the other options are not suitable, go back to the response you generated on your own earlier in this exercise. Evaluate your suggestion in terms of its assertiveness and responsibleness.

Communicating with Clients Who Are Sad or Depressed
Step One: Assessment of the Data

1. Review the following situation and formulate what you think are your client's thoughts and feelings. Indicate what you think your client is requesting from you.

Jim is an 18-year-old client on your orthopedic unit. He has been in traction for several weeks after breaking his leg in a football game. Jim is an all-star athlete who finds it frustrating and boring being cooped up in the hospital. He is only able to do prescribed exercises because of the importance of keeping his traction in perfect tension and alignment. He is worried about getting behind in his school work. This is Jim's final year at high school and his hopes of making the honor list are evaporating. In the last few weeks you have noticed that Jim is becoming less talkative, and that he does not joke with you and the other nurses like he used to. You are worried about these changes in Jim as you enter his room to collect his breakfast tray.

> **You:** "Good morning, Jim. Aren't you hungry? You haven't touched your breakfast this morning."
>
> **Jim:** "No . . . I didn't want it" (looking away from you and sighing).
>
> **You:** "What's happened to your healthy appetite?"
>
> **Jim:** "Oh . . . it's gone like everything else. What's the point of eating? I've got nothing to look forward to. All my plans have gone down the tube." (Jim's voice is flat and he makes no eye contact with you.)

2. Take a piece of paper and write down your assessment of Jim's thoughts and feelings. Indicate what request Jim is making of you, his nurse for the day.
3. Compare your assessment with the one that follows:
Thoughts: Jim thinks that his academic and athletic hopes are not going to be realized this year. He is aware that he must remain in traction for another 6 weeks and at this point in his life this length of time seems like a total disaster.
Feelings: Jim probably has mixed feelings. Right now he feels discouraged and hopeless about his future. It is likely that he is frustrated that his plans have been thwarted, angry that it is his life that has been so affected, and apathetic about doing anything.
Request: Jim wants you to understand how he is feeling. He may also be wanting some help to lift himself out of his depression.
4. Did your assessment reflect an accurate analysis of the facts as they were presented? If not, return to the original data presented in the vignette and reassess the cognitive and affective messages. If so, then proceed with step two.

Step Two: Communication Strategies and Desired Outcomes

5. You have determined that Jim needs understanding and information. On a separate sheet of paper identify what communication behaviors you would use to respond to Jim's requests. Indicate what desired outcomes you expect by using the communication behaviors you have suggested.

6. Compare your suggested strategy with this one:

Jim's requests are reasonable and it is appropriate to respond to them. Warmth and genuineness would convey that you care for Jim. An empathic response would demonstrate that you really understand the unhappy situation he is in. Effective inquiry about his interest in doing something about his situation would be respectful. When he shows interest in doing something constructive about making his situation more bearable you could express your opinions about how he might begin. When talking to Jim it would be important to stop whatever physical activity you are doing (taking away his breakfast tray), face him, and give him your full attention. If his despair generates negative feelings in you (such as hopelessness or anger), relax before you respond. Visualize yourself responding to Jim in a caring and constructive way. If necessary, use your positive self-talk to remind yourself that you can be therapeutic when one of your clients is sad.

This strategy would make Jim feel cared for and give him some hope that he can do something constructive to make his life more bearable while he is confined to a hospital bed. This planned intervention might lift his mood.

Step Three: Implementing and Evaluating Your Communication Strategy

7. Now you must reply to Jim. On a separate sheet of paper write down the response that you have developed. Keep it handy so that you can refer to it later.
8. At this point you get the chance to compare your suggested response with several options listed below. Look over each of the response choices and turn to Appendix A to read a critique of each option.

As you review the following response choices, look for those that are congruent with your assessment of Jim's requests and your desire to communicate in an assertive and responsible way.

CHOICE K "You're young, Jim. It won't be that long until you will be out of traction and getting back in shape again. Come on, Jim, chin up. There's no point getting depressed. You might as well make the best of it. We all have disappointments in life. I've had plenty and you just have to make the best of things and ride through the bad times."

CHOICE B "I'm worried about you, Jim. You're not your happy-go-lucky self in the last few days. You're not thinking of doing anything like harming yourself, are you?"

CHOICE Q "You're really feeling down aren't you? Being stuck in this traction is a drag. Maybe you're afraid you'll have trouble catching up with things in your life. You still have about 6 weeks left in traction, Jim. I'm sure if we put our heads together we could come up with some things you could do to make life more interesting and keep you current with things you feel are slipping out of your grasp. Would you like to brainstorm together?"

CHOICE X "I'm sorry you feel that way, Jim."

9. After you have found the most satisfactory strategy and discovered why the other options are not suitable, go back to the suggested response you generated earlier in the exercise. Evaluate yours in terms of its assertiveness and responsibleness.

Communicating with Colleagues Who Are Sad or Depressed
Step One: Assessment of the Data

1. Read over the following situation and formulate your own assessment of your colleague's thoughts, feelings, and requests.

Petra is a fellow student whom you have come to know and like. The two of you have been in the same class sections in nursing and coincidentally have had the same clinical rotations for the past 1½ years. Now you are working on an oncology unit where many of the clients are dying of cancer. Petra has been quieter and kept more to herself in the past week. She looks wan and lethargic, in sharp contrast to her usual witty and spunky self. At your coffee break one morning you ask Petra how she is feeling and she responds with:

> **Petra:** "I didn't think it was that noticeable. It's the unit we're on now . . . I don't think I can take much more of it. My visions of being a nurse are to cure people—get them well again. All the people we are nursing now are dying and there's no way around it. It's so depressing. How can you stand it yourself? I go home every night and all I can think about is 'Is this all there is to life?' All we do seems so pointless if this is how things end."

2. On a separate sheet of paper write down your assessment of Petra's thoughts and feelings. Indicate what request Petra is making of you, her classmate.
3. Compare your assessment with the assessment that follows:

Thoughts: Petra thinks it's pointless nursing clients to health if they are going to end up dying in a terminal unit in a hospital. She wonders how you cope with the seeming futility of it all, and possibly she wonders if she can continue in nursing with such a hopeless attitude.

Feelings: Petra is feeling discouraged and sad about the death and dying she sees every day on the wards. She is shocked about the apparent hopelessness of nursing, since people end up suffering and dying anyway. She is worried about coming to terms with her feelings so that she can continue nursing. She is dispirited and wants to know how you handle similar feelings.

Request: Petra wants you to understand and accept how she is feeling. She is also asking you for some information about how to handle her feelings so that they do not interfere with her ability to nurse effectively. Indirectly she is asking to be comforted by having some of her sad feelings dissipated.

4. Does your assessment reflect an accurate analysis of the facts as they were presented by Petra? If not, return to the original vignette and re-assess the cognitive and affective messages. If so, then proceed with step two.

Step Two: Communication Strategies and Desired Outcomes

5. You have determined that Petra needs understanding and informa-tion. Identify what communication behaviors you would use to show Petra how you intend to respond to her requests. Indicate the desired outcome of your strategy. Write down your suggestions.

6. Compare your suggested strategy with this one:

It is quite a risk for Petra to reveal her feelings and questions about nursing; therefore it is important to respect and accept the issues she is trying to work through. It is appropriate to respond to Petra's requests, and warmth and respect need to be conveyed to show Petra that you do not harbor negative feelings about her wondering about the purpose of nursing. Accurate, genuine empathy will show her that you understand her disillusionment. To show her you are willing to share how you handle similar feelings you might use an appropriate self-disclosure. If you wish to invite her to explore the whole topic of the meaning of life, you might make a gentle suggestion about how to begin.

This strategy would make Petra feel understood and possibly get her started on finding answers to some crucial questions for her personal and professional life. Her sadness is not likely to lift immediately because she is facing some major philosophical questions, but this strategy may give her some direction about how to find some answers.

Step Three: Implementing and Evaluating Your Communication Strategy

7. Now you must reply to Petra. Develop your own response to Petra and write it down on a separate sheet of paper. Keep it handy so that you can refer to it later.

8. At this point you get the chance to compare your suggested response with several options listed below. Look over each of the response choices and turn to Appendix A to read a critique of each option.

As you review the following choices, look for those that are congruent with your assessment of Petra's requests and your desire to communicate in an assertive and responsible way.

CHOICE W "You're wondering what's the point of nursing if clients end up dying on a unit like this one where everyone is terminally ill. When I feel discouraged, like you are now, I try to adjust my perspective. I have to remind myself that the people we see in here are a small sample of the people in our city. There are lots of older healthy people out there living active lives. Something else I try to do, even though I need to work at it more, is strengthen my belief that dying is part of living. I think we have control over how we adjust to our dying, and I like to think I can help some of our clients upstairs *live* each day until they die. I think of their time on our unit as a very special part of their lives. These thoughts help me feel more hopeful, anyway. What do you think?"

CHOICE C "Well, your sadness *does* show, Petra. Those clients are sad enough without having us add to their misery. Everyone has to die, Petra. You must accept that."

CHOICE L "Boy, you are down about this rotation, Petra. Let's talk about something more pleasant that'll cheer you up. Are you and Gary going to the hockey game on Friday?"

CHOICE P "Petra, I should have picked up that something was really getting to you on this rotation. I knew there was something, and I thought it might have to do with Gary. Gee, I don't know what to say, Petra. These are issues you have to sort out. I know it's hard to accept, Petra, but some of our clients are going to die. Yet some do get better, too. Keep that in mind. You'll feel better when we're on the next rotation on the childrens' ward."

9. After you have found the most satisfactory strategy and discovered why the other options are unsuitable, go back to the suggested response you generated earlier in the exercise. Evaluate yours in terms of its assertiveness and responsibleness.

Communicating with Clients Who Are Crying
Step One: Assessment of the Data

1. Review the following situation and formulate your own assessment of the client's thoughts, feelings, and requests.

   Mrs. Urst is a 35-year-old woman who has just given birth to her second child 2 days ago. Both she and her baby are healthy, and her husband and their 8-year-old son are thrilled with the new addition to their family. You have been Mrs. Urst's nurse for the past 3 days. You have just entered her room with the heat lamp to find her weeping with the curtains pulled. She has gone through several tissues and her eyes are red and swollen.

   You: "Oh. Mrs. Urst. You are really upset. What's troubling you?"

   Mrs. Urst: "Ohhhh . . . (sobs and blows nose; laughs and then starts crying again) I can't stop. It's just dawned on me that I'm now a mother of two. It's ridiculous . . . (sobs) . . . I've known for 9 months, but now I wonder how I'll cope. I've forgotten all the stuff mothers need to know and if I stay at home I'll forget all the stuff secretaries are supposed to know. Why did we get ourselves into this predicament? Oh, I'm sorry to burden you. I guess I've just got the 'baby blues' (blows nose and bites lip to keep from crying anymore)."

2. On a separate sheet of paper write down your assessment of Mrs. Urst's thoughts and feelings. Indicate what request Mrs. Urst is making of you, her nurse for the day.
3. Compare your assessment with the following one:

Thoughts: Mrs. Urst thinks she is going to have difficulty being a mother of two. She wonders if she has made a mistake by having another child. She thinks she might be overburdening you with her disclosure.

Feelings: Mrs. Urst is upset and mixed up. She is overwhelmed by the new responsibilities she will have as mother of a newborn, and she is worried that being away from her job as a secretary will get her out of practice. She is somewhat embarrassed by her outburst and tries to pass it off as "baby blues" to save face.

Request: Mrs. Urst wants you to understand her fears of being overwhelmed but she does not want to delve into her personal life in any great detail, as indicated by her referral to baby blues and her apology that she might be burdening you. She may be indirectly asking you for reassurance that she will manage.

4. Did your assessment reflect an accurate analysis of the facts as they were presented? If not, return to the original data presented in the vignette and reassess the cognitive and affective messages. If so, then proceed with step two.

Step Two: Communication Strategies and Desired Outcomes

5. You have determined that Mrs. Urst needs understanding and comfort. Identify what communication behaviors you would use to show Mrs. Urst that you are prepared to act on her reasonable requests. Indicate the desired outcome of your suggested strategy. Write down these plans on a separate piece of paper.
6. Compare your suggested strategy with this one:

Warmth would be appropriate to show you care about her upset. Respect for her privacy could be demonstrated by nonjudgmental, empathic reference to her struggle between being a mother and a working person. It would be appropriate to express your concurrence that some of her feelings are related to her post-natal hormonal imbalance. Your opinion that she will likely work out a satisfactory schedule would reassure her, once you have convinced her that you understand her feelings.

This strategy would make Mrs. Urst feel understood and diminish her embarrassment. In addition, your reassurance would make her feel hopeful that she can and will manage.

Step Three: Implementing and Evaluating Your Communication Strategy

7. Now you must reply to Mrs. Urst. Develop your own response to her and write it on a separate sheet of paper. Keep it handy so that you can refer to it later.
8. At this point you get the chance to compare your suggested response with several options listed below. Look over each of the response choices and turn to Appendix A to read a critique of each.

As you review the following response choices, look for those that are congruent with your assessment of Mrs. Urst's requests and your desire to communicate in an assertive and responsible way.

CHOICE D "There, there, Mrs. Urst. It's natural for most women to have a crying spell after giving birth. Things will work out; they always do. Most mothers get the 'baby blues.' I see it all the time. Don't feel embarrassed."

CHOICE I "It's too late to be crying over spilt milk, Mrs. Urst. You must have thought about all this when you discovered you were pregnant. I have your heat lamp here. Could you get ready for your treatment? You'll feel better when you are all healed up."

CHOICE R "I'm sorry you're so upset, Mrs. Urst. I'll come back later and see you about your treatment."

CHOICE Y "It's likely that your tears are in part due to 'baby blues,' Mrs. Urst. But your whole world has been upset with the arrival of your new daughter; that's bound to take some time to adjust to. Working out a schedule between two important roles like motherhood and career is complicated. Given time to adjust to your new schedule I'm certain you can work out something that suits you. If you'd like to have a sounding board I'd be glad to fill the role while you're here in hospital."

9. After you have found the most satisfactory strategy and discovered why the other options are unsuitable, go back to the suggested response you generated earlier in the exercise. Evaluate yours in terms of its assertiveness and responsibleness.

Communicating with Colleagues Who Are Crying
Step One: Assessment of the Data

1. Review the following situation and formulate your own assessment of the client's thoughts, feelings, and requests.

Don is a nurse on the geriatric rehabilitation unit where you are working. When you go into the office to collect your purse you find him sitting in a chair with his head in his hands. When he sees you coming in he quickly rubs his eyes and turns in his chair so that you cannot see his face. He gets out a tissue and blows his nose and says:

> **Don:** "Come on in, Kathy. Guess you caught me crying. It's the news about Mr. Kent that's got to me. (Looking at you) I really thought he would make it. I can't believe he's dead. He was making so much progress. I never thought I'd say it, but I'll even miss the way he used to act like the king of the ward."

Don is referring to Mr. Kent, a resident of your rehabilitation unit, who was transferred yesterday to an acute care hospital for an I.V.P. Mr. Kent had been on the unit for 8 months, during which time he made himself known by his lively and sometimes overbearing involvement with all the staff. He was a well-liked, integral part of the life of your unit. Your colleague, Don, had often been assigned as Mr. Kent's nurse because of Mr. Kent's request for a male nurse. Don and Mr. Kent had enjoyed friendly arguments about politics.

2. On a separate sheet of paper write down your assessment of Don's thoughts and feelings. Indicate what request Don is making of you, his co-worker.
3. Compare your assessment with the assessment that follows:

Thoughts: Don is having difficulty believing that Mr. Kent is dead, in view of his progress just before his transfer.

Feelings: Don is shocked and saddened by his client's death. He feels confused and amazed because Mr. Kent seemed to be improving. He misses Mr. Kent, and even longs for his more unpleasant habits.

Request: His invitation for you to enter the room, and his self-disclosure, are evidence that Don is asking you to listen to him. He is asking for understanding and some comfort.

4. Did your assessment reflect an accurate analysis of the facts as they were presented? If not, return to the original data presented in the vignette and reassess the cognitive and affective messages. If so, then proceed with step two.

Step Two: Communication Strategies and Desired Outcomes

5. You have determined that Don needs understanding and comfort. Identify what communication behaviors you would use to show Don how you intend to respond to his reasonable requests. Indicate the desired outcome of your suggested strategy. Write your ideas down on a separate sheet of paper for future reference.
6. Compare your suggested strategy with this one:

An empathic response would show your understanding of Don's bereavement. Expressing your opinion about the comfort Don provided Mr. Kent would be respectful and give Don some comfort. Coming into the room and being with Don would be a warm gesture showing your respect for his feelings. If it felt genuinely comfortable for you, then a gentle touch would also convey your warmth and comfort to Don.

This strategy would make Don feel understood and comforted.

Step Three: Implementing and Evaluating Your Communication Strategy

7. Now you must reply to Don. Develop your own response to Don and write it on a separate sheet of paper. Keep it handy so that you can refer to it later in the chapter.
8. At this point you get the chance to compare your suggested response with several options listed below. Look over each of the response choices and turn to Appendix A to read a critique of each.

As you review the following response choices, look for those that are congruent with your assessment of Don's requests and your desire to communicate in an assertive and responsible way.

CHOICE G (You sit down beside Don.) "I can't believe Mr. Kent is dead either, Don. You and he had such a close relationship that I can see why you are so saddened. You gave him a lot of pleasure with those heavy political discussions. It's so hard to just keep on working when you lose someone as special as Mr. Kent. Can I help you out with your assignment in any way today, Don?"

CHOICE N Continuing to get your purse in the locked drawer, "I'll be out of your way just as soon as I get my purse, Don. It's awful news, isn't it?"

CHOICE U "I can see that you're upset, Don, but we've got to get used to these old people dying. It's true the unit won't be the same without him, but another resident will come along and we'll all get attached to him. Do you want to come to lunch with us? We're going to try that new deli, you know the one Johnson's took over. It'd do you good."

9. After you have found the most satisfactory strategy and discovered why the other options are not suitable, go back to the suggested response you generated earlier in this exercise. Evaluate yours in terms of its assertiveness and responsibleness.

PRACTICING COMMUNICATING ASSERTIVELY AND RESPONSIBLY WITH DISTRESSED CLIENTS AND COLLEAGUES

Exercise 1. For this exercise work in threes. You will need a tape recorder for this exercise. One of you will roleplay a distressed client or colleague and one the listener; the third will give feedback to the listener on her ability to communicate in an assertive and responsible way with the distressed person. The distressed client (or colleague) will communicate to the nurse by being upset, crying, sad, or depressed. The nurse will attempt to respond in an assertive and responsible way. The feedback giver will indicate to the nurse how effective she was in employing an assertive and responsible style. Tape this interaction so that you can use the recording to complete Exercise 2.

Make sure each of you has a turn in each of the roles. Allow enough time to do this exercise, including time for feedback.

After you have each had a turn in all roles, join the rest of your classmates. Together as a group discuss what you have learned about helpful and nonhelpful ways to communicate with distressed clients and colleagues.

Exercise 2. Transcribe into writing 10 paired interactions (what the distressed person said and what you said is one paired interaction) from the tape recorded interview you did in Exercise 1. For each statement that the distressed person made, write down your assessment of his thoughts, feelings, and whether it is appropriate to meet the request he is making. Examine the strategy you used to respond to your "client" or "colleague" and evaluate whether it met his request. If not, generate an alternative response that would be assertive and responsible. This review of your communication will help you develop more effective communication skills with distressed clients and colleagues.

REFERENCES

Gerrard, B. (1978). *Interpersonal skills for health professionals: A review of the literature.* Unpublished manuscript. McMaster University, Hamilton, Ontario, Canada.

SUGGESTIONS FOR FURTHER READING

Arnold, J. (1990). Grieving. *Imprint, 37*(1), 43-46.
Blackburn, F.C., & Copley, R. (1989). One precious moment. *Nursing '89, 19*(9), 52-54.
Coolican, M., Vassar, E., Gragan, J. (1989). Helping survivors survive. *Nursing '89,* 19(8), 51-53.
Getz, W.L., Allen, B., Myers, R.K., & Lindner, R.C. (1983). *Brief counseling with suicidal persons.* Lexington, Mass.: Lexington Books.
Johnson, J.L., & Morse, J.M. (1990). Regaining control: The process of adjustment after myocardial infarction. *Imprint, 19*(2), 126-135.
Leonard, C.V. (1975). Treating the suicidal patient: A communication approach. *Journal of Psychiatric Nursing and Mental Health Services, 13,* 19-22.
Lipkin, G.B., & Cohen, R.G. (1986) *Effective approaches to patients' behavior* (3rd ed.). New York: Springer Publishing Company.
Murphy, S.A. (1983). Theoretical perspectives on bereavement. In P.L. Chinn (Ed.) *Advances in nursing theory development,* (pp. 191-206). Rockville, Md.: Aspen Systems Corporation.
Purdy, A.M. (1990). The disabled patient: The grief that never ends. *Imprint, 37*(1), 68-69.
Rosen, S.L. (1990). Stillbirth: What the nurse should and should not do. *Imprint, 37*(1), 65-67.
Schubert, J. (1990). Comparing the grief reactions of a rehabilitation and a psychiatric patient. *Imprint, 37*(1), 59-62.
Thompson, D.R., Webster, R.A., & Meddis, R. (1990). In hospital counselling for first time myocardial infarction patients and spouses: Effects on satisfaction. *Journal of Advanced Nursing, 15*(9), 1064-1069.
Ufema, J. (1989). Insights on death and dying. *Nursing '89, 19*(8), 24-25.

CHAPTER 21

Communicating Assertively and Responsibly with Aggressive Clients and Colleagues

"When one is a victim of aggression
one does not waste time preparing
the menu for the victory banquet."

Louis Laberge

OBJECTIVES

This chapter is designed to give you practice communicating assertively and responsibly with aggressive clients and colleagues. Some of the reasons nurses have trouble relating to aggressive clients and colleagues will be highlighted so that you can work on overcoming any that apply to you. You will have the chance to compare the effectiveness of your suggested interventions with options that range in helpfulness. This comparison will improve your ability to correctly use the communication behaviors you learned in Parts One and Two. The practice of correcting your interventions will develop your critical ability to continuously improve your communication with aggressive clients and colleagues.

WHY AGGRESSIVE BEHAVIOR IS PROBLEMATIC FOR NURSES

Aggressiveness refers to rejecting, hostile, abusive, and manipulative behaviors. Aggressiveness from our clients and colleagues is a problem for nurses for several reasons. Aggressiveness is unpleasant because it is evidence of the other person's lack of respect for our feelings or right to be treated with courtesy and consideration. Knowledge of this mistreatment hurts and insults us and makes us want to stop this attack on our self-esteem.

Most of us would like to stand up for our right to be treated with respect in a way that is firm, effective (puts a stop to the aggressive behavior), and embarrasses neither us nor the other person; in other words we want to handle the aggression assertively. Our fears are that we will become enraged and lash out at the other person, fueling the fires of escalating aggression, or that we will remain tight-lipped and slink away, carrying around the smoldering wish to more effectively deal with an attacker. Our fears of losing control or embarrassing ourselves, or our insecurity in our ability to communicate assertively and deal with the oppression, keep us from acting effectively.

When we encounter aggressive behavior our self-esteem and physical safety are threatened. This chapter will help you deal with aggression so that you feel confident and comfortable.

Communicating Effectively with Aggressive Clients and Colleagues

Jakubowski and Lange (1978) outlined the following ways of dealing with aggression from others.

Get to the Source of the Problem

Asking for more information—so that you are clear about the reason for your aggressor's discontent—will show him your interest in his reactions and open up dialogue for resolution. Finding out what is causing the aggressor to attack you is a logical place to begin. For example, you might ask your supervisor, who has just reprimanded you for telephoning the intern on call about one of your seriously ill clients, this question:

> **Assertive You:** "I see that you are angry that I phoned Dr. Jones about our client's unstable vital signs. Could you tell me what upsets you about my calling him?"

This respectful acknowledgment of your aggressor's message allows him to clarify the problem. Using an empathic response demonstrates your understanding of the other's feelings and can disarm him enough to deescalate the aggression. The open-ended phrasing of your questions is less threatening than an aggressive approach like: "Why are you trying to stop me?"

Increase Your Aggressor's Awareness of His Abusive Behavior and Its Negative Effects

Asking questions to determine whether your aggressor is aware of the insulting impact of his aggression, or frankly pointing out his oppressiveness, is a technique to heighten the awareness of an aggressor to his ways.

For example, after repeated abuse and criticism from the resident-on-call, you inform him:

Assertive You: "Dr. Smith, when you swear at me and raise your voice when ordering me to get things for you, it makes working with you unpleasant."

Remaining calm and controlled in the face of an aggressor provides a contrast that may help him to realize that his behavior is out of line.

Limit the Aggressive Behavior

Employing a C.A.R.E. confrontation (chapter 12) lets your aggressor know, in no uncertain terms, what bothers you about his behavior and how you want him to change. Or sometimes, ignoring or dismissing the aggression and continuing with your more important agenda takes the wind out of an aggressor's sails and puts the emphasis on more pressing items.

For example, you are giving the end-of-shift report to the evening staff and one evening nurse repeatedly interrupts, quizzing you on an irrelevant matter. You curtail her aggression with:

Assertive You: "Sharon, I'd like to finish the report so please hold your questions and talk to me about it later."

For each aggressor and situation you will have different expected outcomes and want to use different assertive strategies. The important point is that you develop skills for dealing assertively with aggression so that you can maintain your self-respect while being courteous, and that you have "a constructive impact on the other person" (Jakubowski & Lange, 1978, p. 245). As a nurse, you must not tolerate continued aggression against yourself if you intend to preserve your self-esteem and credibility with clients and colleagues.

Improving Your Communication Skill with Aggressive Clients and Colleagues

The work you will do in this chapter will give you practice in dealing assertively with aggression so that in real-life situations you will feel and act more confidently. The forthcoming examples will help you overcome some of the barriers to relating with aggressive clients and colleagues, and generate more effective responses to aggression. You will be given situations involving aggressive clients and colleagues. Your task is to assess each situation, determine the request being made, and choose the most assertive and responsible communication strategy.

Appendix B contains a critique of all the response choices for each situation. It is a good idea to review all of them to learn about the strengths and limitations of each.

Communicating with Rejecting Clients
Step One: Assessment of the Data

1. Review the following situation and formulate your own assessment of the client's thoughts, feelings, and requests.

   Mr. Hunter has been a client on your medical-burn unit for 6 weeks. He has extensive burns to his arms, upper body, and face as a result of trying to rescue his daughter from a house fire. He has been in isolation for the duration of his hospitalization. Chris, your colleague who has been his primary nurse since his admission, has left for a vacation. As the student having your clinical experience on this unit you have been assigned to care for Mr. Hunter in Chris' absence. His wounds require extensive debridement and frequent dressing changes.

   You are changing a dressing on Mr. Hunter's shoulder when this conversation takes place:

   > **You:** "I'm going to let that soak for 5 minutes, Mr. Hunter. Then I'll remove it and do your other shoulder. Your burns are healing nicely."

   > **Mr. Hunter:** "That's thanks to Chris. She's a wonderful nurse. You've replaced her on her days off before and you don't do things like she does. I want you to be careful and do things like they are supposed to be done. You're just a student and I'm going to watch you carefully; if you do anything out of line I'm going to report you to your instructor."

2. On a separate piece of paper write down your assessment of Mr. Hunter's thoughts and feelings. Indicate what request Mr. Hunter is making of you, his "replacement" nurse.
3. Compare your assessment with the one below:

   Thoughts: Mr. Hunter is afraid you might do something to undermine Chris' effective nursing care of his burns. He thinks that because you are a student you might not care for his wounds with the same safety and skill that "his" nurse did.

   Feelings: He misses the consistent care he had from daily interaction with his primary nurse, Chris. He feels threatened and at the mercy of your care, in which he does not have confidence. He is afraid that you might do something to set back the progress of his healing.

   Request: The aggressiveness of his threat tells you how much Mr. Hunter wants you to take precautions to ensure continued healing of his burns. He wants to be reassured by your actions and words that you will give safe nursing care. His requests are for understanding, comfort, and safe burn treatment.

4. Did your assessment reflect an accurate analysis of the facts as they were presented? If not, return to the original vignette and reassess the cognitive and affective messages. If so, then proceed with step two.

Step Two: Communication Strategies and Desired Outcomes

5. You have determined that Mr. Hunter needs to be understood and comforted by your actions and your words. Identify what communication behaviors you would use to respond to Mr. Hunter's requests. Indicate the desired outcome of your strategy. Write your suggestions down on a separate sheet of paper for future reference.

6. Compare your suggested strategy with this one:

    Remaining calm would be important to avoid escalating his aggression. Relaxation will help you focus and avoid hostility yourself. Visualize responding in a compassionate way and use positive self-talk to remember not to explode at his aggressiveness. Empathic acknowledgement of his respect for Chris' care would reassure him that you understand the importance of safe care to ensure continued healing. Informing him that you will give your best care, and explaining what you are doing would dispel his apprehensions about your abilities. Ignoring his threat to report you would likely diminish his hostility.

    These interventions would likely let Mr. Hunter know that you understand both his vulnerability as a client and his longing for the consistent care from his primary nurse. Your directness, confidence, and calmness would likely make him optimistic and hopeful about the quality of care he will receive from you.

Step Three: Implementing and Evaluating Your Communication Strategy

7. Now you must reply to Mr. Hunter. Develop your own response to Mr. Hunter and write it on a separate sheet of paper. Keep it handy so that you can refer to it later.

8. At this point you get the chance to compare your suggested response with several options listed below. Look over each of the response choices and turn to Appendix B to read a critique of each.

    As you review the following response choices, look for those that are congruent with your assessment of Mr. Hunter's requests, and your desire to communicate in an assertive and responsible way.

CHOICE E "Report me if you want to Mr. Hunter. You don't honestly think my clinical instructor would give me the responsibility of caring for you if she didn't think that I could do it, do you? If you'd just give me a chance you'd see what a good nurse I can be."

CHOICE A "If you want a graduate nurse I can arrange to transfer so you can feel safer, Mr. Hunter. It sounds like you want a fully qualified graduate assigned to you."

CHOICE M "You're welcome to watch what I do and ask any questions. I'm sure my way of doing things is a little different from Chris', but I do guarantee that what I'm doing is safe and in keeping with your physician's orders. It is hard when things are done differently by each nurse, and you are likely missing Chris' style since you worked closely together for the 6 weeks you have been here. Do you want to ask me anything about what I've done so far in changing your dressing?"

CHOICE Z "You're just missing Chris, Mr. Hunter, and taking it out on me. I don't want to be compared to another nurse, and I won't have you making threats to report me to my instructor. I am in the top 10 of my class and I don't want you to question my care any more in the future. You had better get used to the idea that I am going to be your nurse."

9. After you have found the most satisfactory strategy and discovered why the other options are not suitable, go back to the suggested response you generated earlier in this exercise. Evaluate yours in terms of its assertiveness and responsibleness.

Communicating with Rejecting Colleagues
Step One: Assessment of the Data

1. Review the following situation and formulate your own assessment of your colleague's thoughts, feelings, and requests.

You are a student nurse in your second year of a diploma program. In the past 6 weeks you have had your clinical experience in the maternity services of the hospital. During that time your clinical instructor has been meticulously thorough in her supervision and teaching of the skills needed for maternity nursing. This area of nursing is one you love and you think you might pursue a career in this field. You feel you are adept at the physical care of both mother and baby, and you have been influential in helping mothers and fathers adjust to caring for their newborns. Your teaching sessions to mothers have been rated as outstanding, and the head nurse in maternity has indicated that she is pleased with your work.

Despite your certainty that you are doing a good job, and positive feedback from clients and staff, you have never received a word of praise from your clinical instructor. In fact, she takes every opportunity to tell you where you could improve and is picayune in her reprimands about your small errors. You are disappointed that your instructor is not more encouraging and enthusiastic about your successes. Today she is meeting with you to give you feedback on the bath class you gave to the fathers. You have had a chance to look over the fathers' evaluation forms and they clearly state that your manner and content were reassuring in their first experience of bathing their newborns. Your instructor has just listed everything you did wrong and made suggestions about how you could improve such a class in the future.

Instructor: ". . . In sum, you need to polish your professionalism. You are much too casual; you always are, for that matter. How do you expect anyone to treat you like a professional if you are lax and don't have a tight rein on things? You need to shape up in that regard and you'll command a lot more respect."

2. On a separate sheet of paper write down your assessment of your instructor's thoughts and feelings. Indicate what request she is making of you, her nursing student.
3. Compare your assessment with that below:

Thoughts: Your instructor thinks you need to be more professional, and that if you could cultivate this demeanor you would gain more respect.

Feelings: She is disappointed in your overall consistent lack of professionalism. It is highly likely that she feels a great responsibility to shape you into her image of a perfectly functioning nurse.

Request: She wants you to change your behavior on a consistent basis to a style of operating that matches her image of professionalism. She expects you to put up with negative feedback in this evaluation, as she has during your complete rotation.

4. Did your assessment reflect an accurate analysis of the facts as they were presented? If not, return to the original data presented in the vignette and reassess the cognitive and affective messages. If so, proceed with step two.

Step Two: Communication Strategies and Desired Outcomes

5. You have determined that your instructor is making an unreasonable request of you. You are disappointed and angry that she continues her unwillingness to give you legitimate praise for the good work you have done. Identify what communication strategies you would use to handle her request. Indicate the desired outcomes of your suggested strategy. Write this information on a separate piece of paper for future reference.
6. Compare your suggested strategy with this one:

It would be important to relax and visualize yourself responding assertively in the wave of such rejecting aggression. A request for specificity would be in order because she has not really explained what she means by being more "professional." It would be appropriate to express your opinion that the evidence you have received from the two classes indicates that you are performing well as a maternity nurse. A C.A.R.E. confrontation would be acceptable to let her know that you are disappointed in the absence of positive feedback and that you would like to receive some from her in your final evaluation as a student on the unit.

Strategies like these would let her clearly know—in a way that respects her as your instructor—that you want a stop to her rejecting aggression.

Step Three: Implementing and Evaluating Your Communication Strategy

7. Now you must reply to your instructor. Develop your own response to her and write it down on a separate sheet of paper. Keep it handy so that you can refer to it later.

8. At this point you get the chance to compare your suggested response with several options listed below. Look over each of the response choices and turn to Appendix B to read a critique of each.

As you review the following response choices look for those that are congruent with your assessment of your instructor's requests and your desire to communicate in an assertive and responsible way.

CHOICE H "I can see you are giving me some advice that you believe is very important, but it's not clear to me. What exactly do you mean by 'professional'? If you explain what you mean it'll be clearer to me so that I will be more likely to improve."

CHOICE B "I'm tired of your suggestions for my improvement. You have never once said anything positive in the 5 weeks I have been here. The staff and clients give me more strokes than you do. I need some positive feedback from you, too."

CHOICE Y "Well, I'll try to do my best to be more professional in the future."

CHOICE J "I know that when you give me all those suggestions about improving you are trying to help me be the best maternity nurse I can be. It's disappointing that you haven't also noted some of the good things I've done and some of the ways in which I've acted professionally. I have received enough super evaluations from the clients and encouraging comments from the staff to support my belief that I am doing some things well. Before I leave this rotation I would like you to give me some positive feedback in addition to your suggestions for improvement. Will you do that for me?"

9. After you have found the most satisfactory strategy and discovered why the other options are not suitable, go back to the suggested response you generated earlier in this exercise. Evaluate yours in terms of its assertiveness and responsibleness.

Communicating with Hostile Clients
Step One: Assessment of the Data

1. Review the following situation and formulate your own assessment of the client's thoughts, feelings and requests.

Debbie is an 18-year-old client on the medical ward where you nurse. She is a recently diagnosed diabetic and is terrified of receiving her insulin injection. When you go to administer it she screams and kicks. It requires two staff members to hold her down securely in order to give the insulin safely. You know that this situation is unsatisfactory because Debbie will have to give her own insulin soon. She will have to overcome her fear and gradually take on more responsibility for her self care.

You decide to talk with Debbie about your desire for her to be more involved in her diabetic care. You have started the conversation by explaining that you have some ideas about how she can overcome her fear and learn to be more confident in giving her insulin. Debbie interrupts you with:

> **Debbie:** "Hold it! (Raising her voice) I'm not, repeat, NOT EVER going to give myself insulin. Get out, you bloodsucking vampire! You enjoy torturing me every morning. Well FORGET IT! GET LOST! Go find someone else to bug. Just get off my back about this insulin jazz." (Debbie comes face to face with you, and looks you right in the eye. She is red in the face and has her fists clenched and raised.)

2. On a separate sheet of paper write down your assessment of Debbie's thoughts and feelings. Indicate what request she is making of you, her nurse.
3. Compare your analysis with the assessment written below:

Thoughts: Debbie thinks you are cruel to "force" her to get more involved in taking her insulin.

Feelings: Because she is terrified of giving herself insulin, and is probably having trouble accepting that she is diabetic, Debbie is enraged and fiercely trying to keep you at bay to protect her denial and fear. Her affrontive attack on you comes from her insecurity.

Request: Her obvious request is for you to leave her alone. The rational part of her (which is overshadowed by her fear) knows that you are right and that she will have to learn to be calmer about her insulin. Directly, Debbie is requesting to be understood and she wants you to act by leaving. Indirectly she is requesting to be comforted.

4. Did your assessment reflect an accurate analysis of the facts as they were presented? If not, return to the original data presented in the vignette and reassess the cognitive and affective messages. If so, then proceed with step two.

Step Two: Communication Strategies and Desired Outcomes

5. You have determined that Debbie is requesting understanding, action, and comfort. Identify the communication behaviors you would use to show Debbie how you intend to respond to her requests. Indicate the desired outcomes of your suggested strategy. Write down your ideas on a separate sheet of paper.
6. Compare your suggested strategy with this one:

It is reasonable to meet Debbie's request for understanding and her implied request for comfort. She has a great adjustment to make as a diabetic and you can help her by showing you understand. It is unreasonable to meet Debbie's request for action by leaving. She is frightened and needs someone to be in control. If you leave by walking away, or become aggressive, her fear and anger will escalate out of control.

Remaining calm will help you think more clearly, and might help calm Debbie. Being calm indicates that you are in control. If it is difficult for you to remain calm in the face of such enraged hostility, you could focus and visualize yourself reacting in a collected way. An empathic response to Debbie's fear and anger about having to take insulin would let her know that you do understand. A firm expression of your opinion — that she needs to learn how to be calmer about receiving her insulin — would indicate that you are in control, want to help her, and will not be put off or reject her because of her angry outburst. A gentle suggestion about how you would like to proceed to help her might make her reconsider your plan and decide that it might not be so terrifying.

This approach would show Debbie that you understand her and that you will stick with her to help her through her fear and anger; it will also give her hope of regaining self-control. She will not likely feel happy for some time, but this response will help diminish her terror.

Step Three: Implementing and Evaluating Your Communication Strategy

7. Now you must reply to Debbie. Develop your own response to Debbie and write it down on a separate sheet of paper. Keep it handy so that you can refer to it later.
8. Here is where you get the chance to compare your suggested response with several options listed below. Look over each of the response choices and turn to Appendix B to read a critique of each.

As you review the following response choices, look for those that are congruent with your assessment of Debbie's requests and your desire to communicate in an assertive and responsible way.

CHOICE C (Reaching out and putting your arm around Debbie's shoulders) "There, there, Debbie. Don't be so angry. It's just a matter of time before you'll feel okay about taking your insulin. I'm just here to help you. You'll see that you'll be feeling calm about the whole thing in a few weeks."

CHOICE K "Don't you talk to me like that, young lady. You'd better show a little more respect for me or you'll be in trouble. I know what's best for you. I've had lots of experience, so if you're smart you'll cooperate."

CHOICE Q "I know it is scary to receive a needle every morning, Debbie. It's a big thing to adjust to, especially for someone as active and as healthy as you. I can help you to feel quite confident, and eventually even comfortable, about taking your insulin. What I'd like you to do is to sit down with me right now and listen to my plan. I want you to hear me out, and then you can ask any questions and consider whether you'd like to try it."

CHOICE X "Debbie, I was only trying to help you" (you say before you leave Debbie's room).

9. After you have found the most satisfactory strategy and discovered why the others are not suitable options, go back to the original suggested strategy you generated earlier in this exercise. Evaluate yours in terms of its assertiveness and responsibleness.

Communicating with Hostile Colleagues
Step One: Assessment of the Data

1. Review the following situation and formulate your own assessment of your colleague's thoughts, feelings, and requests.

You are a nurse working in the psychiatric assessment services in your hospital. There are small interviewing rooms that can be booked for private interviews with clients and their families. In the past 3 days your interviews have been 5 minutes longer than the ½ hour that you had booked. By going over time you have delayed the interviews of others. Your colleague Karen has been annoyed but understanding because you are not usually so inconsiderate.

Today you booked the room for 45 minutes so that you could complete your interview without holding up others. However, your client has just revealed some serious information about her marriage and is upset and crying in the interview room. You know you need about 5 minutes over your time to help your client calm down before vacating the interview room. Karen has booked the room after you. She has knocked on the door twice already to remind you that your time is up. When you come out with your client she blasts you with:

> **Karen:** "It's about time. This is the fourth time this week that I've had to wait for you to leave the room when I've booked it. This has got to stop. My client's family is here on their lunch hour. You aren't the only one with important things to do, you know" (Karen's voice is raised and her hands are on her hips).

2. On a separate sheet of paper write down your assessment of Karen's thoughts and feelings. Indicate what request Karen is making of you, her nurse colleague.
3. Compare your analysis with this assessment:

Thoughts: Karen thinks you are rude and inconsiderate to go beyond your allotted time in the shared interview room.

Feelings: Karen is annoyed because you have eaten into the time she had planned to be in the room. She is feeling pressured because the family she wants to interview only has a limited period of time. She is worried about seeming to be rude to them by not being able to get into the only private room available. Karen is frustrated and disappointed that you have behaved in such an inconsiderate way.

Request: Karen wants you to understand how inconvenienced she and her clients were by your thoughtlessness. She wants you to act more responsibly in the future by vacating the room after your time is up.

4. Did your assessment reflect an accurate analysis of the facts as they were presented? If not, return to the original data presented in the vignette and reassess the cognitive and affective messages. If so, then proceed with step two.

Step Two: Communication Strategies and Desired Outcomes

5. You have determined that Karen wants understanding and action. Identify which communication behaviors you would use to respond to Karen. Indicate the desired outcomes of your strategy. Write your ideas down on a separate sheet of paper so that you can refer to them later.
6. Compare your suggested strategy with this one:

Karen's request for understanding and future consideration are legitimate. It is reasonable to respond to them with an empathic reply and a promise to be more careful in the future. It is unreasonable to accept Karen's hostile aggressiveness, especially since she embarrassed you in front of all three clients and any other staff members in the vicinity. It would be important to stay calm and make a C.A.R.E. confrontation to Karen, asking her to speak more courteously to you about issues that bother her. It would be better to wait until later in the day to speak with Karen, at a time when you both have an opportunity to complete your discussion.

This strategy would make Karen feel assured that you respect her rights and it would make her aware of your rights, too.

Step Three: Implementing and Evaluating Your Communication Strategy

7. Now you must reply to Karen. On a separate sheet of paper develop your own response to Karen and keep it handy.
8. At this point you get the opportunity to compare your suggested response with several options listed below. Look over each of the response choices and turn to Appendix B to read a critique of each.

As you review the following response choices, look for those that are congruent with your assessment of Karen's requests and your desire to communicate in an assertive and responsible way.

CHOICE D (At the time) "I apologize to all of you (looking at Karen and her clients) for this inconvenience." (Later, at a mutually convenient time when you and Karen are alone) "Karen, I'd like to talk with you about how you handled my overstaying my booking time this morning." (Proceeding after Karen agrees to do so) "I will really try not to inconvenience you by going over my booked time in the future. I was very embarrassed that you 'scolded' me in front of our clients in the middle of the hall where everyone could hear. In the future, I would appreciate it if you would ask to talk about any complaints you have in private. Then no one would be embarrassed and we can keep our staff quarrels separate from the clients. Could you do this, Karen?"

CHOICE L (At the time) "Just a minute, Karen. What do you mean? I wouldn't deliberately try to annoy you by overstaying my time. You should know there's a very good reason for my delay. I'm not deliberately trying to inconvenience you. The room is yours now."

CHOICE P (At the time) Getting red in the face and avoiding eye contact with Karen and her clients, you walk right past them. Later, when you have an opportunity to have contact with Karen you avoid her. You refuse to make eye contact and you do not initiate conversation with her even though you do with the rest of the staff.

CHOICE W (At the time) "I'm sorry, Karen."

9. After you have found the most satisfactory strategy and discovered why the other options are not satisfactory, go back to the suggested response you generated earlier in this exercise. Evaluate yours in terms of its assertiveness and responsibleness.

Communicating with Abusive Clients
Step One: Assessment of the Data

1. Review the following situation and formulate your own assessment of your client's thoughts, feelings and requests.

   Mrs. Suit is a 60-year-old client, on your unit for 1 week to have a thorough investigation of multiple health problems including shortness of breath, heart palpitations, and a possible ulcer. She has been very demanding, especially on the days when her husband is unable to get up to visit her. Today she has put her call light on repeatedly and this time she has asked you to bring her some ice water in a glass and a fresh straw. You start out for the kitchen but are waylaid by the distraught son of another client. He is almost in tears and wants to discuss with you the news of his father's cancer and forthcoming surgery. You pause to talk with him before you get Mrs. Suit's ice drink. When you get back to Mrs. Suit's room she lambastes you with:

   > **Mrs. Suit:** "Damnation. You could die here before you get a simple glass of water. Geezus, you're such a smart ass; you probably think I'm just a sick old lady, but I've got just as much right to

service as anybody in this hospital. What in the hell were you do-ing, melting some ice? Gawdamnit. Just give me the straw; you're slower than molasses in January. I'll open it myself. If I let you do it you could take all night. You can go now. You smart-assed nurses think you're so gawdamn important but you can't even get an old lady a drink of water without messing things up."

2. On a separate sheet of paper write down your assessment of Mrs. Suit's thoughts and feelings. Indicate what request Mrs. Suit is making of you, her nurse.
3. Compare your assessment with the one below:

Thoughts: Mrs. Suit thinks you took your time bringing her the ice water because you don't think either she or her request is important.

Feelings: Mrs. Suit's feelings are hurt because of her assumption that your tardiness is associated with lack of respect for her. Her abusiveness is her defense against her hurt feelings of being rejected. It is likely that she is frightened of the numerous tests she is having in the hospital, and lonely today because she did not receive a visit from her husband. These factors may be compounding her attack on you.

Request: Mrs. Suit is asking you to treat her with more respect by following through on her reasonable requests (like getting a glass of water). Indirectly she is asking you to understand that she feels insecure. Obliquely she is requesting comfort from you and reassurance that you care about her. This request for comfort is for present and future inter-actions.

4. Did your assessment reflect an accurate analysis of the facts as they were presented? If not, return to the original data presented in the vi-gnette and reassess the cognitive and affective messages. If so, then proceed with step two.

Step Two: Communication Strategies and Desired Outcomes

5. You have determined that Mrs. Suit needs understanding and comfort. Identify what communication strategy you would use to respond to her requests. Indicate the desired outcomes of your strategy. Write your ideas down so that you can refer to them later.
6. Compare your suggested strategy with this one:

Mrs. Suit's requests are all legitimate. Her way of expressing them is aggressive and irritating and it would be easy to become offended. The best approach is to stay calm and extend warmth to this upset woman. It might be appropriate to explain your delay to prove that you were not dawdling disrespectfully. Some reassurance of your interest in her would be supportive for her. In the future you could make efforts to ensure that she is made to feel important and cared for (taking her to the sunroom, introducing her to other clients).

This strategy would make her feel cared for and respected.

Step Three: Implementing and Evaluating Your Communication Strategy

7. Now you must reply to Mrs. Suit. On a separate sheet of paper develop your own response to Mrs. Suit and keep it for future reference.
8. At this point you get the chance to compare your suggested strategy with several options listed below. Look over each of the response choices and turn to Appendix B to read a critique of each.

As you review the following choices, look for those that are congruent with your assessment of Mrs. Suit's requests and your desire to communicate in an assertive and responsible way.

CHOICE AA "Mrs. Suit, I'm sorry I was so long in coming with your ice water. It's not that I don't care about you. I was delayed by an upset family member who needed to talk about his seriously ill father. I'm sure you can now understand why I was delayed. I am free for a few minutes now, though, if there's anything you'd like to talk about."

CHOICE I "Mrs. Suit, I went out of my way to get you your water. The least you could do is say "thank you' " (turns and leaves).

CHOICE R "Sorry, Mrs. Suit." (Facial expression is flat and you leave after giving her the straw.)

9. After you have found the most satisfactory strategy and discovered why the other options are not suitable, go back to the original response you generated in this exercise. Evaluate yours in terms of its assertiveness and responsibleness.

Communicating with Abusive Colleagues
Step One: Assessment of the Data

1. Review the following situation and formulate your own assessment of your colleague's thoughts, feelings, and requests.

You have been a student nurse on a surgical unit for 3 weeks. For the past 3 days you have been the medication nurse. On this unit the job of giving out medications is particularly difficult and time-consuming. Clients are often downstairs having preoperative tests, dressings changed, or busy at physical therapy; all of these make it difficult to give out the medications smoothly. In addition there are many intravenous drips to be regulated. You find it confusing to keep track of the I.V.s, the regular medications, and clients' requests for postoperative analgesics.

Your clinical instructor has encouraged you by assuring you that you are doing a fine job. She has remarked that you are safe and careful with distributing the medications and informed you that speed will come with practice. The team leader on the floor has not been so supportive. From the first day you took over as medication nurse she has been hostile and insulting. She has said such destructive things as: "I know you students have to learn but we've got sick people here who can't wait all day for their meds. You're going to have to speed things up." and "Look out. Here comes speedy!" (to another nurse at the nursing station). She has undermined you by coming to get the medication keys from you and giving some clients narcotic pain relievers, saying: "If she has to wait for you to get there her pain will have her on the ceiling."

You are just returning to the nursing station after distributing your morning medications. Your hostile team leader is at the station and affronts you with:

> **Team Leader:** "Well, what do you know? You're finally here. While you've been poking along out on the floor I've given three clients their pain killers. I bet you haven't remembered your I.V.s, have you? Well, speedy, I've been keeping my eye on them and you'd better change the bag in room 25. I don't know how you're going to function as a graduate when you don't have someone like me looking over your shoulder."

2. On a separate sheet of paper write down your assessment of your team leader's thoughts and feelings. Indicate what request she is making of you, the student nurse giving medications on this surgical unit.
3. Compare your analysis with that below:

Thoughts: Your team leader thinks you are far too slow as a medication nurse. She has the notion that you are incapable of taking charge of all the medication nurse's responsibilities at this point.

Feelings: She is concerned about those clients who need their postoperative medications, and she is worried that the I.V.s will run dry. She is irritated by your slowness and unwilling to remember that it takes practice to become faster at this complicated task. Her annoyance makes her take out her frustration on you.

Request: Your team leader wants you to be faster as a medication nurse. She wants you to simultaneously keep track of I.V.s, regular medications, and p.r.n. orders for analgesics. *And,* she wants you to develop accurate speed immediately. She is requesting that you understand what she wants and that you comply with it immediately.

4. Did your assessment reflect an accurate analysis of the facts as they were presented? If not, return to the original data presented in the vignette and reassess the cognitive and affective messages. If so, then proceed with step two.

Step Two: Communication Strategies and Desired Outcomes

5. You have determined that the team leader wants understanding and action. Identify what communication behaviors you would use to respond to her requests. Indicate the desired outcome of your strategy. Write down your ideas so that you can refer to them later.
6. Compare your suggested strategy with this one:

Her request for understanding is legitimate but her request for immediate increased speed as medication nurse is unreasonable, given your lack of experience. It would be important to keep calm and remain unflustered so as to respond to your team leader in a clear, direct way. If you get out of control you may be upset for the rest of the day and increase your chances of making an error.

Remain calm, using imagery and positive self-talk to help you stay focused on responding assertively and responsibly to your team leader. It would be appropriate that you thank her for the help she has given you. However, it is also necessary that you ask her to consult you before giving out medications to anybody, to ensure that you as the person in charge of medications are kept informed and that no duplications are made. A C.A.R.E. confrontation to request that she have more patience with your beginning skill would let her know how it would be more helpful for her to relate to you.

This approach will let your team leader know that you do understand the need for speed and accuracy in a medication nurse, but that her request for immediate action is unreasonable. She may not like your assertive response because it will point out to her that she has been aggressive and that you do not intend to tolerate being treated in such a destructive manner. Your strategy may change her behavior in a positive way; however, if she escalates her abusiveness to you, you can confront her again and indicate a more serious consequence (such as reporting her aggressiveness to your clinical instructor).

Step Three: Implementing and Evaluating Your Communication Strategy

7. Now you must reply to your team leader. On a separate sheet of paper develop your own response to her. Keep it for future reference.
8. At this point you get the chance to compare your suggested response with several options listed below. Look over each of the response choices and turn to Appendix B to read a critique of each.

As you review the following response choices look for those that are congruent with your assessment of your team leader's requests and your desire to communicate in an assertive and responsible way.

CHOICE F "I hope when I am a graduate I am more considerate of students than you are. Don't you remember what it was like when you were learning? Your insults aren't helpful at all."

CHOICE N "I guess it's hard for you to sit back and have someone less experienced give out the medications. I understand the concerns you have about the clients receiving their medication on time; however, I have to learn and it will take a few more days before I am faster at this new job. It would be helpful if you would let me know when clients are asking for, or have received, their analgesics so that I can keep track of who's had what. I appreciate your giving the clients their meds these past days but I would like to try to do the whole job of being a medication nurse now that I'm getting the hang of it. Will you let me do that?"

CHOICE S "Oh. I'll go and attend to those I.V.s right away. Sorry I'm so slow; it must drive you crazy."

9. After you have found the most satisfactory strategy and discovered why the other options are not suitable, go back to the suggested response you generated in this exercise. Evaluate yours in terms of its assertiveness and responsibleness.

Communicating with Manipulative Clients
Step One: Assessment of the Data

1. Review the following situation and formulate your own assessment of your client's thoughts, feelings, and requests.

   Mr. Gilmour is a 58-year-old gentleman on your rehabilitative stroke unit. He is a heavy smoker and because he burns holes in his clothing it is the policy to keep his cigarettes at the nursing station, ensure that he wears a nonflammable smoking jacket, and supervise him when he smokes. Mr. Gilmour has a knack of asking for cigarettes at the most inconvenient times. He knows he is supposed to wait until report is over before he asks for a smoke, but he invariably bugs the nursing staff at report time. You are the nurse in charge of the day shift and you want to complete the report to the evening staff so that you can go home. Mr. Gilmour has already interrupted your report three times to ask for a smoke. You gave him a cigarette a ½ hour ago. His fourth manipulative attempt goes like this:

   > **Mr. Gilmour:** "Aw, come on. I'll smoke it right here where you can see me. I promise I won't start a fire. (He moves his wheelchair closer and closer to the small area where you are having report.) It won't hurt you to give me one little smoke. Come on. I haven't had one all afternoon. Give a guy a break. I had to go for that stupid x-ray so I missed my after-lunch smoke. Just one and then I won't bother you again."

2. On a separate sheet of paper write down your assessment of Mr. Gilmour's thoughts and feelings. Indicate what request Mr. Gilmour is making of you, the nurse in charge on days.
3. Compare your analysis with the one below:
Thoughts: Mr. Gilmour thinks he deserves a cigarette and believes that if he bugs you enough he will get what he wants.
Feelings: He is annoyed that you are not giving into his requests. He feels especially justified in persisting because he has not had a cigarette for what he thinks is a few hours.
Request: Mr. Gilmour's request is for understanding (about his craving to have a smoke) and action (you giving him a cigarette).
4. Did your assessment reflect an accurate analysis of the facts as they were presented? If not, return to the original data presented in the vignette and reassess the cognitive and affective messages. If so, proceed with step two.

Step Two: Communication Strategies and Desired Outcomes

5. You have determined that Mr. Gilmour wants understanding and action. Identify what communication behaviors you would use to respond to his requests. Indicate the desired outcomes for your suggested strategy. Write your ideas down for future reference.

6. Compare your suggested strategy to this one:

It would be tempting to lash out aggressively at Mr. Gilmour but this attack would only hurt his feelings, make you feel bad, and embarrass everyone. Even though you are frustrated by Mr. Gilmour's manipulative persistence it is important to stay calm and handle the situation assertively and responsibly. It would be wise to be consistent with the rule the unit has made of refusing cigarettes during report. You know that report will be finished in 5 minutes and that it is not unreasonable for Mr. Gilmour to wait that long. A firm refusal to comply, and a request that Mr. Gilmour leave you in peace to complete your nursing report, would be appropriate. It would be important to ensure that he does get a smoke right after report.

This strategy would demonstrate to Mr. Gilmour that he cannot break a reasonable rule that has been established for a good purpose. Your firmness would respect your own right to finish report without being interrupted and would treat Mr. Gilmour with respect.

Step Three: Implementing and Evaluating Your Communication Strategy

7. Now you must reply to Mr. Gilmour. On a separate sheet of paper develop your own response to Mr. Gilmour and keep it handy for future reference.

8. At this point you get the chance to compare your suggested response with several options listed below. Look over each of the response choices and turn to Appendix B to read a critique of each.

As you review the following response choices look for those that are congruent with your assessment of Mr. Gilmour's requests and your desire to communicate in an assertive and responsible way.

CHOICE G "Get out of here and leave us alone so that we can finish report. As soon as we are finished we will give you a cigarette."

CHOICE U "Mr. Gilmour, please do not interrupt us while we are having report. We will finish in 5 minutes if you stop interrupting us. It's only been a ½ hour since your last cigarette, and when report is finished one of the evening nurses will give you a cigarette. If you do not leave us now, then we will delay giving you a cigarette for another hour."

CHOICE BB "Ohhhh! (exasperated). At this point I'd do anything to get this report over so I can leave. Here's a cigarette."

9. After you have found the most satisfactory strategy and discovered why the other options are unsuitable, go back to the suggested re-

sponse you generated earlier in this exercise. Evaluate your response in terms of its assertiveness and responsibleness.

Communicating with Manipulative Colleagues
Step One: Assessment of the Data

1. Review the following situation and formulate your own assessment of your colleague's thoughts, feelings, and requests.

You are a nurse on the renal dialysis unit in your hospital. It is midway through an uneventful evening shift. Your colleague, Noreen, has suffered a splitting headache all night and she is concerned that it will develop into one of her immobilizing migraine headaches. She approaches you with this request:

> **Noreen:** "Leslie, I can't take this head of mine any longer. I feel like my brain has dried up into a hard ball and it's knocking against my skull. And on the outside it feels like a vise locking in on it. I've already tossed up what little supper I could eat. Leslie, could you give me some IM analgesic for my head? I've used it in the past and it stops me from vomiting and somehow eases my head, too. My doctor would agree to it, I swear; so won't you please help me out of my misery? It's not like it's a narcotic I'm asking for. What do you say? I might be of some help to you for the rest of the night if you give me the analgesic."

2. On a separate sheet of paper write down your assessment of Noreen's thoughts and feelings. Indicate what request Noreen is making of you, her colleague on the evening shift.
3. Compare your analysis with the assessment below:

Thoughts: Noreen thinks that the analgesic will help her to feel better. She thinks it is reasonable for you to give her the analgesic without an order from her physician.

Feelings: Noreen is feeling pretty sick with her impending migraine headache and feels hopeful that you will help her by giving the analgesic.

Request: Noreen is asking you to understand that her head is making her feel violently ill. She is requesting action in the form of you giving her an injection of the analgesic.

4. Did your assessment reflect an accurate analysis of the facts as they were presented? If not, return to the original data presented in the vignette and reassess the cognitive and affective message. If so, then proceed with step two.

Step Two: Communication Strategies and Desired Outcomes

5. You have determined that Noreen wants understanding and action. Identify what communication strategies you would use to respond to her request. Indicate the desired outcomes of your suggested strategy. Write your ideas down so that you can refer to them later.
6. Compare your suggested strategy to this one:

Warmth and an empathic reply would convey your compassion with her severe headache. Her request for you to give her an injection without a physician's order is unreasonable because it puts you in jeopardy of disciplinary action from your professional nursing association. Furthermore, you would be unwise to administer anything that might be damaging to your colleague since she has not been examined by a physician. A firm refusal to comply with her request would be appropriate, as would be a suggestion that she call the nursing supervisor and arrange to leave work to attend to her health.

This strategy would show Noreen you understand and care about how she is feeling, and make it clear that you want her to handle her health problems through the correct channels.

Step Three: Implementing and Evaluating Your Communication Strategy

7. Now you must reply to Noreen. On a separate sheet of paper develop your own response to Noreen and keep it handy for future reference.
8. At this point you get to compare your suggested response with several options listed below. Look over each of the response choices and turn to Appendix B to read a critique of each.

As you review the following response choices look for those that are congruent with your assessment of Noreen's requests and your desire to communicate in an assertive and responsible way.

CHOICE O "Are you serious, Noreen? I can't give you anything from the med cupboard. If you're that sick you'd better go home."

CHOICE T "Well, I guess that would be okay, Noreen. Do you really think so? You're right, it's a drug you have used before. Okay, I'll do it. Do you really think we're doing the right thing?"

CHOICE V "Noreen, you sound terrible. I think if you're that uncomfortable you'd better call the supervisor and arrange to go home. I will not give you any meds from the unit and I don't think you should take anything until you've checked with your doctor. The unit has been quiet and I know I can manage. Would you like me to call the evening supervisor for you?"

9. After you have found the most satisfactory strategy and discovered why the other options were unsuitable, go back to the suggested response you generated earlier in this example. Evaluate yours in terms of its assertiveness and responsibleness.

PRACTICING COMMUNICATING WITH AGGRESSIVE CLIENTS AND COLLEAGUES

Exercise 1. (You will need an audio tape recorder.) For this exercise work in threes. One will roleplay an aggressive client or colleague, another will be the nurse, and the third will give feedback to the nurse. The

aggressive client (or colleague) will communicate to the nurse in a rejecting, hostile, abusive, or manipulative way. The nurse will attempt to respond in an assertive and responsible way. The feedback giver will indicate to the nurse how effective she was in employing an assertive and
responsible style. Tape the dialogue between client (or colleague) and
nurse so that you can use the recording to complete Exercise 2.

Make sure each of you has the chance to roleplay all three roles. After
you have done this exercise in your small groups, rejoin your colleagues
in the rest of the class. Pool together what you have learned about communicating effectively with aggressive clients and colleagues.

Exercise 2. Transcribe into writing 10 paired interactions (what the aggressive person said and what you said is one paired interaction) from the
tape-recorded interview you did in Exercise 1. For each statement that
the aggressive person made write down your assessment of his thoughts
and feelings, and whether it is appropriate to meet the request he is making. Examine the strategy you used to respond to your "client" or "colleague" and evaluate whether it met his request. If not, generate an alternative response that is assertive and responsible. This review will help
you develop more effective communication skills with aggressive clients
and colleagues.

REFERENCES

Jakubowski, P., & Lange, A.J. (1978). *The assertive option: Your rights and responsibilities.*
Champaign, Ill.: Research Press Company.

SUGGESTIONS FOR FURTHER READING

Lipkin, G.B., & Cohen, R.G. (1986). *Effective approaches to patients' behavior* (3rd ed.). New
York: Springer Publishing Company.
Mackay, H. (1990). Beware the office bully. In H. Mackay, *Beware the naked man who offers you
his shirt* (pp. 45-49). New York: Ivy Books.
Medved, R. (1990). Strategies for handling angry patients and their families. *Nursing '90, 21* (4).
Murphy, T.G. (1990). Improving nurse/doctor communications. *Nursing '90, 20* (8), 114-118.
Stuart, G.W., & Sundeen, S.J. (1991). Problems with the expression of anger. In G.W. Stuart &
S.J. Sundeen, *Principles and practice of psychiatric nursing* (4th ed.), (pp. 539-565). St. Louis:
Mosby–Year Book.
Turnbull, J., Aitken, I., Black, L., & Patterson, B. (1990). Turn it around: Short-term manage-
ment for aggression and anger. *Journal of Psychosocial Nursing, 28* (6), 7-14.

CHAPTER 22

Communicating Assertively and Responsibly with Unpopular Clients

*"No man has a right in America
to treat any other man tolerantly,
for tolerance is the assumption
of superiority."*

Wendell Wilkie

OBJECTIVES

This chapter will help you become more aware of how your prejudices about clients' behavior and personality affect how you relate to them. You will become more aware of client characteristics that trigger you to withdraw your caring. This knowledge will alert you to your negative tendencies and remind you to treat all your clients fairly, safely, and in a way that respects their dignity.

The exercises in the chapter will help you communicate more caringly with unpopular clients.

WHO ARE THE UNPOPULAR CLIENTS?

It might shock you to learn that all clients are not thought of or treated similarly. All nurses at some time have clients they do not like (Kus, 1990). Although there is nothing intrinsic to any client that makes them likable or not, there are clients whom a single nurse or groups of nurses externally evaluate as popular or unpopular (p. 554). Before reading what the literature documents as the most popular and unpopular clients, take a moment to discover and examine your own attitudes towards your clients. Answer the following questions as specifically as possible:

• What are the characteristics of those clients whom you have enjoyed nursing?

• What are the features of clients whom you have not enjoyed nursing?

Now, compare your answers with those of your colleagues in your class. Where do your views overlap? In what ways are your preferences and nonpreferences for clients different? What do your collective opinions suggest to you about the client-nurse relationship?

In 1972 Stockwell published the findings of her classic study, *The unpopular patient,* which set out to determine whether there were some clients whom the nursing team enjoyed caring for more than others, and whether there was any measurable difference in the nursing care afforded to the most and least popular clients. Her findings were startling at that time, and still have such potential impact for nurses that they have been republished in a 1984 edition. She discovered that foreign clients, those with more than 3 months hospitalization experience, clients with some type of physical defect, and those with a psychiatric diagnosis figured significantly in the unpopular group. Personality factors of the client played a significant part (sometimes the only one) in accounting for whether they were considered unpopular by the nursing team.

Stockwell's research findings revealed that unpopular clients did not receive individual holistic care, and that nurses withdrew their caring interpersonal communication from these clients. When clients do not fit into our molds we become annoyed and respond to our anger by displacing it onto our clients as dislike (Gerrard, 1978).

Lorber (1975) investigated the reactions of doctors and nurses to the attitudes and behaviors of surgical clients. Nurses and physicians labeled clients who interrupted well-established routines and made extra work for them "problem" clients. Those who minimized the trouble they caused staff by their extraordinary cooperativeness were considered "good."

Characteristics of Unpopular Clients and Effects on Nurses

(Stockwell, 1972; Lorber, 1975; Kus, 1990)

Unpopular clients:

• Grumble or complain.
• Indicate their lack of enjoyment at being in hospital.
• Imply that they are suffering more than nurses believe.
• Suffer from conditions nurses feel could be better cared for in other units or specialized hospitals.
• Take up more time and attention than is deemed warranted.
• Are complaintive, uncooperative, or argumentative.
• Have severe complications, poor prognoses, or difficult diagnoses.
• Require extensive explanations, reassurance, or encouragement.
• Are of low social value.

- Are of low moral worth.
- Have unchosen stigmata (such as sexual orientation, gender, race, or ethnicity).
- Have "own fault" diagnosis (such as alcoholism or lung cancer from heavy smoking).
- Have fear-causing conditions (such as highly contagious or incurable diseases; violent tendencies).
- Engender feelings of incompetence in nurses (have conditions about which nurses know little).

Nurses' Reactions to Unpopular Clients

Nurses feel:
- Frustrated and impatient with "grumblers and moaners."
- Afraid of being trapped or "caught" by complainers.
- Irritated that unpopular clients waste their time.
- Incompetent to provide the necessary care for complicated cases and psychiatric clients.
- Relief when "unmanageables" are transferred.
- Dissatisfaction with their jobs.
- Changes in their health (such as insomnia or anorexia).

Nurses act by:
- Ignoring or avoiding demanding clients.
- Indicating to demanding clients that others need their attention more.
- Labeling demanding clients as nuisances or hypochondriacs.
- Showing reluctance to provide necessary care if clients are thought to be inappropriate.
- Scolding and reprimanding.
- Administering tranquilizers and sedatives to control their behavior.
- Recommending transfer and discharge.
- Requesting psychiatric consultation to manage unruly behavior.
- Extending minimally adequate care.
- Withdrawing from peers.
- Becoming critical of the profession or the institution.
- Withholding pain medication.
- Ignoring clients' lights or call bells.
- Being cool, detached, and insensitive.
- Feeling guilty.

This evidence suggests that nurses and other health professionals have definite ideas of what is acceptable client behavior and what is not. Look at the list you prepared earlier of client characteristics you dislike. How does it compare to the findings from the literature?

In contrast to unpopular clients, popular clients were found to have the following characteristics (Stockwell, 1972; Lorber, 1975). They:
- Were able to converse readily with nurses.
- Knew the nurses' names.
- Were able to joke and laugh with the nurses.

- Were determined to get well again.
- Were cooperative and compliant with therapeutic regimen.
- Were manageable by routine methods.
- Rarely complained of pain or discomfort.
- Minimized the trouble they caused staff by their extraordinary coopera-
  tiveness.

Nurses demonstrated the following reactions to popular clients:

- Enjoyed interacting with clients who were "fun," had a good sense of
  humor, were easy to get along with. and friendly.
- Gave superior care and did more for the popular client in the long run.
- Treated them more leniently.
- Gave them special favors and readily filled ordinary requests.

Look again at your list of appealing client characteristics and compare your reactions to these findings from the literature.

We would all agree that each one of our clients deserves to receive
courteous care regardless of cultural background, chronicity of illness,
personality, and type of illness (including the extent of complications). Is
it not shocking to discover that despite the emphasis on compassion in
our nursing education, we are unable to consistently extend respectful
nursing care to all our clients? It is not humanly possible to like all our
clients. However, it is a professional expectation and responsibility that
we treat each client with courtesy, and provide care that meets standards
for nursing practice, regardless of whether or not we like our client.

To ignore or convey dislike to our clients is antithetic to the policy of
nurturing a therapeutic helping relationship with them. When we show
our dislike to clients, they feel unsupported. The message we convey is
that they are unimportant and that we do not care about them or their
problems. By extending our compassion, administering effective nursing
interventions, and minimizing evidence of our dislike we can be influential in eliminating some of the client behaviors we find problematic.

How to Overcome Negative Attitudes and Antagonistic Behavior Towards Unpopular Clients

You entered nursing so that you could be helpful to others. It is highly
likely that you still hope to achieve that goal. Once you are aware of
when you are less than helpful to clients you consider to be unpopular,
you are in a position to change such behavior. One effective approach is to
try to perceive things from your client's point of view. As trite as this
sounds, it is difficult to do. Our dislikes and biases blind us from considering things from the client's point of view. The approach suggested here
is designed to shift your attitude and help you move to a more adaptive,
less negative view of your client. Changing your attitude will not automatically change your nursing behavior, but the pause to view your client differently will jog your compassion and your desire to show consideration for your clients instead of dishonorable disrespect.

These examples will help illustrate how to achieve this empathic perspective:

Situation One:

Mrs. White is a 48-year-old accountant who has been diabetic since age 17. In the past 3 years she has been hospitalized for circulatory damage to her feet, resulting in amputation of two toes from both feet. She claims that she does not have time for adequate foot care as she is working long hours and is on her feet all day. On this admission she has several lesions on the remaining toes on both feet. If special skin care treatments are ineffective, Mrs. White faces the possibility of further amputations.

Your Possible Negative Attitude and Behavior

Your reaction to Mrs. White's predicament is one of disapproval. You think she is wasting valuable health care resources by occupying a hospital bed when she could have avoided the skin breakdown by a few extra minutes of attention to her feet each day. Taking better care of herself would have meant she would be out in the community leading a productive life instead of taking up expensive nursing services that others need. You resent her being on your unit and find yourself taking your time to answer her call bell, and leaving her alone for long periods. In the back of your mind you think that if she finds her hospital stay uncomfortable, she might take better precautions to avoid admission in the future.

Your awareness of how you are taking out your anger on Mrs. White by treating her disrespectfully (and possibly unsafely) is the first step in changing your behavior.

Seeing the Situation Through the Eyes of Your Client, Mrs. White

To help you change your behavior toward Mrs. White, it helps if you can see things from her point of view. Find a spot where you can think without being interrupted. Mentally put yourself in Mrs. White's position and attempt to understand how she might be thinking and feeling about being in the hospital. Your thoughts might go something like this:

> "I have to wait so long for the nurse to answer the bell. It's not like I overuse the privilege. I wish they would come sooner, especially when I need the bedpan. I feel so helpless in here; I can't do a thing for myself it seems. I'm so used to being independent. I'll do anything to get healed and get out of the hospital. The pain I'm having makes me wish I'd been more stringent about my foot care. I hope they don't have to operate. I don't know if I'd be able to walk without a walker if they remove any more toes. How could I work then?"

Taking the time to imagine how you would feel in Mrs. White's position may open up your compassion for her. Instead of focusing on her neglect, this exercise may help you to pay attention to her distress *here and now*. Your fresh empathic viewpoint may help you treat her more respectfully.

You might now respond to her call bell more quickly and extend your warmth to her. You might seek her out when you have a few extra minutes and explore her reactions to her illness and hospitalization. Instead of aggressively taking out your anger on Mrs. White, you might be more direct and confront her about her noncompliant foot care. Your problem-solving ability and empathic listening skills will help you to assess what prevents her from performing more rigorous skin care. From there you can help her work out a plan to overcome these blocks. By making your interventions more positive you will help her reduce her anxiety about her predicament.

It is responsible to expand your comprehension so that you see the situation from your client's perspective. This fuller vision provides you with more data to complete the nursing process. When you see both sides it is more likely that you will act assertively, taking into account not only your feelings but those of your client.

Situation Two:

Mr. Rogers is a 39-year-old client in terminal stages of cancer. Although he has only been hospitalized on your unit for the past 4 weeks, he has been in and out with exacerbations for the past year. He is weak and most care-givers are certain he will die soon. He is in isolation and requires extensive dressing changes to open areas on his legs. The ulcerated area is draining purulent matter and has a foul odor that is almost suffocating. Mr. Rogers has lost 40 pounds over the last year and is emaciated. The darkened areas under his eyes, sagging skin, and low energy level create the impression that he is barely hanging on to life with each breath he takes.

Your Possible Negative Attitude and Behavior

It is painful for you to even enter his room because you are reminded of the times when he had color in his cheeks and kept you on your toes with his engaging sense of humor. You miss his former self and feel saddened about his impending death. You are distressed because you gag and feel nauseated when you change his dressings. When you gown up and go into his room to administer his care you feel trapped. You are at a loss for what to say and you just want to get your physical nursing care done so that you can leave. You work at top speed and leave as soon as his dressings are done.

Seeing the Situation Through the Eyes of Your Client, Mr. Rogers

Find the time and place to quietly contemplate about how Mr. Rogers thinks and feels. Try to imagine things from his perspective. Your thoughts might go something like this:

> "I'm ready to go. I wish I could just die soon. I'm so uncomfortable, I can't sleep, and I'm bored when I'm awake. I'd really like some company. I must be a sight to look at, though. No wonder everyone looks shocked when they see me. It's lonely waiting."

Taking the opportunity to try to imagine how Mr. Rogers is reacting generates several ways you could intervene to be more helpful. This exercise in empathy helps you to focus on how he is *here and now* as opposed to emphasizing how he *used to be*.

Even though Mr. Rogers does not have much energy to talk, you could arrange to spend time in his room and read to him, or arrange for some music he likes. He might be comforted by a back rub. Reading the paper to him, writing letters for him, or updating him on events are some activities that require minimal energy from him, yet allow him contact with you. Ensuring that his analgesics are administered consistently so that he is pain-free, and reminding him to change his position frequently in the bed, are measures that will increase his ability to relax.

Deodorizing the room frequently would make the environment more pleasant for him, his visitors, and staff. To help you manage through the dressing changes you could wear a mask and increase all the positive stimuli that you can think of (music on, flowers within view, open window). It might help distract your attention from the unpleasant odor if you can start telling him a story when you are doing a dressing change. The activity would keep your mind focused on something more positive.

It is assertive to consider the situation from your client's point of view as well as your own. If we only concentrate on the negative aspects we are likely to act aggressively and only attempt to achieve our own goals. It is responsible to see things from the client's viewpoint so that we generate plans that consider his important perspective. All our clients have the right to feel cared for.

PRACTICING COMMUNICATING ASSERTIVELY AND RESPONSIBLY WITH UNPOPULAR CLIENTS

Exercise 1. Below are six situations depicting unpopular clients. Possible reactions that you might have to these "problem" clients are suggested. Your task is to put yourself in the clients' places and imagine what the situation feels like from their perspective. Then your task is to indicate how these insights would free you to interact in a more caring way with your clients. Be sure that your new approaches are assertive and responsible.

A. A 73-year-old foreign client refuses to eat his hospital food. He is on a special diet and it is important that he ingest only what the nutritionist and physician have ordered. His wife brings him food that is rich in spices and sauces. Both the client and his wife complain when the ethnic food is withdrawn and hospital food is the only choice.

You feel furious that this client is unwilling to abide by the good judgment of the physician and nutritionist. You feel disdain that he has abused his body for so many years, and are amazed that he will not take advantage of the good advice being offered by his caretakers. You avoid eye contact with this client, not speaking to his wife and spending little time with him. You curtly order him to eat the hospital diet when you deliver his meal tray and you make a point of picking up his tray so that you can check how much he ate. When his intake has been less than adequate, you tell him you will not remove his tray until he has eaten more.

- Put yourself in this client's place and imagine what things are like from his perspective.
- With your new insight, how would you act assertively and responsibly towards your client?

B. Betty is a 16-year-old girl on your orthopedic unit. She has been in traction for 2 months after a car accident and has multiple fractures and burns. Her parents' home is over 100 miles away and they only visit Betty every third weekend. Betty is terribly homesick and cries for hours after her parents leave. She hates being in traction and just wants to go home. She is withdrawn and refuses to do any of the occupational therapy projects her therapist provides. She does not encourage any interaction with the other two teenagers on the unit, despite their extensive efforts to divert her attention away from her unhappy situation. With the nursing and physical therapy staff she is curt and stoic, doing the minimum of what is required of her.

You have been Betty's nurse since her admission to the unit. At first you were enthusiastic that you could cheer her up and encourage her to make the best of her situation. When she did not respond positively to your efforts and continued to be morose about being on the unit, you started to withdraw from her. Your once vivacious conversation has become almost nonexistent, and you find yourself talking to the other clients or nurses in the room instead of Betty. When you have a few spare minutes you refrain from spending them with Betty. After her parents leave one night you scold her for "acting like a baby" when you find her crying.

- Put yourself in this client's place and imagine what things are like from her perspective.
- With your new insight, how would you act assertively and responsibly towards Betty?

C. Miss Kerns is a 47-year-old school teacher who was transferred to your medical unit from the psychiatric unit upstairs. Over the past 2 years she has been admitted to psychiatry for bouts of depression of unknown origin. Many modalities (medication, psychotherapy, physical therapies) have been employed without success to treat her depression. She is on your unit for investigation of medical reasons for her low moods. She looks sullen and poorly groomed and mopes around in a house coat instead of getting dressed. She rarely volunteers to speak to any of the staff, and when you initiate a conversation it is a tense situation, because she is slow to respond and often just nods or sighs.

After some time you begin to realize that you have invested little time in getting to know Miss Kerns. You have expended almost no effort finding out about her likes, dislikes and reaction to being in the hospital. It becomes apparent that you are ignoring her because she is not easy to talk to and because you believe she does not belong on the unit. You are a bit frightened of her flattened affect, and the thought that she might be malingering bothers you.

- Put yourself in this client's place and imagine what things are like from her perspective.
- With your new insight, how would you act assertively and responsibly toward Miss Kerns?

D. Mr. Dirk is a 79-year-old client who has just undergone successful cataract surgery. He has been assured that the surgical procedure and immediate postoperative period have passed without complications. Nevertheless, he rings his bell at least every 15 minutes. Most often he only wants to be reassured or have contact with another person. He will ask: "Am I going to be able to see? Has my landlord called? I'm worried about my dog. Could you turn down the radio just a touch?" When his bell has not been answered promptly enough for his liking Mr. Dirk has called out until someone has heard him. He has asked his roommate to go and find you and urge you to come to his room immediately.

Mr. Dirk's demanding behavior is irritating you. You are annoyed that he will not be patient enough to wait until you are free to attend to him. You are adamant that he must understand how busy you are with clients who have undergone major surgery and need your care and attention. Today you told him that he should consider himself lucky to be doing so well, and that your services were needed by much sicker people.

- Put yourself in this client's place and imagine what things are like from his perspective.
- With your new insight, how would you act assertively and responsibly toward Mr. Dirk?

E. Mrs. Pews delivered a healthy 6-pound boy 3 days ago. Although she is an experienced mother (she has a 12-year-old son and an 11-year-old daughter), she acts otherwise. She asks you to supervise every activity she does with her son, such as changing his diaper, situating him on the breast, burping him, and bathing him. Every time you enter her room she questions you about how to do things right for her new baby.

You are feeling burdened and pressed by her constant demands. The attention you give her only temporarily alleviates her anxiety, and you feel like you will never be free from her demands. Now, when she rings her bell, you ask your co-worker to answer it for you. When you are "caught" and cannot avoid her, you find yourself being sharp with her to avoid being barraged.

- Put yourself in Mrs. Pews' place and imagine what things are like from her perspective.
- With your new insight, how would you act assertively and responsibly towards her?

F. A 42-year-old man has been admitted to the emergency ward after taking an overdose of pills. This suicide attempt is his third in the past 3 months. He and his wife separated 6 months ago, and he was left with the responsibility of raising their two teenage sons.

You are shocked that a father with this task could be so selfish and irresponsible. You feel resentful that he is using up costly emergency health services when he should be at home. Your first reaction to his arrival is "Not him again!" You have an urge to tell him that he needs to stop feeling sorry for himself and get on with taking care of his boys. Your anger towards him is smoldering, and at the same time you are uncertain about what to say or how to approach him. Deep down you are frightened by his self-destructiveness.

- Put yourself in this man's place and imagine what things are like from his perspective.
- With your new insight, how would you act assertively and responsibly towards him?

After you have done this exercise by yourself, get together with your colleagues in your class and compare your approaches. What similarities and differences were there in your ideas about how the client in each example viewed things? Check the congruency and diversity of the suggestions you all made for changing your nursing behavior in each of the vignettes.

Exercise 2. Think of a client you are now nursing whom you consider to be unpopular or problematic. Make note of the specific aspects of his behavior which are annoying you. Elaborate on how this client makes you feel and react. Then try to imagine how your client is viewing things. Take time to discover his point of view. Next, think about how your insight can help generate more positive approaches to your unpopular client. After you have done this exercise on your own, share your creative approaches with your colleagues.

Lastly, carry out your more responsible and assertive plan with your client. Note how you feel and how your client reacts to your new approach. Compare experiences with your co-students.

REFERENCES

Gerrard, B. (1978). *Interpersonal skills for health professionals: A review of the literature.* Unpublished manuscript. McMaster University, Hamilton, Ontario, Canada.

Kus, R.F. (1990). Nurses and unpopular clients. In J.C. McCloskey & H.K. Grace (Eds.), *Current issues in nursing* (pp. 554-558). St. Louis: Mosby–Year Book.

Lorber, J. (1975). Good patients and problem patients: conformity and deviance in a general hospital. *Journal of Health and Social Behavior,* 16 (2), pp. 213-225.

Stockwell, F. (1984). *The unpopular patient.* London: Royal College of Nursing. White Friars Press Ltd. (Republished in 1984 by Groom Helm Limited, London.)

SUGGESTIONS FOR FURTHER READING

Barnes, K.E. (1990). An examination of nurses' feelings about patients with specific feeding needs. *Journal of Advanced Nursing, 15* (6), 703-711.

Beebe, L.H. (1990). Reframe your outlook on recidivism. *Journal of Psychosocial Nursing, 28* (9), 31-33).

Boland, B.K. (1990). Fear of AIDS in nursing staff. *Nursing Management, 21* (6), 40-44.

Carey, N., Jones, S.L., & O'Tolle, A.W. (1990). Do your feel powerless when a patient refuses medication? *Journal of Psychosocial Nursing, 28* (10), 19-25.

Clients have the right to refuse medications and this study reports the nursing responses to this behavior. This article expands nurses' understanding of common nursing reactions to medication refusal. The first step in acting differently to unpopular client behavior is to know our own reactions.

Korniewicz, D.M., O'Brien, M.E., Larson, E. (1990). Coping with AIDS and HIV. *Journal of Psychosocial Nursing, 28* (3), 14-21.

Knapp, M.L. (1980). *Essentials of nonverbal communication.* New York: Holt, Rinehart and Winston.

Chapter 5, "The effects of physical appearance and dress," and chapter 6, "The effects of body movement and posture," illustrate nonverbal behavior which conveys like and dislike.

LaClave, L.J., & Brack, G. (1989). Reframing to deal with patient resistance: Practical application. *American Journal of Psychotherapy, XLIII* (1), 68-75.

This article describes the challenges for helpers of clients who have been labelled resistant and describes the process and benefits of reframing to enhance humane ways of approaching them.

Lipkin, G.B., & Cohen, R.G. (1973). *Effective approaches to patients' behavior.* New York: Springer Publishing Company, Inc.

This concisely written nursing text has suggestions for interacting in a number of "unpopular" client situations.

McCloskey, J.C., & Grace, H.K. (Eds.) (1990). *Current issues in nursing.* St. Louis: Mosby–Year Book.

Part Eleven on *Cultural Diversity* provides readers with viewpoints on some of the cross-cultural and gender-related sources of disrespectful attitudes and behavior in nursing. Nurses will benefit from the up-to-date and forthright acknowledgment of these issues.

Myers, I.B. (1980). *Gifts differing.* Palo Alto, Calif.: Consulting Psychologists Press, Inc.

This readable, comprehensive book on personality type describes how our differences in preferences for perceiving and thinking can lead to lack of appreciation and discrimination for others with unfamiliar and different preferences. Guidelines for communicating effectively with different types are outlined.

Purtilo, R. (1990). *Health professional and patient interaction* (4th ed.). Philadelphia: W.B. Saunders Company.

Chapter 10, "Culture, bias, and discrimination," expands nurses' awareness of how cultural variation and personal bias can effect the client-nurse relationship.

CHAPTER 23

Managing Team Conflict
in Assertive and Responsible Ways

*"For souls in growth, great quarrels
are great emancipators."*

Logan Pearsall Smith

OBJECTIVES

There is potential for conflict whenever two people come together. Although conflict is inevitable, it can result in advantageous outcomes. This chapter will increase your knowledge of the nature of conflict and help you develop a positive attitude towards it. You will gain proficiency in handling conflict in assertive and responsible ways through the examples and exercises.

WHAT IS CONFLICT?

"Conflict arises when individuals hold incompatible or seemingly incompatible ideas, interests, or values, but conflict can only occur where interdependency exists. For this reason conflict resolution is necessary to preserve and improve relationships with others as well as meet one's own needs" (Cushnie, 1988).

Cushnie (1988) identifies the following four categories of conflicts intensifying in degree of difficulty from top to bottom:

Facts:

Differences about data. These disagreements can be resolved by terminating debate and seeking information from reliable sources.

Methods:

differences about how something is done. Conflict about methods occurs when there is no absolute standard shared by all parties affected by the issue. Resolving conflicts of this kind includes acknowledging that there is more than one way to accomplish the same goal or task. A way to minimize this type of conflict is to establish criteria for method selection.

Goals:

Differences about desired outcomes. Discussion often reveals that parties share a common concern. If they are able to identify a common goal, this redefinition opens up new opportunities for problem solving.

Values:

Differences in belief systems are the most complex type of conflict, requiring a high level of motivation from involved parties to understand each others' beliefs. If parties can avoid the divisiveness of allocating the other's viewpoint to rigid categories of "right" or "wrong" and find compatible goals, they are on their way to conflict management (Cushnie, 1988, p. 734).

There are several forms of conflict (Kinder, 1981):

- **Intrapersonal conflict** occurs within an individual
- **Interpersonal conflict** occurs between two individuals or among members of a group
- **Intragroup conflict** occurs within an established group
- **Intergroup conflict** is the struggle between groups

The focus of this chapter is on interpersonal conflict in the context of a workplace or school setting.

Health-care teams are composed of people with many different backgrounds. A variety of professional outlooks are found in a team of nurses, physicians, clergy, nutritionists, occupational and physical therapists, social workers, and others. In addition to the differences in socialization that these professionals bring, they carry personal views based on sex, age, cultural origins, socioeconomic situations, and life experience. This potpourri is a potential source of conflict on any health care team.

This variety gives birth to different perceptions about an issue, and the role and obligations each should fulfill. When team members do not see eye-to-eye about the situation or their respective roles, then the potential for conflict is great.

Many times team members have different (or opposing) ideological views on a situation. Their views may come from having different objectives or from endorsing different priorities among the objectives. Conflict results when team members do not agree on what to do, how to do it, and when to do it.

Occasionally conflict will resurface between team members who have had a long history of conflict. The degree of trust and collaboration has been worn down between these people, and their competitiveness is sharpened. Such a situation fuels conflict.

CONFLICT RESOLUTION

You know you cannot avoid conflict. What you can avoid is feeling impotent or uncomfortable when you encounter conflict situations. By now you are familiar with assertiveness and responsibleness. These approaches will help you resolve conflicts in constructive ways.

Resolving a conflict means acting in a way so that an agreement is reached that is acceptable, and even pleasing, to both parties. If both parties cannot agree on a resolution, the conflict will continue. When conflict drags out and team members do not see a hopeful resolution on the horizon, then helplessness prevails. Any health care team that is stuck in this hopeless situation is not working at its full capacity. Client care and morale suffer when conflicts are unresolved.

There are three ways you can approach conflict resolution; one of these approaches is constructive and two are destructive.

The win-win approach to conflict resolution requires you to be assertive and responsible. This approach results in a solution with which you and your colleague(s) are happy. Not only is the outcome satisfactory, but using a win-win approach employs your full creativity and often results in a unique and innovative resolution.

The lose-win approach is one where you allow your colleague(s) to resolve the conflict at your expense. Either you are not happy with the outcome or you permit your colleague(s) to walk all over you. This approach is unassertive and nonresponsible.

The win-lose approach is the opposite of the lose-win approach. You may resolve the conflict in a way satisfying to you, but in the process you bulldoze right over the rights of your colleague(s). This approach is aggressive and nonresponsible.

Any win-lose/lose-win approach creates forces that aggravate the struggle and do little to discover constructive solutions acceptable to all involved (Likert & Likert, 1976). Conflicts have destructive consequences if the participants are dissatisfied with the outcome and feel they have lost (Deutsch, 1973).

A conflict is more constructive when the outcomes are satisfying to all the participants than if it is satisfying only to some. Because conflict is inevitable, it helps to know how to use it as an opportunity to be constructive—because the alternatives have unpleasant consequences.

A win-win conflict management strategy involves covering each of these steps:

1. See the problem in terms of needs (what is required) instead of solutions (what should be done) in order to facilitate a mutual problem solving approach, detach yourself from biases, and stay focused on the actual data.
2. Consider the problem as a **mutual** one to be solved, requiring the active involvement of all affected (not a passive or excluding involvement, as in a lose-win or win-lose struggle).
3. Describe the conflict as specifically as possible, using undistorted data.
4. Identify the differences between concerned parties before attempting to resolve the conflict.
5. See the conflict from the other person's point of view.

6. Use brainstorming to arrive at possible solutions instead of using the first or most convenient idea.
7. Select the solution that best meets both parties' needs and all possible consequences.
8. Reach an agreement about how the conflict is to end and not recur.
9. Plan who will do what and where and when it will be done.
10. After the plan has been implemented, evaluate the problem-solving process and review how well the solution turned out (ANA, 1990).

Table 23-1 summarizes three different approaches to conflict. The assertive/responsible attitude toward conflict and approach to conflict resolution is contrasted with the nonassertive/nonresponsible approaches.

Assertive and Responsible Ways to Overcome Conflict

On health care teams conflict can involve all members or a few. How to manage conflict using a win-win approach in both these instances is explored.

A Conflict Situation Involving the Whole Health Care Team

1. Before you can do anything to resolve a conflict you need to fully understand the conflict, including your thoughts and feelings about the situation, as well as the thoughts of your colleagues. If you try to resolve a conflict without completing an assessment you will probably overlook some important factor that could result in an unsatisfactory resolution.

Example: You believe that clients have the right to be informed about any untoward side-effects they might experience when taking a prescribed medication. On your unit few clients are told in advance of the potential side-effects. This omission is incompatible with your beliefs about good nursing care and client rights. You discover that many of your colleagues, the other nurses and physicians on your team, prefer to keep knowledge of side-effects from clients so that they will be more likely to comply with taking the medication. Here the conflict is incompatible activities (informing/not informing) and beliefs (autonomy/dependency) about clients' rights.

2. To fully understand your side of the conflict, you need to take time to examine your thoughts and feelings. You cannot complete this step in a hurry. You need to sit down (with paper and pencil if you need it) and discover your answers to the following questions:

What Is It about This Conflict That Bothers Me?

In thinking about the conflict you might have some of the following thoughts:

"It bothers me that clients are not warned about side-effects they might get from the medications."

Table 23-1 ASSERTIVE/RESPONSIBLE VERSUS NONASSERTIVE/NONRESPONSIBLE WAYS OF HANDLING TEAM CONFLICT

Characteristic	Win-win	Lose-win	Win-lose
Attitude Toward Conflict	Assumes conflict is inevitable and occurs whenever people work together Assumes conflict can be managed so that creative solutions are achieved Assumes controversy involves everyone in the issue and increases members' commitment Assumes conflict can be resolved in ways that are satisfying to all team members	Assumes conflicts are sent to try us Assumes in a conflict the other person always wins Assumes it's a foregone conclusion that the plan to resolve the conflict will satisfy only others Wonders why there must be conflict in every workplace	Sees conflict as a challenge to be won Considers manipulation needed to win Conflicts are never ceasing and thinks fighting is required to get what you want Feels the other guy is trying his best to win
Approach to Conflict Resolution	Employs a systematic problem-solving approach	Decides in advance that the other person will win and gives up	Keeps fighting with biased information that supports own viewpoint
Data Collection	Examines own thoughts and feelings objectively Listens empathically to colleagues' point of view	Prematurely closes data collection Assumes it is hopeless to collect data because of irrational belief that others	Only seeks, examines, and submits data that supports own desired resolution

	Seeks relevant information from appropriate resources (literature, consultants) Shares knowledge of conflict with all others involved Does not make inferences in data collection phase Remains objective	will win regardless Dwells on how bad things will be when the conflict is resolved in her "opponent's" favor Passively participates in information sharing	
Assessment	Formulates an accurate definition of the conflict Shares her assessment with colleagues Acknowledges colleagues' perceptions of the conflict	Defines conflict in terms of how it affects her colleagues Gives up defining the conflict from her point of view	Does not seek out colleagues' assessment of the conflict Overwhelmingly argues her assessment of the conflict
Resolution Generating	Considers resolutions that satisfy all involved Chooses resolutions which maximize the benefits and minimize the drawbacks	Contributes little to this planning because she assumes she will be told what to do by the winner	Only considers or supports plans that agree with her interpretation of the conflict Sabotages plans that oppose her view
Evaluation	Maintains vigilance to ensure that resolution continues to satisfy herself and colleagues on the team	Complains that she knew the resolution would never be successful; is disgruntled	Ignores the fact that others are not satisfied with the resolution

"It's not right that they don't have full knowledge of the treatment, and that they are choosing to take the pills without fully understanding the implications."

"I feel that it is dishonest to withhold information about side-effects from clients."

"I believe that people have the responsibility to decide what they should do about their health. By withholding information we are keeping the control of clients' health in our hands."

Answering this question makes it clearer what the conflict means to you. You have a strong value that clients should be given the information they need to make the best decision about what health behavior to adopt.

Our initial reaction to a conflict situation is often influenced more by emotion than intellect. The tension or anxiety creates a "fight or flight" stress response, and the intensity of the stress response varies in relation to the degree of threat perceived (Cushnie, 1988). Taking time to sort out your emotional reactions as you just did helps to control your emotions and facilitate your effectiveness in conflict management.

What Would Be a Satisfactory Resolution to This Conflict for Me?

In thinking about how you would like to have the conflict resolved you come up with the following idea:

"The most satisfactory resolution for me would be to institute a policy that all clients will be informed in advance about any possible side-effects of any medication prescribed for them."

It is important to answer this question. Often we know there is a conflict but we are uncertain about how we want it resolved. The clearer you can be in answering these questions, the more articulate you will be to others about your stand on the issue.

3. Discover what your colleagues' responses are to the same two questions you just answered yourself. This step requires you to invest time and energy, but you need this information to have a complete understanding of the conflict. The best approach is to arrange a time to sit down with your colleagues and find out:

What Is It about the Conflict That Bothers Them?

Your colleagues may come up with some of the following ideas:

"If we told every client about possible side-effects it would take too much time."

"If clients knew all the possible side-effects, they might not take the medications and then they'd never benefit from them."

"I believe that we should not scare clients by telling them everything that can go wrong. After all, they're already sick. Why add to their worries?"

You are learning that your colleagues have their clients' interests at heart when they avoid telling them about the side-effects. They have raised a significant point about the time factor as well. Discovering alternative viewpoints will expand your awareness of conflict you encounter.

What Is a Satisfactory Resolution to the Conflict for Your Colleagues?

These are some examples of what your colleagues might tell you:

> "The only solution I can see is to tell only those clients who ask about the side-effects."

> "I think we should only give out information about the most common and significant side-effects so that clients will be inclined to take their medication."

> "I think we should continue as usual. I've never known any client who was upset about not knowing the side-effects of the medications. They need the medications to get well again."

These suggestions from your colleagues tell you that they value something more than client autonomy: they value compliance and recovery from illness. You have learned that some of your colleagues are agreeable to informing clients about side-effects under certain circumstances.

Finding the answers to these questions will take your best interpersonal communication skills. When you are invested in an issue it becomes harder to see other points of view. In a conflict situation it is important to listen actively to what your colleagues have to say and check out that you have understood their side of the issue.

4. In addition to information obtained from the thoughts and feelings of the people involved in the conflict, you may need information from other sources. In this example you could seek the counsel of the hospital's legal advisor about the rights of your clients. There may be a Clients' Rights Committee which could advise you.

For example, your legal counsel may advise you that:

> "Clients have the right by law to be informed of any likely untoward effects of any treatment regimen, unless such information would be considered by the care-givers to be threatening to the client's well-being."

A guideline like this is sufficiently nonspecific that your health care team would have to make its own interpretation of its application.

5. Once you have fully explored how you and your colleagues feel about the conflict, and acquired any other relevant information, the next step is to search for a resolution that will be satisfactory to all of you. This is no easy feat; the win-win approach takes time and effort.

One creative approach at this stage is to brainstorm ideas. Out of brainstorming is likely to come a creative and original resolution to your conflict (D'Zurilla & Goldfried, 1971). It is important that everyone involved in the conflict situation have an opportunity to contribute ideas about how to resolve it. In this example there should be representation from nurses, physicians, and clients.

In the brainstorming process it is important that every idea be considered, and that no ideas are ridiculed or deleted. Using this rule means that team members must acknowledge and respect each other's ideas. This action of listening to one other will help to diffuse any hostility that may have arisen as the conflict grew. In a conflict situation competitiveness often reigns, with individuals wanting to get their own way; brainstorming ensures that team members communicate in a cooperative way.

In this situation the following suggestions for resolution of the conflict were put forward:

- Give information about side-effects only to clients who ask for it.
- Before any client starts on a medication he must be able to recite its benefits and side-effects.
- Leave a copy of the drug description manual in the clients' common room so that any who wish to check on the side-effects can do so.
- Give clients copies of the telephone numbers of the pharmaceutical companies so that they can call a representative and find out any information about drugs that are prescribed for them.
- Have the pharmacist prepare information sheets about the side-effects of clients' drugs that would be available for them to keep and review.
- Give a card to every client when he is admitted to the unit that advises him that he has the right to know the side-effects of treatments and medications and only needs to ask the staff to receive this information.
- Wait until clients experience side-effects and then clearly explain them to the clients.
- Nurses and physicians should initiate a policy of inviting questions from clients about the side-effects of a medication when they are started on it.

You can see that the suggestions represent a variety of points of view.
6. The next step is to choose an acceptable resolution from the many suggestions put forth. The most expedient action to take on this unit is to form a committee composed of staff members representing both sides of the conflict, as well as clients and administrators of the unit.

You are selected as a member who favors informed consent. Another nurse—with the point of view that informing clients can cause unnecessary problems—is also selected. The head nurse, one physician, and a representative from the Clients' Rights Committee complete the membership.

This committee has the responsibility to develop a policy about what information to give clients concerning side-effects of their medication. The decision it makes must meet certain criteria in a win-win approach to conflict resolution. It must satisfy both points of view, be feasible to carry out on the unit (in terms of cost, staffing abilities), and be legally sound.

7. The next step is to systematically review the pros and cons of the eligible resolutions remaining. At this stage team members must remain open to each others' points of view, and give all members a chance to defend or refute points. When a group is trying to reach the best decision it must create a climate that allows members to speak freely.

When the atmosphere is competitive the communication between parties is unreliable (Deutsch, 1973). Members sabotage each other by providing misleading or biased information that leads to mistrust. When the communication breaks down this way it is unlikely that the best decision will be chosen because the data base will be incomplete and inaccurate. It takes a concerted effort by members and leader to ensure that all points of view are encouraged and respected.

8. After considerable discussion the group narrowed down the choices for resolution to the following:

- Give a card to every client when he is admitted to the unit that advises him that he has the right to know the side-effects of any medications, and that he only needs to ask the staff to receive this information.
- Nurses and physicians should initiate a policy of inviting questions from clients about the side-effects of their medications at the time a client is started on a new medication.
- Before any client starts on a medication he must be able to recite its benefits and side-effects.

After much deliberation the committee decided that distributing cards for clients would be too expensive. The members came up with the idea of adding the following paragraph to the "Permission For Treatment" sheet that all clients must sign on admission:

> I am aware that all treatments, including medications, have benefits as well as potential untoward effects. I am aware that I have the right to ask my care-givers about these possible negative effects, and that I can expect to have any information explained to me in language that I am able to understand. I am aware that, if after careful consideration I refuse to comply fully with the suggested regimen (treatments and medications), this action will in no way jeopardize the care I receive by the health-care team in this hospital.
>
> Date_____Signature_____
> Witness_____

This action appealed to all members of the committee. They felt it would inform clients of their rights at the beginning of their hospital stay and instill the idea that their questions would be welcomed and answered in a clear way.

The second decision made by the committee was to endorse as unit policy the following suggestion:

- Each time a client starts on a new medication he will be informed of the benefits and untoward effects in a simple, clear way. At this time he will be invited and encouraged to ask any questions.

It took the committee much time to arrive at this decision. None of the committee members had difficulty with the suggestion of telling clients about the benefits of medications, but they were reluctant to explain the potential hazards. After looking at the issue from many angles, all members agreed that it was unfair to give only half of the picture to clients. A compromise was drawn whereby all concurred that only the most likely side-effects would be explained to clients and the probability of their occurrence would be specified. Any known corrective action would also be made known to clients (such as laxative for constipation; extra fluids and chewing gum for dryness in the mouth; avoiding abrupt movements for vertigo).

Committee members agreed that the workload for launching this new policy would be shared between physicians and nurses. Whenever a physician prescribed a new medication he would be responsible for explaining the rationale, benefits, and risks to his clients, and he would invite questions. This delegation would mean that nurses would not solely incur the extra time that implementing this policy would demand.

In addition, it was decided that the medication nurse would follow up the physician's explanation when she administered the first dosage of the medication. At that time she would find out what the client understood about the benefits and risks. She would confirm the facts, correct the errors, and invite any further questions. Sharing the responsibility between physicians and nurses made the time commitment feasible for both parties.

The committee stressed that no health professional was expected to remember the side effects of a multitude of medications. Referring to the Pharmaceutical Index and consulting with the hospital pharmacist would be encouraged.

The resolutions arrived at by the committee were satisfactory to all team members and were feasible from an administrative point of view.

8. The process does not stop at the point of agreeing on a resolution. Once the plan is implemented a follow-up evaluation must be carried out to determine if the health care team remains satisfied with the implementation of the resolution. Some questions to complete this evaluation would be:

- Do those who felt strongly that clients have a right to know about side-effects feel that clients are being correctly informed?

- Do those who objected because it could be time consuming and frightening for clients feel that the new plan avoids these negative consequences?

- Are clients of the opinion that their rights are being respected?
- Is the resolution being carried out without undue drawbacks in terms of cost-effectiveness and staffing patterns?

In this example the committee decided to meet 6 weeks after the resolution had been adopted so as to evaluate its effectiveness.

This health care team handled its conflict using a win-win conflict resolution strategy. All sides were asked to contribute their opinions in order to resolve the conflict. This action was assertive because it prevented any one side from coloring the picture or totally biasing the issue. It was responsible because it considered all the data available in the conflict situation: thoughts and feelings of both parties and objective data from a legal perspective.

A Conflict Situation Involving Two Team Members

In contrast to the situation above, conflict situations can be isolated to a small segment of the health care team. An example in which two team members are in conflict will be examined.

Example: You and Jayne are two nursing students on the same medical unit in a general hospital. You are a first-year student and Jayne is in her graduating year. You are studying the concept of loss and its effects on body image. You wish to have Mr. Jones as your client because he has recently had a severe myocardial infarction and it is unlikely that he will be able to resume his former job. Because he has suffered a loss in physical function that affects other areas of his life he would make an excellent candidate for your assignment.

Jayne has been assigned as Mr. Jones' nurse and has been nursing him for the past 3 days. When you ask Jayne if she would switch and let you take on Mr. Jones' care, Jayne refuses on the grounds that she needs to learn about postcardiac care for an assignment she is doing.

At the moment Mr. Jones is the most suitable candidate for both these students. There is a conflict over limited resources in this situation. **1.** The first step to take is to uncover all the information about the conflict. Accomplishing this task involves being open and listening actively. One technique for ensuring that you really understand the conflict from the other's point of view is to reflect empathically to each statement your colleague makes. Here is an example:

> **Jayne:** "I think we have a problem here because I need to continue my care of Mr. Jones to understand how postcardiac clients adjust to the limited activity level and cope with the fear of resuming normal functioning. I can't change with you."

At this point it would be tempting for you to justify that you too need to study Mr. Jones' recovery to understand his loss. Such a defensive approach would escalate your conflict. Instead, to understand the conflict from Jayne's point of view, all you are allowed to do at this point is to empathically reflect her thoughts and feelings. You will soon get your turn to state things from your point of view.

> **You:** "You want to continue nursing Mr. Jones for a longer period of time so that you will really understand the reaction of postcardiac patients to changes in their activity levels."

This response allows your colleague to feel understood and encourages her to reveal more of her point of view.

> **Jayne:** "This is one of my last assignments before I graduate and I'm afraid if I give up Mr. Jones now I would not find another post-cardiac client on whom to do my assignment."

> **You:** "I can see why you do not wish to switch with me. You're concerned that Mr. Jones may turn out to be the last client with postcardiac regimen who you encounter before graduation, and you need this experience."

Besides allowing Jayne to feel understood, reflecting empathically obliges you to fully understand the conflict from her point of view. Without this information you could not come up with the most effective resolution.

You are entitled to describe the conflict from your point of view, and you therefore explain to Jayne the importance of Mr. Jones to your own client assignment. You have no control over whether Jayne will listen empathically to your side of the conflict, but your previous active listening will augment the chances.

2. Once you understand the conflict the next step is to work out a satisfactory resolution. The resolution most acceptable to both you and Jayne (to have Mr. Jones as sole client) is mutually incompatible. You need to generate another suitable resolution. Unlike the first example, there is limited time in which to do so. You propose the following suggestions to Jayne:

- When she is off you will take over as the nurse in charge of Mr. Jones' care.
- You offer to share with her any information you have on loss, as it applies to the postcardiac client, in return for being able to ask her questions about Mr. Jones' adjustment.

Jayne accepts your suggestions and offers the following ones that might be helpful to you:

- You can be present when she is talking to Mr. Jones (if he agrees) so that you can apply some of what she gleans to your study of the concepts of loss and body image.
- She informs you about Mrs. Tenn, a diabetic client on the unit, who is upset that her diabetes prevents her from becoming pregnant again. Jayne suggests that Mrs. Tenn might make a suitable client for your study of loss.
- She offers you a copy of her paper when it is completed, since your topics overlap and you might find it helpful.

This brainstorming has generated several possible resolutions that have benefits for both of you. If you and Jayne adopt all the suggestions, both of you will gain more than you could have if you each went your separate ways. In addition to achieving your learning goals, you both will have the opportunity to learn from each other and possibly develop a closer collegiality.

3. After adopting any resolution to a conflict, it is important to check to see if the plan continues to meet your expectations. The bottom line in this situation is that both you and Jayne complete your assignments. Any additional happenings will be bonuses.

You can see that two of the important processes in effective conflict resolution are empathy and problem-solving. Ensuring that these two strategies are influential in your conflict resolution approach ensures that you will be assertive and responsible.

CONFLICT RESOLUTION AND THE NURSING PROFESSION

Johnson (1990) points out that conflict can be a positive force for nursing if it is used to foster growth-producing change in the profession and in the organizations where nurses work. But she cautions that nurses must know how to use conflict effectively if these benefits are to be realized. In addition to being knowledgeable about managing conflicts, nurses must develop a positive attitude toward conflict by recognizing the potential gains to be realized from conflict (p. 510). Nurses need to become more astute at predicting potential conflicts.

Shifts in power are taking place in the health care system that will be accompanied by more options for conflict resolution. The history of a power differential between nursing and medicine has made it difficult for collaboration to be used as an effective conflict management tool, as collaboration rarely works well where there is a wide difference in power between the groups involved. Johnson advises nursing as a discipline to be concerned about empowering all nurses in the work setting in preparation for handling workplace conflicts.

PRACTICING RESOLVING CONFLICTS

Exercise 1. Work in threes for this exercise. One acts as "pro" and one "con" the issue; the third person acts as coach. You will be presented with a conflict situation and it is the task of "pro" and "con" to resolve the conflict in an assertive and responsible way. The coach will help "pro" and "con" to resolve the issue using the win-win approach.

Guidelines for "Pro" and "Con":

1. Use a systematic problem-solving approach to the conflict you are attempting to resolve.
2. In the data collection phase remember to delve into your own, as well as each others', thoughts and feelings about the conflict.

3. In the resolution-generating phase remember to allow as many suggestions to surface as possible before you make your final decision.
4. The resolution you choose must be one agreeable to both. "Pro" and "con" must agree that the resolution satisfies both parties.
5. For the purposes of this exercise you must follow one additional rule: Whenever your colleague speaks you must empathically reflect what she has said so that she will know you fully understand her point of view.

Guidelines for the Coach:

1. It is your job to remind "pro" and "con" to use a win-win problem-solving approach in their attempts to resolve the conflict.
2. You have the responsibility to remind "pro" and "con" to use empathic responses with each other after each speaks. Do not let them proceed with their negotiation until the listener has used empathy to show she understands the other's position. (For instance, if "con" has just argued against "pro's" point of view, before "pro" can defend her position she must acknowledge "con's" perspective.)

   Here are three situations involving conflict. So that each of you has the opportunity to be "pro," "con," and the coach, each of you will take a different role in the three conflict situations.

Situation One: A Conflict of Methods

You are both nurses working on a medical unit in your hospital. Problem-oriented charting is employed on your unit, and you also use a Kardex system which contains identifying data about clients and the nursing care plan.

"Pro's" Position: You think your unit should do away with the Kardex system. You claim that the nursing care plans are never kept up to date on the Kardexes and you have to refer to the chart to get the most accurate information on the client.

"Con's" Position: You think it is important to keep the Kardexes. They are a handy reference for obtaining an update of the client's situation. Kardexes are especially useful for relief staff or staff returning from days off. You believe that it would be inconvenient to have to refer to the chart each time you wanted to check a client's care plan. Furthermore, the charts are often unavailable because they are being used by other personnel.

Situation Two: A Conflict of Values Compounded by Limited Resources

You are two members of the Awards Selection Committee for your school of nursing. You have one task remaining: to select the student nurse in your class who has demonstrated the best clinical nursing practice. You have narrowed the choice down to two candidates; however, there is only one prize for this category and you must agree on one student nurse.

"Pro's" Position: You believe the prize should go to Ms. James because she has consistently demonstrated excellent charting and made useful suggestions about the management of her clients' care at case conferences. She is motivated to encourage her clients and she has given them consistently courteous, caring nursing.

"Con's" Position: You disagree with your colleague's choice and would like to see this prize awarded to Ms. Timms, who you feel has gone beyond the call of duty in her nursing care. She has helped clients write letters and has spent time supporting family members of her clients. She is highly regarded by the nurses on the units for her ability to work in a cooperative manner.

Situation Three: A Conflict of Goals

You work on a surgical unit in your hospital. There is a movement afoot to allow clients to read their own charts. All staff on your unit have been asked to put forth their views on this proposed policy. You and your colleague have opposing opinions.

"Pro's" Position: You have a strong belief that clients should be permitted to see anything written on their charts. You are convinced that the chart is really the property of the client; after all, it is *his* health that is being charted about. You would like to have access to your chart if you were a client.

"Con's" Position: You think it is absolutely unreasonable that clients should have access to their charts. You think it would lead to all kinds of problems. For one thing, clients would not comprehend the medical jargon and might misinterpret information in their charts. Considerable time would be wasted trying to write in a way that clients would understand. In your view nurses and physicians are the experts and clients should have some faith that they will create an accurate document of their care.

Debriefing Questions

1. What was the most difficult aspect of using the win-win conflict resolution approach?
2. What benefits are there to the win-win approach to resolving conflicts?

Exercise 2. The whole class can participate in this exercise. The goal of this exercise is to resolve a conflict which involves the whole health care team.

Your psychiatric unit has been asked to participate in an investigation to study the effects of a newly developed antidepressant. This mood-elevating drug is not yet available on the market because it requires the final phase of testing with human subjects. Your unit has been asked to participate in a study in which half of the depressed clients will be given this new experimental drug and the others will receive a placebo. Researchers will document the effects (benefits and untoward reactions) of the drugs on your client population. Your health care team must decide today if it will agree to participate in this study.

Six volunteers are needed to roleplay the following positions on the health care team:

Head Nurse: is totally against doing research on human subjects. She is adamant that the clients on her unit should not be requested to participate in this study. "We are in the business to help people, not experiment on them. Our credibility in the eyes of our consumers will be in question if we get involved in this experiment."

Physician: is all for research. "The only way to achieve new frontiers of excellence in client care is through research."

Staff Nurse 1: is dubious about asking clients to participate in research. "When people are depressed they cannot make the best informed decisions. They might think they have to volunteer in order to get good health care from us."

Staff Nurse 2: supports research in psychiatry and believes your unit should set an example by completing this study. "Wonderful cures have come from clinical research. Psychiatric research has taken a back seat too long to medical research."

Occupational Therapist: sees so many immobilized depressed clients who take so long to recover from depression that she welcomes any research that might discover more effective treatment for depression. "We should try anything that will help our depressed clients."

Social Worker: is dubious about putting the clients and their families under one more stress at an already stressful time. "We don't know if this new drug will do any good, and it might do harm. Why should our clients and their families have that possibility to worry about?"

This team has opposing points of view about whether to engage in the drug research. This controversy represents a conflict of values.

The task of the team is to resolve the conflict using the win-win approach. As a team you must use the problem-solving approach and each member must attempt to be assertive in her negotiations.

The rest of the class will observe the team in its deliberations and be prepared to make comments on their conflict resolution procedure.

The team will take 30 to 40 minutes to complete its resolution.

These questions will help you debrief after the exercise:

1. What factors enhanced the team's ability to use a win-win approach to resolve this conflict?
2. What factors made it difficult for the team to use an assertive and responsible approach to resolving this conflict?
3. Was the team able to decide on a resolution that was satisfactory to all team members?
4. If the team did not get to the point of resolving the conflict in the 40

minutes of the roleplay, how would you rate its progress in terms of assertiveness and responsibleness?

If you would like more practice attempting to resolve conflicts that involve the whole team, use the following situations (or develop your own) and take different roles and points of view on the issue.

Situation One:

There is a 48-year-old married man on your unit who has been diagnosed with terminal cancer. There is lack of agreement on your team about whether to inform the client that he is dying. Some members take the view that he will give up hope and become depressed if he is told he is dying. Others claim that he has a right to know his prognosis because he needs the opportunity to get his life affairs in order and say his good-byes to his wife and teenagers.

Situation Two:

Your team is undecided about whether to give a 38-year-old depressed woman on your psychiatric unit a weekend pass. She has made a successful recovery from a suicide attempt 2 weeks ago. The marital problems that were largely responsible for her suicide attempt are being worked out. Some members of the team think that she should wait a week before going home because she is still fragile. They point out that she has the energy to repeat a suicide attempt, and may be so inclined if the visit home is unsuccessful. Other team members think she should be discharged because she needs to get home to where the real problems are so that she and her husband can work on them. The added strain of her husband caring for their children and paying for babysitters when he comes in for conjoint appointments is causing too much unnecessary stress on their family.

REFERENCES

American Nurses' Association. (1990). *Survival skills in the workplace: What every nurse should know.* Kansas City, Mo., The Association.

Cohen, S., & McQuade, K. (1984). Programmed Instruction: Resolving Conflicts. *American Journal of Nursing, 84*(4), pp. 475-489.

Cushnie, P. (1988). Conflict: Developing resolution skills. *American Operating Room Nurses Journal, 47*(3), 732-742.

D'Zurilla, T., & Goldfried, M. (1971). Problem-solving and behavior modification. *Journal of Abnormal Psychology, 78,* pp. 107-126.

Johnson, M. (1990). Use of conflict as a positive force. In J.C. McClosky, & H.K. Grace, (Eds.) *Current issues in nursing,* (pp. 506-511). St. Louis: Mosby–Year Book.

Kinder, J.S. (1981). Conflict and diploma nursing education. In *Management of conflict,* National League for Nursing. New York: Publication No. 16-1859, pp. 10-23.

Likert, R. & Likert, J.G. (1976). *New ways of managing conflict.* New York: McGraw-Hill Book Company.

Muniz, P. (1981). Conflict and strategies for conflict management. In *Management of conflict,* National League for Nursing. New York: Publication No. 16-1859, pp. 1-9.

SUGGESTIONS FOR FURTHER READING

American Nurses' Association. (1990). *Survival skills in the workplace: What every nurse should know.* Kansas City, Mo., Author.

The concise chapter on learning to manage workplace conflicts challenges nurses to ask themselves how they foster a positive workplace environment. The chapter includes an excellent review of an effective problem solving process for resolving workplace conflicts, and apprises readers of the connection between change in organizations and conflict.

Arnold, E., & Boggs, K. (1989). *Interpersonal relationships: Professional communication skills for nurses.* Philadelphia: W.B. Saunders Company.

The authors offer a useful perspective on resolving conflict in the nurse-client relationship. Readers are invited to identify what aspect of nurse-client conflict is more difficult for them. This enlightment helps to understand one's reactions to conflict.

Northouse, P.G., & Northouse, L.L. (1985). *Health communication: A handbook for health professionals.* Englewood Cliffs, N.J.: Prentice-Hall, Inc.

In the chapter on "Conflict and Communication in Health Care Settings" the authors include an overview of the benefits and limitations of the most common styles of approaching interpersonal communication. The review stresses that the conflict-handling style that meets the needs of the particpants, while also fitting the demands of the situation, will be most effective in resolving conflict.

Articles

Adams, R.H., & Applegeet, C.J. (1987). Managing conflict: Techniques managers can use. *American Operating Room Nurses Journal, 46*(6), 1116-1120.

Bream, T., & Schapiro, A. (1989). Nurse-physician networks: A focus for retention. *Nursing Management, 20*(5), 74-77.

Marsden, C. (1990). Ethics of the "doctor-nurse game." *Heart & Lung, 19*(4), 422-424.

CHAPTER 24

Good-Bye
and Good Luck

"The road to wisdom?—Well, it's
plain and simple to express:
Err and err and err again
but less and less and less."

Piet Hein, *Grooks*

THE IMPORTANCE OF EFFECTIVE INTERPERSONAL COMMUNICATION

Our experience tells us that effective interpersonal communication has a positive influence on our well-being. Scientific data supports the belief that good interpersonal communication benefits clients. Gerrard (1978) reviewed the literature of the relationship between health professionals' interpersonal communication skills and client outcome indices. His findings revealed that:

• Clinicians' overall competence was judged by their interpersonal skills.
• Clinicians' good interpersonal communication skills resulted in increased client satisfaction with the health care service.
• Increased client satisfaction led to increased compliance with therapeutic regimen.

Clearly the communication component of the helping relationship is a key factor in clients' perception and evaluation of the health care services we deliver.

Hopefully, you are convinced of the importance of good interpersonal communication. The power of your conviction will be evidenced by the effectiveness of your day-to-day interactions. May you have success in communicating assertively and responsibly with your clients and colleagues.

"Deautomatizing" Ineffective Communication Habits

By actively studying this book you have advanced your cognitive, affective, and psychomotor communication abilities. Your increased knowledge of interpersonal communication has likely prompted some changes in the way you relate to your clients and colleagues. There is one more aspect of behavior we all need to change in order to improve the effectiveness of our interpersonal communication with others: *habits*.

Automatically communicating the same way whenever a situation arises in which that way of relating has become established through repeated use is a habit (Woodruff, 1961, p. 87). Meichenbaum (1977) suggested that factors such as time, mental effort, and the redundancy of social interactions cause habit to be a much more common determinant of social behavior than cognition (p. 210). He advised that if we want to change a behavior, then we must think before we act in order to "deautomatize" ineffective ways. In terms of interpersonal communication, if we think before we speak, we are more likely to avoid using a negative habit and replace it with more enlightened, therapeutic communication.

Developing Your Own Style

Now that you have tackled all three parts of this book, you have learned the basic ingredients to developing and maintaining helpful interactions with your clients and colleagues. At first you probably felt as if you were "trying out" a new way of talking to others. Your efforts to change may have felt stilted and awkward. This stage is a normal part of integrating changes in communication into your style. It is essential to develop your own style, to have a strong sense of what fits comfortably for you. If you incorporate the communication behaviors into your repertoire in a way that you feel natural, then your comfort will come through to others.

You are surrounded by role models such as your teachers and colleagues, and examples drawn from communication textbooks. You can use these references to influence the shaping of your own communication style. The process will be facilitated by noting what feels "like you," and eliminating what does not feel natural. By noticing what phrasing, timing, use of humor, nonverbal gestures, and other facets of communication satisfy you, your own style will emerge and flourish.

Others may be taken aback as you make changes to communicate more assertively and responsibly. It is wise to be prepared for their reactions, be patient with their adjustment, and persevere with your changes!

Continuing Your Development as an Effective Communicator

Expanding your understanding of interpersonal communication does not stop with finishing this book or completing an interpersonal communication skills course. "The vast store of knowledge today, and its continuing exponential growth, precludes a nurse from being an effective professional for long if he or she attempts to function only on the information acquired in school" (Schank, 1990). To continue to be an effective communicator you can expand your knowledge through additional courses, reading, and practice. Another way you can refine what you have learned, and make your knowledge more significant, is through a process of what Moch (1990) calls "personal knowing," or what Schon (1983) calls "reflection-in-action." Using yourself—your observations, feelings, and reflections—and being concerned with your inner experience when communicating can take you to a new level of understanding about interpersonal relationships with clients and colleagues.

Personal knowing is a discovery of self-and-other arrived at through reflection, synthesis of perceptions, and connection with what is known (Moch, 1990). Any encounter with a client (or colleague), or any nursing event, is an opportunity for personal knowing; but you must attempt to eliminate preconceived notions and cultivate an openess, heightened awareness, and a questioning frame of mind. "When someone reflects-in-action, he becomes a researcher in the practice context. He is not dependent on the categories of established theory and technique, but constructs a new theory of the unique case" (Schon, 1983, pp. 68-69). In this phenomenological process "knowing is not acquiring facts, but rather making meaning and giving meaning. To explain is to clarify common meanings and authenicate experiences" (Diekelmann, 1988). Using this method "knowledge is not nomologic—that is, facts, laws, theories—rather it is situational meaning" (p. 143).

Moch (1990) and Schon (1983) suggest that you can advance your knowledge of communication if you enter interpersonal situations with an attitude that seeks answers to questions like these:

• What features do I notice when I come in contact with this client? this colleague? this nursing situation?
• What am I experiencing at this moment while teaching this client? while completing this client health assessment? while presenting this case at the team conference?
• How am I framing this problem that I am trying to solve?
• What is guiding me in knowing what to do in relation to this client or colleague?
• What are the criteria by which I make this judgment?
• What awareness evolved through this nursing encounter?

There is a lot you can learn about interpersonal communication through this process of reflection-in-action. In your career there will be many puzzling, troubling, or interesting aspects of your relationships with clients and colleagues that you try to make sense of and handle. Using a process of attending you can focus on your self, the other person, and the relationship through an awareness of sensations, emotions, cognitions, and spiritual elements. While totally attending to the present experience and the present moment with a client you can evolve to new levels of knowing.

This knowledge will enhance your practice. Through your reflection you will learn something new about communicating that you can call upon and refine in the future. Personal knowing is demanded of professionals focusing on interpersonal processes while blending artistic and scientific components within practice (Moch, 1990). Two of the characteristics of an exceptional nurse are self-awareness and critical thinking (Huston, 1990). These two qualities are essential for reflecting on your interpersonal communication skill with clients and colleagues to advance your personal knowing.

Contributing to Excellence in Your Workplace

Underlining the encouragement for reflection-in-action as a way of developing personal knowing as a nurse professional is the basis of the argument Curtin (1990) put forth: "Neither competence nor compassion is learned from a book. They are behaviors—characteristics of professional practice—which are demonstrated rather than taught. One sees them in action and chooses to (or not to) adopt them as one's own" (p. 7). It is the very act of choosing that is part of personal knowing, and that builds your practice base and your communication repertoire. When you communicate in a certain way because you know through deliberate selection that it is most effective, you are coming from a place of your own truth as a professional. This truth is based on more than theory and facts. It is your synthesis of theory and contemplated experience.

Nurses working in an environment of nursing excellence strive and grow to the level demonstrated by their peers, just as nurses placed in a unit where nursing practice is poor will descend to the lowest common denominator on the floor (Curtin, 1990). "Nurses affect one another so profoundly that they actually influence one another's value choices" (p. 7). If it's true that a nurse's professional character consists of the sum total of the value choices made in professional practice, then it behooves you to share with your colleagues quality demonstrations of your personal knowing about effective interpersonal communication. Your demonstrations of assertive and responsible communication in your workplace relationships serve as role models for your colleagues' adoption (or non-adoption). Communicating effectively, and sharing your personal knowing about interpersonal communication with your nurse colleagues, creates a professional bond (Curtin, 1990) and contributes to excellence in your workplace.

REFERENCES

Curtin, L.L. (1990). The excellence within. *Nursing management, 21*(10), 7.

Diekelmann, N. (1988). Curriculum revolution: A theoretical and philosophical mandate for change. In National League for Nursing, *Curriculum revolution: Mandate for change* (pp. 137-157). New York: National League for Nursing.

Gerrard, B. (1978). *Interpersonal skills for health professionals: A review of the literature.* Unpublished manuscript. McMaster University, Hamilton, Ontario, Canada.

Huston, C.J., What makes the difference? Attributes of the exceptional nurse. *Nursing '90, 20*(5), 170-173.

Meichenbaum, D. (1977). *Cognitive-behavior modification: An integrative approach*. New York: Plenum Press.

Moch, S.D. (1990). Personal knowing: Evolving research and practice. *Scholarly Inquiry for Nursing Practice: An International Journal,* 4(2), 155-170.

Schank, M.J. (1990). Wanted: Nurses with critical thinking skills. *The Journal of Continuing Education in Nursing, 21*(2), 86-89.

Schon, D.A. (1983). *The reflective practitioner: How professionals think in action*. New York: Basic Books, Inc.

Woodruff, A.D. (1961). *Basic concepts of teaching* (concise edition). Scranton, Pa.: Chandler Publishing Company; An Intext Publisher.

Choices of Responses to Distressed Clients and Colleagues

CHOICE A You are defensive and hostile in this response. You have taken Mr. James' remarks as a personal insult, when they were only a release of his intense frustration and worry. By retorting so aggressively you have escalated bad feelings between you and your client and not respected your right to communicate in a caring way. You have not shown Mr. James that you understand his feelings and that you care about his predicament. Although you did not meet his request for understanding, you did meet his request for the action of getting the telephone. This response is not assertive; it is aggressive. Mr. James would likely feel angry and embarrassed by your outburst, not understood or comforted. The only responsible part of this response is your offer to get the telephone.

CHOICE B Your opening words show that you are concerned about the changes you have observed in Jim over the past week; however, by beginning this way you have put the emphasis on yourself instead of on Jim. It is an aggressive approach because it puts your feelings first, at the expense of your client's. Your reflection that Jim is not like his old self is aggressive in its undertone of disappointment and scolding. By asking Jim if he is contemplating harming himself you are reading more into his symptoms than he presented. Jim might suspect that you are more worried about yourself (should he be seriously considering harming himself) than you are about his misery. As well as being aggressive, this response is not responsible because it does not pick up on the data Jim presented; it exaggerates and goes beyond the facts. Jim would likely not feel understood or helped by this response. He would likely be cautious about revealing any further information to you because your words suggest that you do not want to get involved if there is any sign of trouble.

CHOICE C Petra is likely to feel judged and reprimanded by this approach. Your confrontation would likely sting. It is judgmental and puts down your colleague. You proceed to lay on a lot of guilt about how she should hide her feelings to protect her clients, without giving her the right to have the feelings that she does. This approach is aggressive and uncaring. By not picking up on both her requests you have used an irresponsible strategy.

CHOICE D This strategy is not responsible because it tunes in neither to the information Mrs. Urst gave about her conflict between career and motherhood, nor her stark realization that she is now the mother of two. Your patronizing choice of words is aggressive and demeaning. Mrs. Urst would not likely feel understood or comforted by this response. She might feel that you are insensitive to her concerns. She might feel like a child that has just been dismissed.

CHOICE F This response is assertive and responsible. Your warmth and slight teasing shows Joe that you forgive him for his lack of consideration. By quickly focusing on his reason for being upset you show him that you understand his situation. Your empathic remarks about his feelings are accurate and specific, leaving Joe no doubt that you understand him. Your self-disclosure is appropriate because Joe wants to be a parent, and your own experience will likely give him hope that he will adjust. Joe would probably feel accepted and reassured by these words.

CHOICE G By sitting down you showed respect for the importance of Don's feelings. Your self-disclosure let Don know that you understood his feelings of shock at the news of this resident's death. Your acknowledgment of the joy that Don brought to Mr. Kent would be pleasing to Don. Your offer to help him with his work for today was respectfully offered because of the gentle phrasing. Your response is assertive because it offers Don helpful communication while respecting your right to be helpful, and it is responsible because it tunes in to all the data Don presented.

CHOICE I This choice is aggressive because it judges and punishes Mrs. Urst for having normal doubts and fears. It is not a responsible strategy because it misses out on the data about her conflict of roles and her shock about being the mother of two. Mrs. Urst would likely feel insulted that you question her decision making and angry that you did not give her a chance to respond before unilaterally controlling the situation (by pushing to get the treatment done). Your insensitive suggestion that she will see things differently when she is feeling better is arrogant and would likely frustrate Mrs. Urst. You have not respected your right to communicate in a caring way.

CHOICE J By not saying anything you have lost the opportunity to show Mr. James that you understand how he feels about his situation. Your unassertive actions of blushing and looking flustered make you feel disappointed that you concentrated on your feelings without conveying any compassion to your client. Although you missed out meeting his request for understanding, you did offer him the telephone. Mr. James would likely be more discomforted, and possibly embarrassed, that he upset you. This response is not assertive and is only minimally responsible.

CHOICE K This choice is irresponsible because it does not acknowledge Jim's feelings of lethargy and disappointment in a therapeutic way. This response is judgmental and demanding. Jim is not accepted for feeling the way he does. This aggressive approach bulldozes over Jim's sadness. It protects neither his right to feel the way he does nor your right to relate to your client in a sensitive and caring way. Jim would not feel understood by this strategy, and it is unlikely he would look to you for advice on how to get himself out of his unhappy state. He has received the facile message from you that it is easy to stay happy: just keep your chin up in the face of any troubles.

CHOICE L Petra would likely feel ignored by this strategy. By diverting the conversation from your classmate's important self-disclosure you have minimized the importance of what she is saying, and you have overruled her right to be understood and respected. By avoiding the sensitive area of her feelings you have been unassertive; neither her rights nor yours have been attended to with this reply. This response is irresponsible because it does not pick up on the information embodied in Petra's plea.

CHOICE N This is an unassertive and irresponsible response. By not pausing to show consideration for Don's reaction you evaded giving him the support he could have appreciated. Your opening remarks are inappropriately focused on you, and they could indicate that the whole situation is embarrassing. This self-centeredness is not helpful. Your vague references to Mr. Kent's death are disrespectful in their lack of specificity. This strategy would leave Don feeling uncomfortable and hurt by your lack of respect for both him and his client.

CHOICE O You have met Joe's request for forgiveness and you have made an attempt to reassure him that you think he will adjust to the situation. Your attempt is unassertive because it does not acknowledge the specific feelings that Joe raised when he related his troubles to you. This choice is glib and is not responsible because it is not a specific reflection of the data presented. Joe would not likely feel you really understood the depth and turbulence of his reactions.

CHOICE P Petra would likely feel understood, and somewhat admonished, by this strategy. At the beginning your focus is more on your guilty feelings about not picking up on Petra's changes. This self-disclosure is irrelevant. It is aggressive because it suggests that Petra's sadness is so blatant that it would be obvious to anyone. Your suggestion that she needs to work out her concerns is obvious and unhelpful. It is glib to suggest that she will feel better in the next rotation. She is likely hoping for a more personal disclosure about how you, a colleague, would handle these important issues in a similar situation. Your reply is partially responsible.

CHOICE Q This strategy is responsible because it picks up on all the data presented in Jim's opener. His feelings that there is nothing to look forward to was acknowledged. It was wise to point out that he still has 6 more weeks in traction so that he might want to consider some ways to make his forced immobility more interesting and useful. It was assertive to suggest that you could work out a remedy to his despair together, and it was respectful to ask if he was ready to talk about plans. This response is assertive because it meets his request for help and employs your skills in a helpful way. It is responsible because it attends to the verbal and nonverbal data about Jim's thoughts and feelings. Jim would likely feel that you understood his situation and consequently he might consider working with you in some way to make his confinement less wasteful and bleak.

CHOICE R This self-disclosure could have been a beautiful introduction to an empathic response; however, by itself it is inadequate. Mrs. Urst would be left to wonder why you are sorry. Is it because you do not know how to handle her crying; or because you think she should be able to snap back to her gay self; or because you care about her and are sad that she is distressed? It is unassertive to leave your intentions dangling and to leave Mrs. Urst without asking if you could be of some help. This response is not responsible because it does not reflect the data Mrs. Urst supplied.

CHOICE S This response is the most assertive and responsible. It shows respect for his thoughts about having to reach home and secure his glasses, and you have conveyed your understanding of his frustration at being in a strange place. Furthermore, you have offered to help him cope until his glasses arrive. Your offer is respectful because it allows him to dictate when he will need help so that he can maintain maximum independence. You offered to bring the telephone early in the response, thereby showing him you understand the importance of having contact with his wife. You can feel good about your response. You have met your client's requests and responded in keeping with your professional and caring image of yourself. It is likely that Mr. James would feel comforted by your words.

CHOICE T Joe is likely to feel dismissed by this reply. You have forgiven Joe and thereby met his request for action. You have not demonstrated your understanding of his situation with your vague reference to the fact that we all get upset at times. This response would not lead Joe to feel you understand his serious and important situation. This communication strategy is unassertive because it does not meet your colleague's right to be understood, and it does not demonstrate your ability to communicate in a caring way. Accepting his apology is responsible, but failure to act on all the data is irresponsible.

CHOICE U This reply is aggressive and irresponsible. It indicates that you see Don is upset, but you neglect to show any compassion for his feelings. Your aggressive style of rushing him to consider new residents at this point is premature and disrespectful. Your invitation for lunch is intended to convey kindness but your judgmental authoritarian approach takes the caring out of it. Your style is aggressive and would likely make Don feel angry and misunderstood. Your reply is partially responsible because you pick up that he is sad, but you have not shown understanding for the depth of Don's feelings in his bereavement.

CHOICE V Although you forgive Joe for his thoughtlessness, you are somewhat stern given his special circumstances and considering that it was not his usual way of doing things. Your warning about the future is aggressive and detracts from your forgiveness. Your exuberance about the news of the pregnancy is insensitive, given Joe's reaction. Your enthusiasm is aggressive because it puts pressure on Joe to feel happy when he really feels quite desperate. This communication strategy is aggressive and irresponsible. Joe would likely feel misunderstood and judged.

CHOICE W Petra would likely feel understood and accepted by your reply, and have some alternative and more hopeful ways of viewing the situation on her nursing unit. Right at the beginning you acknowledged Petra's feelings of despair so that she would know that you understood her. This approach is assertive because it attends to her right to receive helpful communication, and it meets your expectations that you will reach out to your colleagues in a caring way. By responding to her request for respectful understanding, and offering her some insights about how you sort out your feelings, you are responding to the information she gave you. In doing so you are communicating in a responsible way. You did not force your coping methods onto her; rather, you revealed how they were helpful for you and asked for her opinions. This approach is respectful of her individual style of handling events. Your self-disclosure—revealing that you have not sorted out all your thoughts on these important issues—would likely make Petra feel that she is not alone in trying to come to terms with the purpose of nursing (and life).

CHOICE X This reply is unassertive. It does not respect Jim's right to receive your helpful comments, and it deprives you of the right to communicate effectively. By not picking up on the specific information Jim gave you in his statement, and linking that to the changes you have observed in Jim in the past few weeks, you have responded without using half of the data. This reply is superficial and Jim would likely feel that the weight of his sadness had fully escaped you. He would not likely feel that he could confide any further in you after receiving this insensitive remark.

CHOICE Y This response is assertive because it demonstrates your ability to communicate sensitively to Mrs. Urst. Your agreement that her tears were in part due to postnatal blues allowed her to feel less embarrassed, yet you did not ignore her real worries about juggling her roles. You did not give her advice that would have been premature, but you gave her the option of talking more about her feelings with you if she would like. This invitation allows her to choose if and when she would like to talk, and is respectful of her privacy. Your accurate use of empathy would let her know you understand her confusion and ambivalence. Your style is assertive and your words are responsible. Mrs. Urst's requests would be met with this response.

CHOICE Z   This response is only partially assertive and responsible. It comes closer to filling his request for understanding than other options. You have conveyed understanding of his discomfort at being in a strange place, and you have offered to get the telephone for him. Your attempt at self-disclosure is incomplete and unspecific, and therefore would not convey the understanding you intended. What is missing is your acknowledgment of his frustration at not being able to function without his glasses, and his strong desire to contact his wife. Mr. James would probably feel somewhat comforted by your attempt to understand him, but he would be left wondering how you could possibly understand his unique predicament. This response is only partially assertive and responsible.

Choices of Responses to Aggressive Clients and Colleagues

***

CHOICE A   This is an unassertive reply. You have acknowledged Mr. Hunter's need for secure, safe, nursing care, but you have not given any credit to your ability to provide this care. You have not respected your own skills and abilities. Mr. Hunter may feel reassured that he can get a registered nurse instead of you, a student nurse, but he would not be impressed with your lack of confidence in your own abilities. This response is not responsible because you missed data about his difficulty adjusting to his primary nurse's absence. This strategy might make Mr. Hunter wonder about his safety in your hands, and it might embarrass him that you so easily crumbled under his attack.

CHOICE B   This response is aggressive and hostile to your instructor. You have harbored resentment about her lack of positive feedback for 5 weeks and have not appropriately brought it up at an earlier time. Today your buildup of anger and disappointment has come crashing out against her. Although this response protects your right to speak up, it overrides her right to have her feelings respected. Not only would this response make her feel threatened and angry, but it might result in a discipline case with your school of nursing. This response in no way guarantees that you will receive positive feedback from your instructor in the future.

CHOICE C   This approach is aggressive in style. There is arrogance in your touching Debbie and telling her not to feel the way she does. Your response is not sensitive to her right to her feelings. This response is irresponsible because it does not pick up on the obvious data that Debbie refuses to be rushed to accept her diabetes and need for insulin. It may escalate Debbie's fury to touch her at this point. Debbie would likely feel talked down to and disregarded.

CHOICE D   This strategy is assertive. Your apology to Karen and her clients was timely and respected their legitimate rights. Its brevity and promptness deescalated any further hostility between your two parties. This approach is responsible because it acknowledges your role in inconveniencing others. All concerned would be satisfied with this reply. Waiting until a moment when you and Karen could talk privately and freely about how she embarrassed you was considerate and respected your right to talk out this important issue. Your request to talk to Karen, and your honesty about the issue, helped to focus on the problem right away. Starting with an apology reassured her of your sincerity. Waiting for her permission to pursue your agenda was respectful. Your C.A.R.E. confrontation spelled out clearly what bothered you and how you want your colleague to behave in the future. Karen would feel that you understood her beef with your overstaying in the room, and she would easily be able to receive your feedback about her rudeness.

CHOICE E   This response is aggressive and almost taunting. It would only serve to escalate the anger building between you. It attacks Mr. Hunter's vulnerability. He has no control over who nurses him and you have threatened his security by implying that reporting you would be futile. Your sauciness about the decision of your instructor would only make Mr. Hunter feel less secure. This response is irresponsible because it does not attend to the data about Mr. Hunter's feelings of insecurity and his desire to heal without relapse. It shows no sensitivity to his feelings of missing his primary nurse. This response would likely make Mr. Hunter feel insecure and threatened himself.

CHOICE F   This response is aggressive. It is a direct, insulting attack on your team leader. It does nothing to respect your right to communicate in a caring way, and it ignores her concerns about your slowness. This style of responding would only make your team leader want to retaliate by being more aggressive with you in the future.

CHOICE G   You have responsibly acknowledged Mr. Gilmour's need for a cigarette, but your style is aggressive and rude. It does not respect your right to communicate assertively and would likely make everyone a little embarrassed.

CHOICE H   This response is assertive because it puts the onus on your instructor for more specificity in her suggestion about how you should change. It is her responsibility to clarify her meaning. This response is also responsible because it picks up on the data you have been given about her intention to transform you into a professional nurse. This response would likely make your instructor clarify her meaning of "professional" to your satisfaction. With this information you could then decide whether to point out any evidence you have about your professional demeanor. If she cannot be clear in her expectations, then you have the right to ask her to withdraw the accusation that you are unprofessional.

The issue of your right to receive some positive feedback from your instructor has not been dealt with in this response. Including such a request would augment the assertiveness of your response.

CHOICE I This reply is irresponsible because it does not take into account Mrs. Suit's worry or anxiety. It is aggressive because it sarcastically insults her and does not respect your right to communicate in a caring way. This reply would put down Mrs. Suit and make her feel angry and embarrassed.

CHOICE J This is an assertive response. You have pointed out in a C.A.R.E. confrontation exactly what bothers you and how you want her to change. Your specificity and courteous manner would protect her self-respect while you stand up for your legitimate rights. This strategy is also responsible because your instructor can pick up your hint about giving you feedback in an effort to improve your performance, and you remind her of some data she has overlooked. It is likely that this gentle confrontation will invite your instructor to look at her omissions and try to rectify the situation by being more accepting of your abilities as a maternity nurse.

CHOICE K This aggressive approach would likely increase Debbie's anger. At the least, it would dissolve any rapport or trust you had developed. You have not respected her right to be treated with respect and compassion. Irresponsibly, you have not attended to the data about her fear or her need to go slowly in her acceptance. You have not respected your right to communicate in a caring way. Debbie would likely feel even more angry and helpless because you are "pulling rank" on her. It would take a long time to repair the bad feelings generated by this response.

CHOICE L This choice is aggressive in style. Your opening phrase attacks Karen and escalates the hostility between the two of you. Your defensiveness embarrasses everyone—staff and clients. This response is irresponsible in its lack of attention to Karen's request for understanding and an apology.

CHOICE M This reply is assertive because it confidently assures him that you know what you are doing and invites him to make any inquiries about your nursing care. Your agreement about differences between nurses might reduce his anxiety over apparent variations in nursing styles. Your acknowledgment of his missing his primary nurse would show him you understand the mutuality that they had developed. Your assurance that your care is safe and congruent with doctor's orders would reassure him that you understand his urgency to be well cared for. This responsible and assertive response would make Mr. Hunter feel understood and comforted.

CHOICE N This reply is assertive and responsible. It stands up for your right to be given a chance to learn, and it shows respect for your team leader. You have acknowledged her legitimate concerns about the clients and requested her help in facilitating your development as a medication nurse. This response would make it clear what behavior you expect in a way that makes it easy for her to comply.

CHOICE O   This response is aggressive. It blasts Noreen without showing any compassion for how she is feeling; however, it does respect your right to nurse within the limits of the law and your own convictions. Noreen would likely feel attacked, but she would definitely get the message that she should go off duty.

CHOICE P   This is an unassertive approach. You have not acknowledged Karen's feelings nor have you spoken to her about your own anger at her aggressiveness. You have irresponsibly ignored Karen's legitimate requests. By sulking and avoiding her you are harboring bad feelings, instead of dealing with them in a forthright manner. You, Karen, and other staff members would all feel uptight with this strategy.

CHOICE Q   This response is assertive because it acknowledges both Debbie's right to be understood, and your right to communicate caringly and offer Debbie a way to desensitize herself to insulin. It is responsible because it picks up on her need to have her fear understood. You have comforted her by taking control and offering her a plan that might help her. Leaving or getting angry would have removed your supportive backing from Debbie. This response would make Debbie feel secure that you understand her fear, but you have the willingness and interest in her to help her through it.

CHOICE R   This is an irresponsible and unassertive response. You have neither attended to her request to be treated with respect nor showed you understand her feelings of helplessness. You have not respected your own rights as a nurse on the unit; you had another important task to accomplish that delayed you and you have the right and responsibility to communicate in a caring way to all your clients. Mrs. Suit may have felt important that you apologized, but your manner indicated only that you wanted to get out of her presence as soon as possible. Your lack of warmth and genuine respect would let Mrs. Suit know that you did not really care for her.

CHOICE S   This response is unassertive. You deserve to be bullied when you encourage it with such a meek reply. You have not respected your right to be treated in a patient manner. Your passivity has invited further putdowns.

CHOICE T   Clearly you are doubtful about the ethics of giving her the medication, but you unassertively give in. In so doing you lose your right to act safely and you may do your colleague some unintended harm. You have not acted responsibly because you did not follow up on the data she provided about her migraines, not did you show much compassion for her misery.

CHOICE U   This firm, clear reply is assertive: it respects Mr. Gilmour's dignity and your right to communicate in a respectful way. Your inclusion of a negative consequence demonstrates that you are serious about your request for him to stop bothering you during report. This reply is responsible because it takes into account that Mr. Gilmour had a smoke recently, that there is a well established rule about the times for his smoking, and that you have a right to finish work on time. Although Mr. Gilmour will likely be displeased by your reply he will know you are definite.

CHOICE V   This reply is assertive and responsible. You acknowledged Noreen's extreme discomfort and wisely suggested that she go home. You protected your right to avoid legal problems and your colleague's right to be properly examined before taking medication by refusing to give her anything. You did not leave her stranded but offered to call the evening supervisor and reassured her that you would manage the shift without her. Noreen might wish to try again to persuade you to give her something for her nausea but that possibility is unlikely given your firmness.

CHOICE W   This is an unassertive response. You have not protected your right to relate to your colleague in a caring way. She requested understanding and a promise that you would not repeat your inconsiderate actions in the future, and you have ignored both these requests by this unspecific response. Karen would feel minimally understood. This reply ignores your responsibility to defend your right to be treated respectfully by your colleague Karen.

CHOICE X   This is an unassertive response. You respected neither Debbie's right to be understood nor your own to communicate in a helpful way. Your reply focuses only on your feelings and misses the important data about Debbie's fear and need for guidance. Debbie would likely feel misunderstood and unsupported with this response.

CHOICE Y   This choice is unassertive. You have buckled under to accept an unreasonable request. Not only is her request unclear, but it does not correspond with how you feel about your work and the feedback you have been getting. This response is unlikely to stop any further aggression from your instructor. It is neither assertive nor responsible.

CHOICE Z   This response is an aggressive overreaction to Mr. Hunter. Returning aggressiveness with aggressiveness only escalates the feud. If Mr. Hunter had been repeatedly comparing your care to Chris' and putting you down, it would then be appropriate to ask him to stop this line of attack. At this point it is irresponsible to do so, because it puts the attention on your feelings rather than his feelings of vulnerability and loss. This is not a helpful response, and would leave Mr. Hunter embarrassed and discomforted.

CHOICE AA   This is an assertive response. You calmly and kindly reassured Mrs. Suit that your delay was not out of disrespect for her. The directness and conciseness of your explanation was not overly apologetic (which would have been unassertive), nor overly defensive (which would have been aggressive). Your reply was responsible because it picked up on her need to be treated with respect. Your offer to stay with her and talk demonstrated that you truly do care about her feelings. The strategy of overlooking her coarse abusive language was probably appropriate in this situation. Her anger stems from her fear and, if you help her cope with some of her legitimate worries, her abusiveness will likely diminish. If not, you could assertively request that she refrain from using abusive language with you.

CHOICE BB   This is an unassertive response. You have given in to Mr. Gilmour's unreasonable request and in the process made it difficult for other staff members to uphold the rule. You have taught Mr. Gilmour that if he persists long enough you will bend the rules. This reply would make you feel badly that you didn't stick to your decision. It irresponsibly ignores the data that he had a cigarette recently.

Index